NEUROLOGICAL EXAMINATION
A Structured Approach

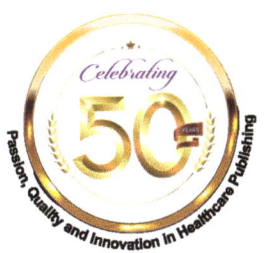

NEUROLOGICAL EXAMINATION
A Structured Approach

GRK Sarma MD DM
Professor
Department of Neurology
St. John's Medical College Hospital
Bengaluru, Karnataka, India

Foreword

P Satishchandra

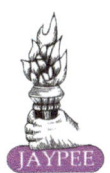

JAYPEE BROTHERS MEDICAL PUBLISHERS
The Health Sciences Publisher
New Delhi | London | Panama

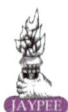 **Jaypee Brothers Medical Publishers (P) Ltd**

Headquarters

Jaypee Brothers Medical Publishers (P) Ltd
4838/24, Ansari Road, Daryaganj
New Delhi 110 002, India
Phone: +91-11-43574357
Fax: +91-11-43574314
Email: jaypee@jaypeebrothers.com

Overseas Offices

J.P. Medical Ltd
83 Victoria Street, London
SW1H 0HW (UK)
Phone: +44 20 3170 8910
Fax: +44 (0)20 3008 6180
Email: info@jpmedpub.com

Jaypee-Highlights Medical Publishers Inc
City of Knowledge, Bld. 235, 2nd Floor, Clayton
Panama City, Panama
Phone: +1 507-301-0496
Fax: +1 507-301-0499
Email: cservice@jphmedical.com

Jaypee Brothers Medical Publishers (P) Ltd
Bhotahity, Kathmandu, Nepal
Phone: +977-9741283608
Email: kathmandu@jaypeebrothers.com

Website: www.jaypeebrothers.com
Website: www.jaypeedigital.com

© 2019, Jaypee Brothers Medical Publishers

The views and opinions expressed in this book are solely those of the original contributor(s)/author(s) and do not necessarily represent those of editor(s) of the book.

All rights reserved by the author. No part of this publication may be reproduced, stored or transmitted in any form or by any means, electronic, mechanical, photocopying, recording or otherwise, without the prior permission in writing of the publishers.

All brand names and product names used in this book are trade names, service marks, trademarks or registered trademarks of their respective owners. The publisher is not associated with any product or vendor mentioned in this book.

Medical knowledge and practice change constantly. This book is designed to provide accurate, authoritative information about the subject matter in question. However, readers are advised to check the most current information available on procedures included and check information from the manufacturer of each product to be administered, to verify the recommended dose, formula, method and duration of administration, adverse effects and contraindications. It is the responsibility of the practitioner to take all appropriate safety precautions. Neither the publisher nor the author(s)/editor(s) assume any liability for any injury and/or damage to persons or property arising from or related to use of material in this book.

This book is sold on the understanding that the publisher is not engaged in providing professional medical services. If such advice or services are required, the services of a competent medical professional should be sought.

Every effort has been made where necessary to contact holders of copyright to obtain permission to reproduce copyright material. If any have been inadvertently overlooked, the publisher will be pleased to make the necessary arrangements at the first opportunity. The **CD/DVD-ROM** (if any) provided in the sealed envelope with this book is complimentary and free of cost. **It is Not meant for sale.**

Inquiries for bulk sales may be solicited at: jaypee@jaypeebrothers.com

Neurological Examination: A Structured Approach

First Edition: **2019**

ISBN: 978-93-5270-516-0

Dedicated to

The Human Mind ………..In Its Quest to Know Itself

Contributors

Chandrakala BS
Associate Professor
Department of Neonatology
St. John's Medical College Hospital
Bengaluru, Karnataka, India

Elisabeth Hartl
Resident
Epilepsy Center
Department of Neurology
University of Munich
Munich, Germany

GRK Sarma
Professor
Department of Neurology
St. John's Medical College Hospital
Bengaluru, Karnataka, India

Madhusudanan M
Professor and Head
Department of Neurology
Pushpagiri Medical College
Thiruvalla, Kerala, India
Former Professor and Head
Department of Neurology
Medical College
Kottayam, Kerala, India

Raghunandan Nadig
Associate Professor
Department of Neurology
St. John's Medical College Hospital
Bengaluru, Karnataka, India

Ranjini Srinivasan
Assistant Professor
Department of Pediatrics
St. John's Medical College Hospital
Bengaluru, Karnataka, India

Seshu Babu G
Ophthalmologist and
Research Consultant
Eye Care Centre
Visakhapatnam
Andhra Pradesh, India

Soheyl Noachtar
Head
Epilepsy Center
Department of Neurology
University of Munich
Munich, Germany

Sushma K
Senior Resident
Department of Pediatrics
St. John's Medical College Hospital
Bengaluru, Karnataka, India

Thomas Mathew
Professor
Department of Neurology
St. John's Medical College Hospital
Bengaluru, Karnataka, India

Foreword

In this era of technological revolution with day-to-day advancement of imaging modalities, clinical examination has become a rarity. However, in the nervous system examination, a good clinician with systematic approach, backed by good history can localize and make proper diagnosis. One should be able to answer two questions at the end of the clinical examination of any case: Where is the lesion? and What is the lesion? Subsequently, one should seek appropriate investigations to confirm the clinical localization. For this, the clinician should approach the case in a systematic way. Taking this cue, Professor GRK Sarma has brought out this important book *Neurological Examination: A Structured Approach*, consisting of 18 chapters, starting from higher mental function assessment and going on from head-to-toe examination.

The most impressive aspect of this book is pictorial presentation, physiological explanation, and clinical tips to elicit the signs brought out in a simple English. It is well written and brought out with clear emphasis on structured clinical case-based approach. Professor GRK Sarma being an excellent clinician and a teacher himself, understanding the lacunae in the present-day teaching has brought out this hand book, which is a must for every medical student both at undergraduate and postgraduate levels. This book in addition, has two chapters on Neurological Examination of a Neonate and Pediatric Neurological Examination at the end. GRK Sarma has recognized that it is very difficult to perform neurological examination for this segment of population and requires special skills.

I have great pleasure in writing the foreword to this book authored by one of my favorites, intelligent students. I am sure this book would become part and parcel of every medical student's bag and they should follow this systematic approach while examining a neurological case to elicit the signs and make excellent clinical diagnosis. I wish this book would make neurological clinical examination simple and enjoyable, so that clinical examination gets back its prime position, even in the days of electrophysiological and imaging revolution.

P Satishchandra
MBBS DM (Neurology) FAMS FIAN FRCP (London)
Advisor and Senior Consultant, Department of Neurology
Apollo Institute of Neurosciences, Jayanagar, Bengaluru, India
Honorary Professor, University of Liverpool, UK

Formerly, Director, Vice-Chancellor and Senior Professor
Department of Neurology
National Institute of Mental Health and Neurosciences (NIMHANS)
Bengaluru, Karnataka, India

Preface

Clinical neurology has received a well-deserved attention in the recent years, with reputed journals discussing and debating its relevance in modern neurology. It suffices here to say that a neurologist with inadequate clinical skills, working with powerful investigative tools like magnetic resonance imaging (MRI), neurogenetics, molecular biology, and neuroimmunology, is like a "rudderless boat in the midst of a tempest". He is certain to be blown in all directions.

There are some excellent and authoritative books on neurological examination. However, the variability and inconsistency in the methods of neurological examination and interpretation among clinicians and trainees is remarkable. This book is an attempt to present neurological examination in a fixed, structured format that minimizes this variability and to encourage uniformity. This book can be used by neurologists, neurosurgeons, physicians, pediatricians as well as postgraduate trainees from these fields. This book is not written with qualifying board examinations alone in mind because, the real test for the clinician is the patient in front of him and there are no shortcuts to success in this real world test.

The following salient features of this book guide the reader in optimally utilizing its contents:

- A good number of neglected topics have been included. These are of immense value in day-to-day practice and are usually not covered in the standard books. These include: Evaluation of seizure semiology, neurological examination of neonates, infants and children, examination of cervical spine and lumbosacral spine, assessment of trigger points and myofascial pain, examination of various joints whose pain overlaps with neurological pain syndromes, and bedside autonomic function tests.
- Many chapters begin with a "pictorial pretest" and end with answers to this test to drive home a fine, teaching point. It is more fruitful to read the chapter and work out the answers instead of jumping to the answer page.
- Each chapter is divided into 4 fixed components. These represent the 4 levels where clinical errors can creep in.

1. Physiological basis: It contains the most relevant neuroanatomical and physiological principles. This section is not a substitute to a more detailed study of these subjects from textbooks.

2. Methodology: It contains the step-by-step description of examination techniques. It is to be understood that there could be many more different methods of examination than what is included here. However, the methods included here have been chosen because either they are the most preferred methods in the standard books or they have been evaluated systematically in various published papers.

3. **Interpretation**: It describes the clinical significance of the results of examination. Clinicians often err at this level and emphasis has been laid on minimizing these errors.

4. **Caveats**: It describes various possible scenarios in which one could go wrong during neurological examination and interpretation.

- The reader, using this fixed format, can quickly access the component of neurological examination that is of interest to him.
- This fixed format also trains one's mind to work in the same logical way while examining the patients in day-to-day practice, instead of mechanically performing the examination. This is one of the primary objectives of this book.
- The bulleted format and direct language used in this book hopefully resonate well with the current generation.
- A list of "Bibliography" is provided in each chapter. The reader can be assured that the contents of this book are all from authoritative sources and not personal opinions and preferences of the author(s).
- The best way of learning examination methods is by reading and doing and then by repeating this sequence again and again. The simple format of this book is meant to facilitate this repetitive reading. Most topics do not take more than 15 minutes to review.

Obviously, a feedback from the readers is the best way to know if this book has done what it set out to do. Any constructive comments and suggestions are most welcome and will be immensely helpful in making this book more synchronized to your needs. Please mail them to sarma.grk@gmail.com and will be discussed in the Google+ page dedicated to this book.

GRK Sarma

Acknowledgments

I sincerely and gratefully acknowledge the following for their support and contribution to this work:
- The management at the St. John's Medical College Hospital, Bengaluru, for permitting me to carry out this work at the institute.
- The Institutional Ethics Review Board (IERB), at the St. John's Medical College Hospital, Bengaluru, for approving this work.
- The patients for consenting to be examined and to be clinically photographed.
- My teachers and senior colleagues for inspiring me to pursue and enjoy an academic career.
- My colleagues who supported and encouraged this work and for sharing their clinical material where necessary.
- The postgraduate trainees at St. John's who played a big role in taking clinical photographs and neuroimages. They also participated in stimulating bedside discussions which improved the contents of this book.
- All the contributing authors, who shared their vast knowledge and experience in their respective areas of expertise by providing excellent write ups and clinical material.
- Dr P Satishchandra, my teacher and Formerly, Director, Vice-Chancellor and Senior Professor, National Institute of Mental Health and Neurosciences (NIMHNS), Bengaluru, for kindly sparing time from his busy schedule to go through the book and writing the foreword for the book. It is an honor and privilege to receive his opinion on this book.
- I am thankful to Shri Jitendar P Vij (Group Chairman), Mr Ankit Vij (Managing Director), Mr MS Mani (Group President), Ms Pooja Bhandari (Production Head), Ms Sunita Katla (Executive Assistant to Group Chairman and Publishing Manager), Mr Rajesh Sharma (Production Coordinator), Ms Seema Dogra (Cover Visualizer), Ms Uma Adhikari (Typesetter), Ms Geeta Rani (Proofreader), Mr Ankush Sharma (Graphic Designer) and team members of M/s Jaypee Brothers Medical Publishers (P) Ltd, New Delhi, India, for all their support to work in this project and make it a success.
- Last, and most importantly, my parents, Smt Sitamahalakshmi and Sri Satyanarayana Murthy for everything; my wife, Dr Prasanthi for her unflinching support and encouragement; children, Sravya and Saketh for being great stress-busters; my brother, Dr Seshu Babu G, sisters, and all my family members for their guidance and valuable advice.

Contents

1. **Assessment of Higher Mental Functions** — 1
   GRK Sarma, Madhusudanan M
   Overview of Mental Status Examination 1
   Assessment of State Functions 3
   Pictorial Pretest 3; Physiological Basis 3; Methodology and Observations 6; Interpretation 8; Caveats 8; Answers to the Pretest 8
   Language Disorders 9
   Definitions Important in Language Assessment 9; Physiologic Basis 10; Methodology 11; Observations 13; Interpretation 14
   The Apraxias 19
   Pictorial Pretest 19; Physiological Basis 20; Methodology 25; Interpretation 25; Answers to the Pretest 26
   Calculations 28
   Calculations and Related Parietal Lobe Functions (Finger Identification, Right-Left Orientation) 28
   The Agnosias 31
   Physiologic Basis 31; Methodology 33; Interpretation 35; Caveats 36
   Memory 38
   Pretest 38; Physiologic Basis 39; Methodology 40; Interpretation 43; Caveats 44; Answers to the Pretest 44
   Construction and Dressing 45
   Pictorial Pretest 45; Construction 45; Dressing 47; Answer to the Pretest 48
   Tests for Higher Order Thinking (Reasoning, Abstraction, Judgment, and Executive Functions) 49
   Physiologic Basis 49; Methodology 49; Judgment, Insight, and Social Appropriateness 50
   Mini-mental Status Examination 51
   Methodology 51; Interpretation 53; Caveats 53

2. **Examination of a Patient in Coma** — 60
   Raghunandan Nadig, GRK Sarma
   Pictorial Pretest 60; Physiological Basis 62; Examination of the Comatose Patient 63; Level of Consciousness 64; Breathing 65; Circulation 66; Motor Response to Stimulus 72; Answers to the Pretest 75

3. **Cranial Nerves** — 76
   GRK Sarma, Seshu Babu G
   The Olfactory Nerve (I N) 76
   Physiologic Basis 76; Definitions 77; Methodology 77; History 77; Examination Technique 78; Interpretation 78; Caveats 79

The Optic Nerve (II N) 80
Physiologic Basis 80;   Methodology 82;   Answers to the Pretest 93;   Clinical Interpretation 99
Ocular Motor Nerves (III, IV and VI) 104
Pictorial Pretest 104;   Ocular Motor Nerves 104;   Physiologic Basis of Ocular Motor System 106;   Certain Terms and Rules 108;   Answers to the Pretest 116;   Examination of Pupils and Lids 117;   The Pupils 119;   Eyelids 133;   Answers to the Pretest 1 135;   Answers to the Pretest 2 136;   Answers to the Pretest 3 137
Examination of Gaze Disorders 138
Pretest 138
Saccades 139
Physiologic Basis 140;   Methodology 143;   Interpretation 144;   Answers to the Pretest 147
The Pursuit System 148
Smooth Pursuit System 150
Vergence System 152
Physiologic Basis 152;   Methodology 153;   Interpretation 153
Nystagmus 154
Physiologic Basis 154;   Methodology and Observations 158;   Interpretation 161;   Caveats 162
Trigeminal Nerve (V N) 163
Pictorial Pretest 163;   Physiological Basis 163;   Motor Nucleus 166;   Sensory Portion 167;   Trigeminal Nerve Divisions 167;   Examination Method 171;   Answers to the Pretest 174
The Facial Nerve (VII N) 176
Methodology 177;   Interpretation 179;   Caveats 180
Vestibulocochlear Nerve (VIII N) 181
Physiological Basics 181;   Cochlear Nerve 183;   Vestibular Nerve 185;   Nystagmus in Vestibular Lesion 188;   Some Practical Points 189
Glossopharyngeal Nerve (IX N) 191
Physiologic Basis 191;   Methodology 192;   Interpretation 193;   Caveats 193
Vagus Nerve (X N) 194
Physiologic Basis 194;   Methodology 197;   Interpretation 197
Accessory Cranial Nerve (XI N) 200
Pictorial Pretest 200;   Physiological Basis 200;   Methodology 203;   Interpretation 203;   Caveats 204;   Answers to the Pretest 204
Hypoglossal Nerve (XII N) 206
Pictorial Pretest 206;   Answer to the Pretest 211

4. **Motor System** 212
   GRK Sarma

   Muscle Tone 214;   Assessment of Muscle Power—General Principles 223
   Scapular Movements 228
   Scapular Abduction and Forward Rotation 229;   Scapular Elevation 231;   Scapular Adduction 232;   Scapular Depression and Adduction 233;   Shoulder Flexion 235;   Shoulder Abduction 239;   Shoulder Internal Rotation 243

Examination of Forearm and Hand 244
Elbow Flexion 244;   Forearm Supination 247;   Forearm Pronation 248;   Wrist Flexion 249;   Metacarpophalangeal Extension 252;   Finger Flexion at Proximal and Distal Interphalangeal Joints 253;   Testing of Distal Interphalangeal Flexion 254;   Finger Metacarpophalangeal Extension 255;   Finger Abduction 256;   Finger Adduction 257;   Thumb Movements 258;   Thumb Extension 260;   Thumb Abduction 261;   Thumb Adduction 263;   Thumb Opposition 264;   Little Finger Opposition 265
Examination of Power of Lower Limb Muscles 266
Hip Flexion 266;   Hip Extension 267;   Hip Adduction 268;   Hip Abduction 269;   Hip External Rotation 270;   Hip Internal Rotation 271;   Knee Flexion 272;   Knee Extension 273;   Ankle Plantar Flexion 275;   Foot Dorsiflexion and Inversion 276;   Foot Inversion 277;   Foot Eversion 278;   Toe Metatarsophalangeal Flexion 279;   Toes Plantar and Distal Interphalanges Flexion 280;   Toe Dorsiflexion 281

5. Examination of the Sensory System   283
GRK Sarma

Proprioception 284
Physiologic Basis 284;   Methodology 285;   Other Tests 286;   Interpretation 287
Vibration 287
Physiologic Basis 287;   Methodology 288;   Interpretation 289
Tactile Sensation 291
Methodology 291;   Pain and Temperature 292;   Segmental Localization of Sensory Loss 294

6. Reflexes   299
GRK Sarma

Deep Tendon Reflexes 299;   Superficial Reflexes 307;   Superficial Abdominal Reflex 307;   Superficial Anal Reflex 308;   Bulbocavernosus Reflex 308;   Cremasteric Reflex 309;   Plantar Reflex and the Babinski Sign 309;   Pathologic or Primitive Reflexes 314;   Pictorial Pretest 314;   Primitive Reflexes 315;   Grasp Reflex 315;   Primitive Oral Reflexes 317;   Palmomental Reflex 318;   Answers to the Pretest 319

7. Examination of Coordination   320
GRK Sarma

Basic Principles 321;   Testing of Station/Stance 323;   Past Pointing 325;   Position Holding 326;   Finger-to-Nose Test 327;   Heel-Knee-Toe Test 328;   Dysdiadochokinesis 329;   Rebound Test 330

8. Examination of Gait   332
GRK Sarma

Gait Assessment 332;   Interpretation 335;   Caveats 338

9. Examination of Movement Disorders   339
GRK Sarma

General Approach to Movement Disorders 339;   Tremor 344;

Archimedes Spiral Drawing (Spirography) 350;
Dystonia 353; Chorea 359; Myoclonus 364; Tics 371

10. Clinical Evaluation of Seizures and Epilepsies — 376
Elisabeth Hartl, Soheyl Noachtar

Seizure Semiology 376
Pictorial Pretest 376; Physiological Basis 378; Answers to the Pretest 386

11. Examination of a Patient with Vertigo — 388
GRK Sarma, Thomas Mathew

Physiologic Basis 389; Ocular Alignment and Ocular Tilt Reaction 390; Subjective Visual Vertical (Bucket Test) 391; Head Heave Test 393; Examination of Eye Movements 393; Gaze-evoked Nystagmus 394; Head-Shaking Nystagmus 395; Hyperventilation-induced Nystagmus 396; Vibration-induced Nystagmus 397; Valsalva-induced Nystagmus 397; Positional Testing 398; The Vestibulo-ocular Reflex 402; Head Heave Test (Translational VOR) 404

12. Autonomic Nervous System — 407
GRK Sarma

Pictorial Pretest 407; Introduction 408; Heart Rate Response to Breathing 411; Bedside Orthostatic Test (Active Standing) 412; Valsalva Maneuver 414; Answers to the Pretest 415

13. Examination of a Patient with Neck Pain — 417
GRK Sarma

Pictorial Pretest 417; Examination of a Patient with Neck and Arm Pain 418; Answers to Pretest 425

14. Examination of a Patient with Low Back Pain — 426
GRK Sarma

Physiological Basis 426; Examination 431; Interpretation 433

15. Examination of Other Joints — 436
GRK Sarma

Shoulder Joint 436; Sacroiliac Joint 440; Knee Joint 443

16. Examination of Trigger Points — 451
GRK Sarma

Myofascial Pain 451

17. Neurological Examination of a Neonate — 458
Chandrakala BS

General Examination 460; Posture 460; Involuntary and Spontaneous Movements 461; Neurobehavioral Items 462; Fontanelles, Sutures and Head Circumference 463; Tone 464; Reflexes 470; Central versus Neuromuscular Hypotonia 473; Cranial Nerve Examination 473; Summary of Age Related Neurological Examination Findings in Neonates 475

18. Pediatric Neurological Examination — 477
Sushma K, Ranjini Srinivasan

General Principles of Pediatric Neurological Examination 477; General Physical Examination in Pediatric Neurology 478

Index — 497

CHAPTER 1

Assessment of Higher Mental Functions

GRK Sarma

OVERVIEW OF MENTAL STATUS EXAMINATION

While performing and interpreting the mental status examination (MSE), it is important to be aware of certain principles so that erroneous conclusions are not reached. MSE is not as straightforward as one wishes it to be and the relationship between the deficits and lesions is not always one to one. It is advisable to first perform the MSE without jumping to localization, note the observations and at the end, put together the pieces of the puzzle to come up with a hypothesis regarding the lesion location. The following principles help one to approach the MSE from a realistic and balanced view point (Box 1.1):

- Functional imaging studies have demonstrated that many mental tasks require activation of "networks" rather than "discrete centers"
- Many tasks that are assessed in MSE are interdependent. So, abnormality in one domain must be interpreted in the light of performance in related domains (e.g. impaired calculation may actually be due to impaired attention or language)
- Most tests that are used therefore assess multiple domains in addition to the target domain
- The mental status test results are usually not diagnostic of a particular disease. Instead, they may yield certain characteristic patterns, which suggest possible anatomical location of the lesion
- Cerebral plasticity may confound the anatomical localization based on MSE. This is especially well-known in language dominance in early onset epilepsy
- Many tests used in the MSE do not have normative data, especially taking into account the multiple variables that influence the performance (e.g. age, race, education, cultural background, etc.)
- Each test has a floor and ceiling effect. In a patient with severe disease, the test may be too difficult to be administered (floor effect). Conversely, in high functional individuals with mild disease, the test may be too simple to be sensitive (ceiling effect). Identifying tasks that a patient can perform with 75% accuracy may avoid these effects
- The performance in each of the tests depends on the integrity of the input route, processing stage and the output route. Therefore, one should not prematurely attribute a deficit in a particular domain to the processing stage. For example, a patient might have poor memory retention which

may be due to severe inattention. In such a patient, one can only label the retentive memory as "not assessable" instead of "impaired". Similar situation is encountered in motor aphasic patient ("output" route)
- The MSE is classified into two broad categories:
  - *State functions:* These include arousal, attention, motivation, mood, and are dependent on integrity of frontal networks and the ascending reticular activating system (ARAS). Deficits in these functions result in deficits in multiple other domains and thus do not have much localizing value. Frontal lobe lesions, multifocal lesions, toxic and metabolic encephalopathies typically result in abnormalities in state functions.
  - *Channel functions:* These include language, explicit memory and perceptual disorders are examples of deficits in channel functions. These require more discrete anatomical networks and have better localizing value
- A number of mental status examination scales are available. The mini-mental status examination (MMSE) scale is widely used as a screening tool. We also use the Montreal Cognitive Assessment (MOCA) tool at our institute for a more detailed, yet rapid, screening
- However, these scales are only a starting point of MSE. In a patient with cognitive symptoms or signs, one has to go beyond these screening tools, dig deeper in selected domains to get a more complete and accurate picture of the impairments. For example, in a patient with language impairment, MMSE and MOCA would provide the clue, but a detailed evaluation is required to qualify and quantify the deficits accurately
- In the subsequent sections, each of the cognitive domains is elaborated to facilitate a detailed assessment. MMSE is presented and discussed separately
- A summary of MSE of a dementia patient and the essential tool kit required are provided at the end of the chapter. These guide the clinician to perform a complete bedside examination of the patient, covering all the cognitive domains.

> **Box 1.1:** The following sequential strategy of MSE is based on the above general principles.

- Detailed history (not elaborated further)
- Behavioral observations during the interview
- State functions:
  - Level of arousal
  - Attention, executive functions
  - Mood
  - Motivation
- Channel dependent functions:
  - Language
  - Praxis
  - Calculations, right-left orientation, finger identification
  - Visual and auditory perception
  - Explicit memory—verbal and nonverbal
  - Construction
  - Judgment, reasoning, abstract thinking, planning, insight
- Classify the deficits into primary and secondary deficits
- Hypothesize on lesion location.

ASSESSMENT OF STATE FUNCTIONS

GRK Sarma

PICTORIAL PRETEST

A 65-year-old man was given the following tests A and B (Fig. 1.1).
1. What are the tests called?
2. What are they aimed at?
3. How do you interpret these test results of this patient?

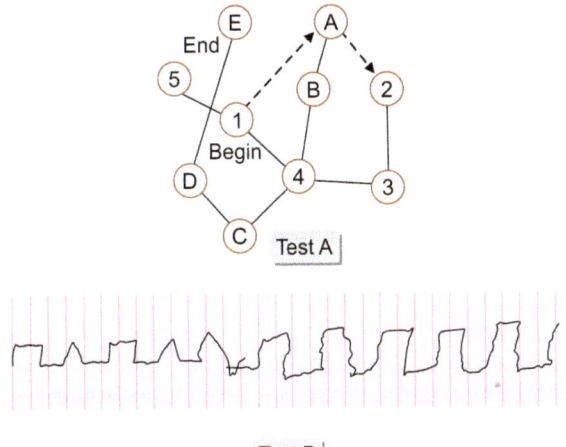

Fig. 1.1: Pictorial pretest.

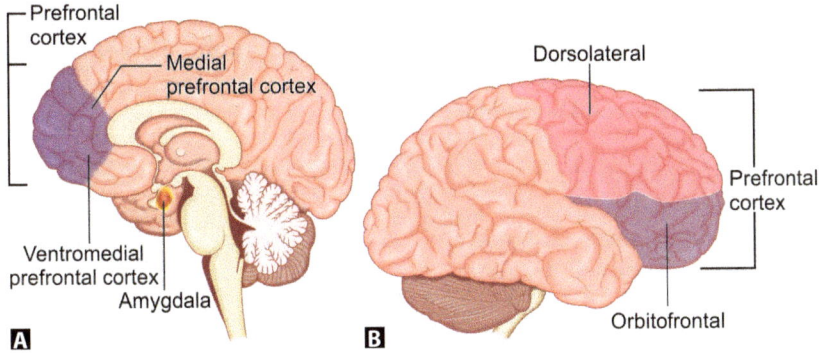

Figs. 1.2A and B: Prefrontal cortex. (A) Medial; (B) Lateral view.

PHYSIOLOGICAL BASIS

Definitions

- **Vigilance:** A state of arousal (alertness) in which, the patient can respond to any environmental stimulus. Arousal and alertness are described in the

chapter "Evaluation of patients in coma". This chapter focuses on the rest of the state functions.
- **Attention:** It is the ability to respond to a specific stimulus without being distracted by internal or external stimulus. A patient may be vigilant, but not necessarily attentive.
- **Sustained attention**: An ability to attend to a specific stimulus over an extended time.
- The part of the frontal lobe anterior to areas 6, 8 and motor language area is called the **prefrontal cortex**. It is subdivided into three regions: dorsolateral prefrontal cortex (**DLPFC**), orbitofrontal cortex (**OFC**) and the medial prefrontal cortex (**MPFC**).
- As with other cognitive functions, the state functions are also believed to be "network" functions comprising of frontal-striatal-thalamic-frontal circuits.

Medial Prefrontal Cortex

- To achieve a particular movement, there has to be an intent and a motivation to move, and a selection of movement pattern that is appropriate to the context and to the emotional content of the stimulus. The various components of the MPFC achieve these functions as follows:
    - The area anterior to the supplementary motor area (**pre-SMA**) in the superior frontal gyrus is related to **the intention to move**, imitation and learning of motor patterns
    - The anterior **cingulate gyrus**, is a part of the limbic circuit. It modulates appropriate **movement selection** and **response to noxious** stimuli
    - The cingulate gyrus assesses the **motivational** content of the external and internal stimuli and regulates the **context dependent** behaviors
    - The cingulate gyrus also modulates the autonomic activity and internal **emotional responses.**
- Syndrome of medial prefrontal circuit:
    - Apathy
    - Akinetic mutism
    - Amotivation
    - Poor response inhibition
    - Diminished self-awareness
    - Depression
    - Reduced responses to pain
    - Aberrant social behavior.

Orbitofrontal Cortex

- It is interconnected to the limbic system and to the ARAS.
- It is activated with the **emotions** of anger and fear.
- It is also activated in response to adverse stimuli.
- It plays a role in **inhibiting** inappropriate responses and behavior, both **emotional** and **motor**.

- Syndrome of orbitofrontal circuit:
  - Mood disorder
  - Obsessive compulsive disorder
  - Irritability
  - Antisocial behavior
  - Undue familiarity
  - Emotional incontinence
  - Inappropriate jocularity, euphoria
  - Distractibility
  - Environmental dependency
  - Poor judgment and insight.

Dorsolateral Prefrontal Cortex

- It has extensive connections with other parts of the prefrontal cortex as well as widespread brain regions. Its functions have been understood based on lesion studies.
- It is important in the organization of self-generated tasks, working memory, and executive functions.

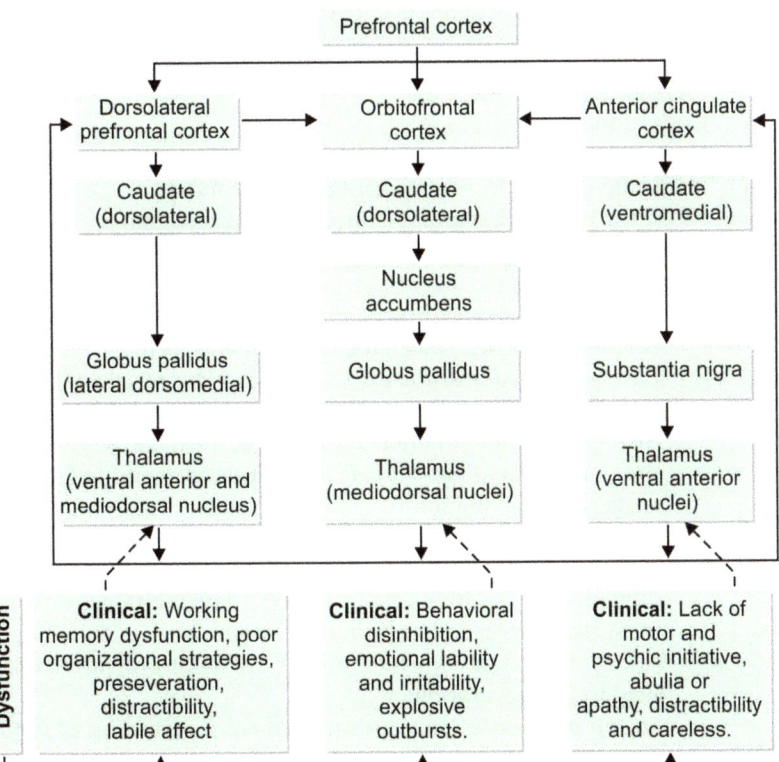

Flowchart 1.1: Prefrontal cortex connections and dysfunctions.

- The frontal executive functions include: decision making, planning, organization, implementation, and monitoring a series of goal-directed actions.
- It also includes, abstraction, judgment, learning, problem-solving, and cognitive flexibility, personality.
- Syndrome of dorsolateral circuit:
  - Poor organizational strategies
  - Poor memory search strategies
  - Stimulus bound behavior
  - Environmental dependency
  - Impaired set shifting.

METHODOLOGY AND OBSERVATIONS

A. **Arousal:** Assessment of level of consciousness is discussed in detail in the chapter "Evaluation of patients in coma".
B. **Attention/orientation/working memory:**
   - Orientation to time (day, date, time, month, season, year), place (country, state, city, hospital name, floor) and person (relatives, friends, caregivers). If the patient gives wrong answers, tell him the correct answer and ask these questions after several minutes to check, if new learning has occurred
   - Digit span: Present a random number containing increasing number of digits, at one digit per second, and ask the patient to repeat the number. Patient is asked to repeat the number forward (normal 7 ± 2) and backward (normal 5± 2). Start with 2 or 3 digit numbers and increase if patient succeeds
   - Count 1 to 20
   - Count 20 to 1
   - Name the months forward (normal: 5–8 seconds)
   - Name the months backward (normal: 10–16 seconds)
   - Recite alphabets in reverse order
   - Distractibility and perseveration:
     - Repetitive alteration of a sequence of 3 hand postures—like tapping the table sequentially with the fist-palm-edge of the hand.
     - *Luria alternating sequence test:* The patient is asked to copy a short segment of alternate open squares and triangles and then extend the sequence to the end of the page, without lifting the pencil. If patient repeats only squares or only triangles, it suggests perseveration
     - *Trail making test:* Patient is presented with an irregular array of circled numbers and is asked to join them in sequence. At a more difficult level, numbers are intermixed with alphabets and these must be connected in alternating sequence (1-a-2-b-3-c- and so on). If patient connects only numbers or only alphabets, it suggests perseveration
     - *Stroop procedure:* In this, names of colors are printed in non-matching colors and patient is asked to name the color of the

text, inhibiting the strong and more automatic tendency to read the word. Errors of commission, i.e. a tendency to read the word suggests an inability to inhibit unwanted responses.
- Vigilance (sustained attention): Continuous performance test using "d" test, in which letter d is mixed with distracting alphabets (like p, b) and numbers. Patient is asked to cross out the target letter "d". This test assesses attention, perseveration and distractibility which manifest as errors of commission and omission
- This test can also be done by reading out a mixture of letters and asking the patient to indicate whenever the target letter (e.g. A) is read out. The letters are read at 1 per second for 1 minute. Normal persons complete the test without errors
- FAS list generation: Patient is asked to generate as many words that start with letter F or A or S as possible over 3 minutes (normal: 36-40 words over 3 minutes)
- Semantic list generation: Patient is asked to generate words of a particular category like animals over a 60 seconds period (normal: 13-23 animals over 60 seconds).

C. **Mood:**
- Observation during the interview
- General questions (how is your mood, do you feel hopeless, do you enjoy activities, death wishes, somatic complaints like fatigue, insomnia, anorexia, etc.)
- Standard questionnaires like Beck depression inventory, Hamilton depression rating scale, etc.

D. **Motivation:**
- Cooperation with the examiner
- Spontaneous demonstration of initiative
- Delayed responses to questions
- Negative curt responses (like "I do not know").

E. **Behavioral changes:** A number of behavioral changes might be reported by the relatives or caregivers and could be observed during the interview sessions by the examiner. It is important to look for and ask for such changes while evaluating patients with cognitive disorders, both from diagnostic and management points of view:
- Outbursts of crying, anger, laughter
- Depression, euphoria
- Facetiousness
- Silliness, inappropriate jocularity
- Apathy, emotional flatness, poor personal hygiene
- Social withdrawal
- Impaired judgment in social or ethical situations
- Disinhibition, inappropriate and careless dressing
- Sexual promiscuity
- Impaired recent memory, new learning
- Inability to solve problems, and plan finances.

INTERPRETATION

- Significant impairment in attention is typically seen in toxic, metabolic encephalopathies and in frontal lobe lesions (especially the prefrontal cortex including posterior cingulated region). It is usually not a feature of dementias
- Orientation to time is impaired earlier than to place and person in encephalopathies
- Reduced digit span suggests impaired working memory (dorsolateral frontal function)
- Impaired counting backward and forward: Mild to severe impairment in attention, and executive function
- Impaired recollection of months and alphabets: Same significance as impaired counting
- Impairment on sequential hand postures (fist-palm-side): Impaired set shifting (executive function). Errors of omission and commission can occur
- Luria's test: Errors of omission and commission can occur. Indicate impaired executive function
- Trail test: Errors can occur due to inattention and perseveration
- Errors of omission indicate distractibility
- Errors of commission indicate perseveration
- Stroop test errors: Indicate inability to suppress unwanted responses, which requires both anterior cingulated cortex and dorsolateral frontal region to be intact
- Impaired word generation suggests retrieval deficit and lack of fund of information, usually with dorsolateral frontal lesions
- Significant change in mood is seen with orbitofrontal lesions and anterior cingulate lesions and includes depression, mania
- Impaired motivation is seen with medial frontal lesions.

CAVEATS

- Digit span cannot be tested in aphasic patients
- Letter A cancellation test cannot be done in aphasic patients
- Anxious patients may perform poorly on sustained attention tests
- Depressed patients may also perform poorly on these tests.

ANSWERS TO THE PRETEST

1. The test A is called trail making test and test B is called Luria test.
2. These tests are aimed at assessing frontal executive functions.
3. In test A, the patient fails to shift from alphabets and numerals as is actually required. This set shifting is a function of dorsolateral frontal cortex and the test result indicates its dysfunction.

   In test B, the patient continues to draw rectangles suggestive of perseveration, which suggests dorsolateral prefrontal dysfunction.

LANGUAGE DISORDERS

GRK Sarma

DEFINITIONS IMPORTANT IN LANGUAGE ASSESSMENT

- **Language:** It is a complex system of communication symbols and rules for their use.
- **Speech morphology:** It is the study of internal structure of words in language.
- **Word:** The smallest **independent** unit of language. Example: "work".
- **Morpheme:** The smallest unit of language with meaning. Example: -er, can be derived by breaking the word "worker". "-er" is dependent on "work", so it cannot be called a word. But, it does have a meaning, hence it is a morpheme. Similarly, "kindness" can be split to produce morpheme "-ness".
- **Phoneme:** A smallest sound that may bring about a change of meaning. As an example, meaning of the word kiss changes to kill by substitution of /s/ by /l/. Thus /s/ and /l/ are two different phonemes.
- **Semantics:** Semantics is the subfield that is devoted to the study of meaning, as inherent at the levels of words, phrases, sentences, and larger units of discourse. The two main areas are *logical semantics*, concerned with matters such as sense and reference and presupposition and implication, and *lexical semantics*, concerned with the analysis of word meanings and relations between them.
- **Syntax:** It is the grammatical construction of phrases and sentences.
- **Pragmatics:** The proper use of speech and language that is appropriate in a given conversational setting. Pragmatics studies how the transmission of meaning depends not only on structural and linguistic knowledge (e.g. grammar, lexicon, etc.) of the speaker and listener, but also on the context of the utterance, any pre-existing knowledge about those involved, the inferred intent of the speaker, and other factors.
- **Aphasia:** An **acquired** language disorder secondary to brain damage
- **Dysphasia:** A **congenital** or developmental language disorder
- **Dysarthria:** A mechanical articulation disorder for single sounds
- **Apraxia:** A misarticulation of phonemes due to inability to translate conscious speech plans into motor plans
- **Muteness:** Total loss of speech of varied etiology, including severe aphasia/anarthria/akinetic mutism/laryngeal disorders/psychogenic causes
- **Anomia:** Inability to produce a specific name. It is characterized by circumlocution and word finding pauses
- **Paraphasia:** It is a phenomenon of substitutions in speech components. This may be literal paraphasia (substitution of one phoneme for another; e.g. foon for spoon) or semantic paraphasia (substitution of one word for another; e.g. pan for spoon)
- **Perseveration:** Inappropriate repetition of previous responses
- **Neologisms:** Use of non-existent words

- **Jargon speech:** A completely meaningless speech containing neologisms and paraphasias.

A recent language network model that recognizes multiple brain regions.

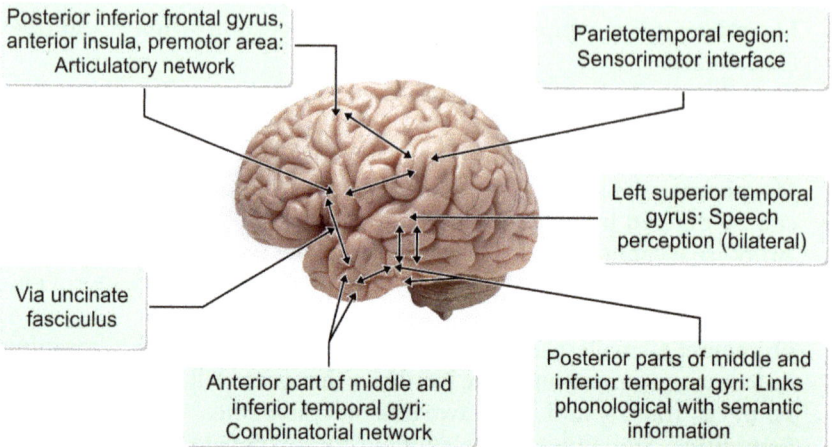

Fig. 1.3: Dual stream model of language network. This has been proposed by Hickok and Poeppel and incorporates the recent evidence provided by functional neuroimaging. This model explains complex manifestations of various brain lesions better than the original, simplistic model put forward by Wernicke. (The double headed arrows indicate the network between various areas).

PHYSIOLOGIC BASIS

Brain Regions Involved in Language

- The **classical model** proposed by **Wernicke** has been expanded and modified by recent evidences, especially from functional neuroimaging studies.
- The current models recognize a larger number of brain regions as important in the language networks. For example, the middle and inferior temporal gyri, the premotor regions and the parietotemporal region at the tip of the sylvian fissure, are all included in the **dual stream model of Hickok and Poeppel**, which has gained wide acceptance (Fig. 1.3).
- Some of the components of language and their anatomical correlates are listed below.
    - *Spoken speech processing:* Heschl's gyrus (bilateral superior temporal gyrus)
    - *Decoding of sounds into language information:* Wernicke's area (area 22), in the left superior temporal gyrus in its posterior part, as well as posterior parts of middle and inferior temporal gyri
    - *Phoneme processing:* Inferior parietal lobule, especially the supramarginal gyrus
    - *Reading comprehension:* Parieto-occipital cortex, especially the angular gyrus

- *Spontaneous speech output:* Broca's area in the posterior inferior frontal gyrus (areas 44, 45), and the premotor cortex which program the motor cortex to produce the sounds.
- *Speech repetition:* Communication between the posterior and anterior speech regions via the arcuate fasciculus and uncinate fasciculus
- *Alerting the language networks:* Anterior thalamus, basal ganglia.

METHODOLOGY

- There are a number of aphasia batteries like Western aphasia battery, Boston aphasia battery, Mississippi aphasia test, etc.
- These are **quantitative tools** that are used by neuropsychologists and speech pathologists and are most useful in the follow-up of aphasic patients
- In neurological practice, to identify the type of aphasia, such quantitative measures may not be required. A careful assessment and correct interpretation of the deficits should suffice.
- Language has to be assessed in six domains as follows:
  1. Spontaneous speech
  2. Naming
  3. Comprehension
  4. Repetition
  5. Reading
  6. Writing

Domain 1: Spontaneous Speech

- **Observe** the speech and language during the routine conversation.
- Ask an open ended question. Example:
  - Why have you come to the hospital?
  - Describe the nature of your job.
- If the patient is not communicative try recitation list. For example:
  - List the days of a week
  - List the months of the year
  - Name some wild animals.

Domain 2: Naming

- Show different categories like objects, body parts, colors, pictures of animals. For example:
  - Pen
  - Watch
  - Key
  - Hand
  - Thumb
  - Elbow
  - Dog
  - Cat

- Crow
- Red color
- Blue color
- Yellow color
- Names of familiar people (relatives/friends, sports persons, politicians).

Domain 3: Auditory Comprehension
- One step commands (beware of apraxias):
  - Stick out your tongue
  - Point to your nose
  - Open your mouth
- Two step commands (beware of body part agnosias, right left disorientation)
  - With your right hand, point to your left ear
  - Point to the ceiling and then to the floor
  - Raise your hand and close your eyes
- Yes or no responses (inform that patient should just say yes or no):
  - Is your name xxx ? (use a wrong name)
  - Is your name zzz? (use patient's correct name)
  - Do you live in xxx? (use a wrong place)
  - Do you live in zzz? (use the correct place of patient's residence)
  - Is this my ear? (point to your nose)
  - Does Sunday come after Saturday?
  - Do you eat every hour?

Domain 4: Repetition
- Single words:
  - Brown
  - Chair
  - Five hundred and fifty five
  - Rajagopalachari
- Sentence repetition (there should be no errors of omission or commission)
  - It is 4 o' clock
  - He locked the doors
  - He searched for keys in his pocket
  - No ifs, ands or buts
  - He opened the sports page of the newspaper for cricket score

Domain 5: Reading
- Simple letters and words:
  - Alphabets (G, C, K, M, etc.)
  - Numbers (3, 8, 6, 9, etc.)
  - Simple words (ear, ant, car, etc.)
- Obeying written commands (carry cards with these commands written):
  - Make a fist
  - Open your mouth

- Point to the floor then point to the ceiling
- With your right hand, point to the left knee
- Reading aloud with comprehension:
  - Ask patient to read a newspaper item and ask him relevant questions.

Domain 6: Writing

- Ask patient to write few sentences about why he has come to the hospital or
- Ask him to write about his job/ business or
- Show him a picture and ask him to write few sentences about it
- If patient has right hemiparesis, ask him to use left hand but allow for some clumsiness.

OBSERVATIONS

- **Spontaneous speech**
  - Initiation difficulty
  - Articulation
  - Fluency (approximate number of words produced per minute. Word finding pauses should be excluded from the timing duration)
  - Prosody (the melodic intonation)
  - Grammatical correctness (agrammatic speech sounds like telegraphic language)
  - Paraphasias: If present, literal or semantic?
  - Neologisms
  - Word finding pauses, circumlocutions.
- **Naming**
  - Impaired naming, in spite of recognition of the object or the person
  - Impaired naming restricted to certain category (s)
  - Confabulation
  - Word finding difficulty, pauses, circumlocution.
- **Comprehension**
  - Impaired comprehension to spoken commands
  - If apraxia/body part agnosia interferes with body part commands, impaired "yes/ no" responses.
- **Repetition**
  - Impaired for difficult consonants in dysarthria
  - Impaired for complex grammatical sentences in aphasia.
- **Reading and writing**
  - Impaired letter formation
  - Spelling errors (most useful in mild Wernicke's aphasia)
  - Impaired grammar
  - Impaired reading comprehension, in spite of good speech comprehension in Broca's aphasia
  - Relatively preserved reading comprehension in spite of impaired auditory comprehension in Wernicke's aphasia

- Impaired reading aloud with preserved reading comprehension in conduction aphasia (reading equivalent of speech repetition).

INTERPRETATION

Interpretation of language assessment is discussed in Table 1.1.

Table 1.1: Interpretation of language assessment.

Broca's Aphasia

Domain	Observation
Spontaneous speech	Non-fluent, telegraphic, agrammatic, dysarthric, literal paraphasias
Naming	Impaired
Comprehension	Intact for yes/no questions and object pointing commands
	Apraxia can mimic comprehension defect for body part commands
	Mild impairment of complex sentences
Repetition	Impaired
Reading	Impaired (with preserved speech comprehension), especially for syntax ("third alexia")
Writing	Impaired, poor letter formation and poor grammar
Associated signs	Right hemiparesis, apraxia of left limbs
Psychiatric symptoms	Depression

Wernicke's Aphasia

Domain	Observation
Spontaneous speech	Fluent, semantic paraphasias, neologism, jargon speech, sometimes logorrhea, no dysarthria
Naming	Impaired, with paraphasias
Comprehension	Impaired even for simple sentences
Repetition	Impaired
Reading	Impaired, but sometimes relatively preserved (opposite of Broca's aphasia)
Writing	Impaired, good letter formation, spelling errors and poor grammar
Associated signs	Visual field defect
Psychiatric symptoms	Agitation

Global Aphasia

Domain	Observation
Spontaneous speech	Mute or non-fluent
Naming	Impaired
Comprehension	Impaired
Repetition	Impaired
Reading	Impaired
Writing	Impaired
Associated signs	Right hemiparesis, hemisensory loss, hemianopia

Contd...

Contd...

Conduction Aphasia

Domain	Observation
Spontaneous speech	Fluent, some literal paraphasias
Naming	Impaired
Comprehension	Intact
Repetition	Severely impaired
Reading	Inability to read aloud, reading comprehension relatively intact
Writing	Impaired variably
Associated signs	Mild right hemiparesis, apraxia of left limbs, right hemisensory Loss, visual field defect

Transcortical Motor Aphasia (similar to Broca's aphasia but with repetition preserved)

Domain	Observation
Spontaneous speech	Non-fluent
Naming	Impaired
Comprehension	Intact
Repetition	Intact
Reading	May or may not be intact
Writing	May or may not be intact

Transcortical Sensory Aphasia (similar to Wernicke's aphasia but with preserved repetition)

Domain	Observation
Spontaneous speech	Fluent, echolalia
Naming	Impaired
Comprehension	Impaired
Repetition	Intact
Reading	Impaired
Writing	Impaired

Transcortical Mixed Aphasia/Isolation of Speech Areas (similar to global aphasia with preserved repetition)

Domain	Observation
Spontaneous speech	Non-fluent, echolalia
Naming	Impaired
Comprehension	Impaired
Repetition	Intact
Reading	Impaired
Writing	Impaired

Contd...

Contd...

Alexia without Agraphia

Domain	Observation
Spontaneous speech	Normal
Naming	Impaired especially for colors
Comprehension	Normal
Repetition	Intact
Reading	Impaired
Writing	Intact
Associated signs	Right hemianopia

Alexia with Agraphia

Domain	Observation
Spontaneous speech	Fluent, some paraphasias
Naming	Impaired
Comprehension	Preserved for spoken language
Repetition	Intact
Reading	Severely impaired
Writing	Severely impaired
Associated signs	Right hemianopia, Gerstmann syndrome

Anomic Aphasia

Domain	Observation
Spontaneous speech	Fluent, word finding pauses, circumlocution
Naming	Impaired
Comprehension	Intact
Repetition	Intact
Reading	Intact
Writing	Intact, but has anomia

Thalamic Aphasia (probably results from impaired alerting of Wernicke's aphasia)

Domain	Observation
Spontaneous speech	Fluent, with prominent fluctuations (language worsens as alertness decreases)
Naming	Impaired
Comprehension	Impaired to a lesser extent than in Wernicke's aphasia
Repetition	Impaired
Reading	Impaired
Writing	Impaired

Contd...

Contd...

Basal Ganglia Lesions (left anterior putamen, caudate, anterior limb of internal capsule)	
Domain	**Observation**
Spontaneous speech	Non-fluent, echolalia, prominent dysarthria
Naming	Impaired
Comprehension	Impaired variably (can mimic Broca's or global aphasia)
Repetition	Intact
Reading	Impaired
Writing	Impaired

Lesion Localization

- **Transcortical motor aphasia:** Left frontal lobe anterior to Broca's area, frontal deep white matter, medial frontal region near SMA (in the anterior cerebral artery territory)
- **Transcortical sensory aphasia:** Left temporo-occipital region
- **Transcortical mixed aphasia:** Large watershed infarctions in the left hemisphere, sparing the perisylvian cortex, but disconnecting them from other cortical regions
- **Conduction aphasia:** Lesion involving **either** the arcuate fasciculus **or** the superior temporal gyrus **or** the inferior parietal region (supramarginal gyrus)
- **Wernicke's aphasia:** Lesion involving Wernicke's area and adjacent temporoparietal region (inferior parietal lobule, superior temporal gyrus). Blood supply is by the inferior division of the MCA
- **Single word comprehension defect:** Lesion limited to Wernicke's area
- **Broca's aphasia:** Lesion involving the Broca's area and adjacent cortex and subcortical white matter
- **Isolated speech initiation defects:** Lesion restricted to Broca's area
- **Global aphasia:** Large lesion involving the left frontal, temporal and parietal lobes. Blood supply: left MCA
- **Anomic aphasia:** Non-localizing left hemispheric disease. Usually superior temporal gyrus, but also frontal or parietal lobe near angular gyrus
- **Alexia with agraphia:** Left angular gyrus lesions
- **Alexia without agraphia:** Disconnection (of language areas from right occipital cortex) by splenial lesion pus left occipital lesion. Patient has intact left hemifield, but written information presented in that hemifield is not conveyed from right occipital cortex to the language areas
- **Third alexia:** Impaired reading comprehension in Broca's aphasia
- **Speech apraxia:** Left frontal or insular lesion.

BIBLIOGRAPHY

1. Brooks DN, Deelman BG, van Zomeren AH, et al. Problems in measuring cognitive recovery after acute brain injury. Journal of Clinical Neuropsychology. 1984;6(1): 71-85.
2. Hickok G, Poeppel D. The cortical organization of speech processing. Nature Reviews Neuroscience. 2007;393-402.
3. Kertesz A, McCabe P. Recovery patterns and prognosis in aphasia. Brain. 1977;100: 1-18.
4. Kertesz A. Western Aphasia Battery Test Manual. The Psychological Corporation. 1982.
5. Kirshner HS. Aphasia and Aphasic syndromes. In: Bradley WG, Daroff RB, Fenichel GM, Jankovic J (Eds). Neurology in Clinical practice, 5th edition, Butterworth Heinemann publication 2008.
6. Nakase-Thompson R, et al. Brief assessment of severe language impairments: initial validation of the Mississippi aphasia screening test. Brain Inj. 2005;19(9): 685-91.
7. Nakase-Thompson R, Manning E, Sherer M, et al. Bedside screen of language disturbance among acute care admissions: initial psychometrics of the Mississippi aphasia screening test. Archives of Clinical Neuropsychology. 2002;17(8):848.
8. Nakase-Thompson R, Manning E, Sherer M, et al. Brief assessment of severe language impairments: Initial validation of the Mississippi Aphasia Screening Test. Brain Injury. 2005;19:685-91.
9. Nakase-Thompson R, Sherer M, Yablon SA, et al. (manuscript in preparation). Divergent and Convergent Validity of the Mississippi Aphasia Screening Test Among Neurorehabilitation Admissions.
10. Nakase-Thompson R, Sherer M, Yablon SA, et al. Assessment of language among neurorehabilitation admissions: convergent and divergent validity of the MAST (ABSTRACT, 2003). Journal of the International Neuropsychological Society. 2003;9:303.
11. Tate RL, Lulyham JM, Broe GA, et al. Psychosocial outcome for the survivors of severe blunt head injury: the result from consecutive series of 100 patients. Journal of Neurology, Neurosurgery & Psychiatry. 1989;52:1128-34.
12. Uzzell BP, Zimmerman RA, Dolinskas CA, et al. Lateralized psychological impairment associated with CT lesions in head injured patients. Cortex. 1979;15:391-401.
13. Wise RJS. Language systems in normal and aphasic human subjects: functional imaging studies and inferences from animal studies. Br Med Bull. 2003;65:95-119.

Assessment of Higher Mental Functions

THE APRAXIAS

GRK Sarma

PICTORIAL PRETEST

Case 1

A 50-year-old man presented with acute right hemiplegia and global aphasia. After the comprehension improved significantly, he was asked to demonstrate how he would use a tooth brush. His response is captured in Figure 1.4A.

He was given his tooth brush and was asked to demonstrate how he would use it. His response was captured in Figure 1.4B.

1. What is the patient's neurological deficit?
2. Where is the lesion?

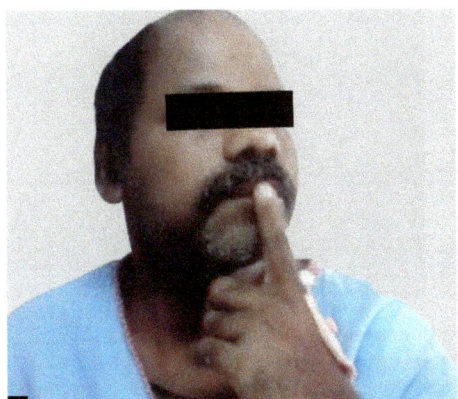 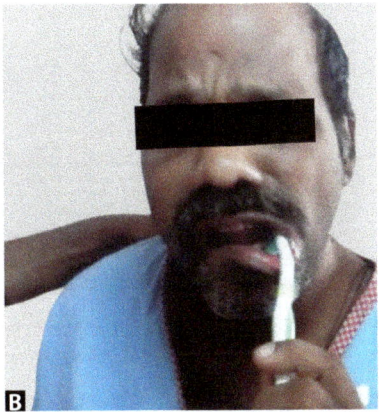

Figs. 1.4A and B: Patient with acute right hemiplegia and global aphasia.

Case 2

This 53-year-old lady was brought with left sided "weakness" following coronary artery bypass graft (CABG). She was not using her left hand for many of her daily activities. She was unable make a fist (Fig. 1.5A) or wave her left hand (Fig. 1.5B) on command. When asked to imitate the examiner's thumbs up gesture, both her hands responded well (Fig. 1.5C). When asked to remove and put on her sweater, her left hand moved quite smoothly to complete the act (Fig. 1.5D).

1. What is this patient's deficit?
2. Where is the localization of lesion?

Answers and discussions are given at the end of the chapter.

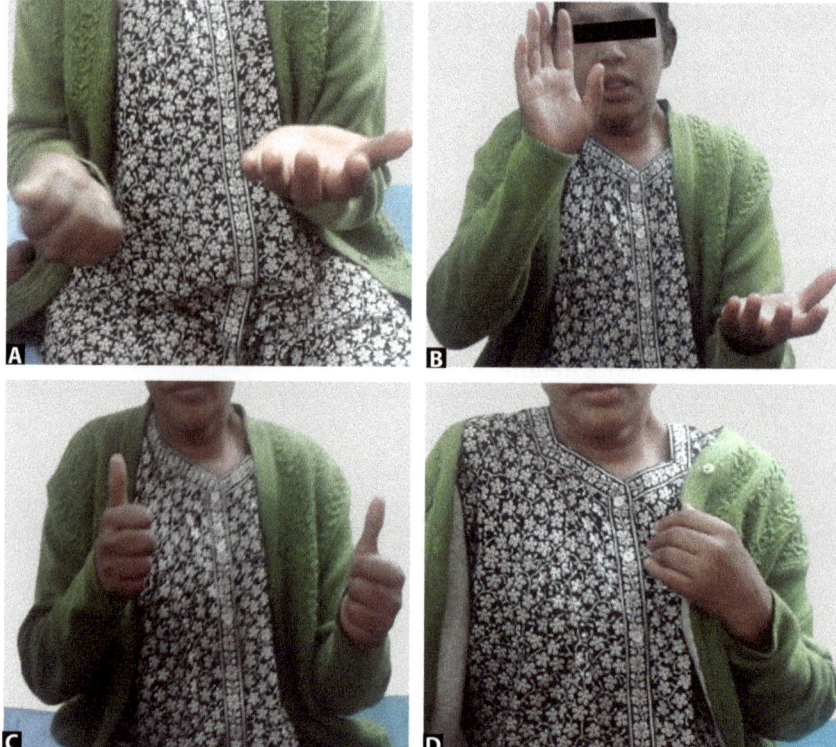

Figs. 1.5A to D: Patient with left-sided "weakness" following coronary artery bypass graft.

PHYSIOLOGICAL BASIS (FIG. 1.6)

- Definition: Apraxia is defined as inability of the patient to **perform, on request,** a learned motor act in the **absence of:**
  - Altered sensorium
  - Inadequate attention
  - Impaired comprehension
  - Significant weakness
  - Sensory loss
  - In-coordination
- The network of structures underlying praxis is thought to include the frontal and parietal cortex, basal ganglia, and white matter tracts containing projections between these areas
- Current neuropsychological models propose the following components of neural networks involved in praxis:
  - Left parietal lobe (around the intraparietal sulcus, including angular gyrus, marginal gyrus, inferior parietal lobule): **Stores program templates** for generation of sequence of movements involved in a particular complex act.

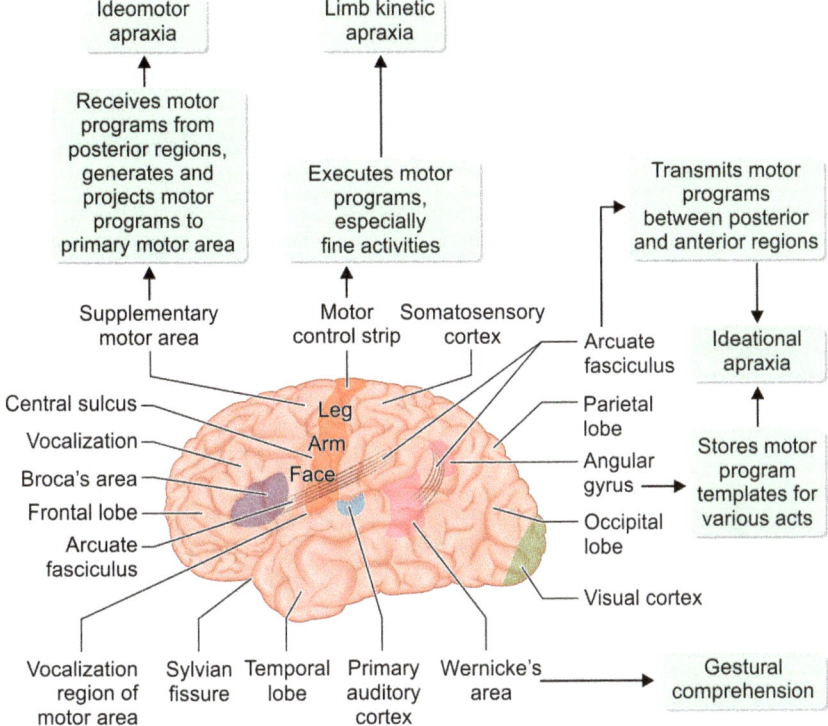

Fig. 1.6: The simplified apraxia network.

- Left parietal lobe also helps in **gestural comprehension**, whereas frontal lobe is required for **gestural production**
- Frontal lobe (middle frontal gyrus, supplementary area) converts these movement programs into movement commands
- Frontal primary motor cortex receives these commands and produces the actual movement, especially **fine distal movements**
- **Basal ganglia** fine tunes these movements
- **Superior longitudinal fasciculus** is important in networking the anterior and posterior regions (frontal and parietal regions)
- **Corpus callosum** is important in networking left and right cortical regions involved in a motor act (e.g. left hand motor act on verbal command requires inter hemispheric transfer of movement commands from left frontoparietal to right frontal regions).
- Apraxias are classified based on the **task involved** and the **body part affected** (Table 1.2):
    - Limb kinetic apraxia
    - Ideomotor apraxia
    - Ideational apraxia
    - Buccofacial apraxia
    - Constructional apraxia
    - Dressing apraxia

- Apraxia of speech
- Apraxia of eyelid opening.

Table 1.2: Evaluation of apraxia.

Types of apraxia	Method	Observation
Apraxia of eyelid opening	Ask the patient to open his closed eyes	Patient has difficulty to open his eyes. Thrusts his head up or manually opens the eyelids
Apraxia of speech	Ask patient to speak certain words on command, compare with spontaneous speech compare his spoken versus written language	Patient has near normal automatic speech. When speaking on command, he may have substitutions, repetitions, additions or prolongations. He may grope for the correct articulatory posture. His written language is spared (in contrast to aphasia)
Orofacial apraxia	Ask patient to pantomime • Blowing a candle • Sniffing a flower • Sucking through a straw • Lick his lips • Protrude the tongue If he fails, show the objects and repeat the commands If he fails, give the objects and repeat the commands	Patient produces inappropriate action. For example, he may blow out when asked to suck
Ideomotor apraxia	*Transitive gestures:* Ask patient to show how he uses a comb/key/ brush/ kicks a ball If he fails, show him or give him the objects and repeat the commands *Intransitive gestures:* Ask him how he salutes/ waves good bye/ snaps fingers/ make a fist. Check if he knows what gesture is being shown to him (e.g. salute)	Patient may produce inappropriate movement, may substitute his finger for the object. There may be temporal and spatial errors affecting timing, sequencing, amplitude, configuration, and limb position in space His performance may or may not improve when the actual object is given (voluntary-automatic dissociation) Patient may/may not identify the meaningful gesture like salute (gestural comprehension). He may comprehend the gesture, but fail to reproduce it
Ideational apraxia	Ask patient to demonstrate how to light a candle using a match box, how to write and post a letter	Patient fails to produce the correct sequence of movements to complete the act. Performance does not improve even if the objects are given

Contd...

Contd...

Types of apraxia	Method	Observation
Limb-kinetic apraxia	Ask patient to pick a small pin or needle from the table top. Ask him to turn over a coin placed near the finger tips so that heads and tails are reversed	The finger movements are slow, clumsy and labored
Constructional apraxia	Ask patient to draw a • Flower • Clock with specified time • Copy a cube • Copy Rey-Osterrieth figure	There may be: • Over-simplification of the picture • Closing-in phenomenon • Multiple perpendicular lines • Hemineglect in flower/ clock • Loss of spatial orientation among the various parts of the picture
Dressing apraxia	Ask patient to remove his shirt/jacket. Then pull a sleeve inside out and ask him to wear again	Patient may ignore the left side, may find it difficult to set right the inverted sleeve and to button the dress accurately
Apraxia of gait	Ask patient to walk	Patient has difficulty in lifting the feet off the ground and move forward (magnetic gait). He may produce repeated labored efforts to produce the desired act. He drags the feet in short steps

Ideomotor apraxia: The motor planning in the **left premotor/ supplementary motor** areas is impaired and not conveyed to the primary motor area. Patients have difficulty in performing individual motor acts on command. They may do better when the object is given and automatically perform these acts in their daily life, the so called **voluntary-automatic dissociation.** It is diagnosed when patient cannot perform one or more of the following:
- **Transitive gestures (involving objects):** Patients fail to:
    - Pantomime an action involving an object (e.g. using a toothbrush or comb)
    - Perform the appropriate action in response to a visually presented object
    - Carry out a movement using the actual object.
- **Intransitive gestures (not involving objects):** Patient fails to:
    - Perform a meaningful gesture with a limb
    - Imitate another person's gesture.

Ideational apraxia: Patient's templates of motor programs to carry out a series of actions are impaired due to lesion in the **dominant posterior region**. In this apraxia:
- Patients have difficulty carrying out a sequence of actions in performance of a complex, multistep task (e.g. making a cup of tea)

- Ideational apraxia is often seen in patients with extensive left hemisphere damage, dementia, or delirium
- This deficit may be due to a combination of executive, language, and memory limitations, or to a general limitation in cognitive resources in addition to higher order motor programming
- Unlike ideomotor apraxia, patient's day to day life is usually affected by ideational apraxia.

Limb-kinetic apraxia
- Described as inaccurate or **clumsy** distal limb movements
- Limb-kinetic apraxia is often seen in the limb contralateral to the affected hemisphere **(frontal lesions) and parkinsonism**
- It is independent of modality (e.g. verbal command versus imitation)
- There is no voluntary-automatic dissociation unlike ideomotor apraxia.

Orofacial apraxia
- There is impairment of skilled movements involving the face, mouth, tongue, larynx, and pharynx
- It has been associated with **left parietal, inferior frontal, deep frontal white matter, insula, and basal ganglia lesions**
- Automatic movements of the same muscles are often preserved (as in ideomotor limb apraxia)
- However, orofacial and limb apraxia can be dissociated, suggesting that the neural systems underlying these disorders are at least partially separable.

Constructional apraxia
- Is an inability to put together the different components of a spatial array
- Can manifest with different features in right hemispheric/left hemispheric/diffuse diseases
- With **right parietal** lesions, the structural complexity is maintained, but the spatial relationship among the various components is disturbed and there is a tendency for neglect of left half of the figure. This is especially brought out in clock or flower drawing
- With left-sided lesion, the figures are oversimplified, without a tendency for neglect. There is a tendency to draw lines perpendicular to those already drawn
- With diffuse lesions as in late dementia, the patients place their drawing close to the model or superimpose on the model (closing-in phenomenon).

Apraxia of eyelid opening
- Characterized by an inability to voluntarily open the closed eyes
- Normally, the orbicularis oculi (OOc) and the levator palpebri superioris (LPS) perform the opposite functions and are reciprocally inhibited while closing and opening the eyes. If the LPS is inappropriately inhibited or the OOc is inappropriately activated, apraxia of eyelid opening results.
- This is seen in right hemispheric or bilateral hemispheric lesions and in basal ganglia diseases (Box 1.2).

Assessment of Higher Mental Functions

Box 1.2: Causes of apraxia of eyelid opening.
- Right hemispheric lesions
- Bilateral hemispheric lesions
- Extrapyramidal diseases:
  - Parkinson's disease
  - Progressive supranuclear palsy (PSP)
  - Huntington's disease
  - Multiple system atrophy (MSA)
  - Cortical basal ganglionic degeneration (CBGD)
  - Hallervorden-Spatz disease
  - Wilson's disease
  - Neuroacanthocytosis
- Motor neuron disease
- Bilateral subthalamic lesions [as in deep brain stimulation (DBS) for Parkinson's disease]

Dressing apraxia
- Seen in right parietal lesions
- Results from a combination of hemineglect, and impaired visuospatial and tactile coordination.

METHODOLOGY

- Assess attention, concentration, comprehension before embarking on apraxia assessment
- Inform the patient's attendant not to interfere in the exam by gesturing to the patient (many attenders believe they are helping the examiner by gesturing the patient during apraxia testing)
- Assess each type of apraxia by different tests. The tests are presented here in "head to toe" order so that a complete examination can be performed.

INTERPRETATION

Clues to Apraxia Localization

- Right hand weakness, left hand apraxia: Left frontal lesion
- No weakness on any side, bilateral limb apraxia: Left parietal lesion
- No weakness on any side, left hand apraxia: Callosal lesion
- Gestural comprehension deficit: Left posterior lesion
- Gestural production deficit: Left anterior lesion
- Apraxia of eyelid opening: Right hemispheric or bilateral hemispheric lesions and basal ganglia diseases (Box 1.2)
- Orofacial apraxia: Left parietal, inferior frontal, deep frontal white matter, insula, and basal ganglia lesions
- Limb-kinetic apraxia: Contralateral primary motor cortex lesion
- Dressing apraxia: Right parietal lesions
- Constructional apraxia: Right or left hemispheric disease or diffuse disease

- Ideational apraxia: Left parietal (especially angular gyrus) lesion or extensive left hemispheric lesion
- Apraxia of speech: Left inferior frontal lesion
- Gait apraxia: Bilateral medial frontal lesions (as in multiple infarcts or hydrocephalus).

BIBLIOGRAPHY

1. Damasio AR, Tranel D, Rizzo M. Disorders of complex visual processing. In: Mesulam MM (Ed). Principles of behavioral and cognitive neurology. New York: Oxford University Press; 2000. pp. 362-3.
2. Geschwind N. The apraxias: neural mechanisms of disorders of learned movement. Am Sci. 1975;63:188-95.
3. Gross RG, Grossman M. Update on apraxias. Curr Neurol Neurosci Rep. 2008;8(6): 490-6.
4. Haaland KY, Harrington DL, Knight RT. Neural representations of skilled movement. Brain. 2000;123 (Pt 11):2306-13.
5. Heilman KM, Rothi LJ, Valenstein E. Two forms of ideomotor apraxia. Neurology. 1982;32:342-6.
6. Heilman KM, Rothi LJG. Apraxia. In: Heilman KM, Valenstein E, (Eds). Clinical Neuropsychology. New York: Oxford University Press 2003. pp. 215-35.
7. Leiguarda RC, Marsden CD. Limb apraxias: Higher-order disorders of sensorimotor integration. Brain. 2000;123.
8. Ozsancak C, Auzou P, Dujardin K, et al. Orofacial apraxia in corticobasal degeneration, progressive supranuclear palsy, multiple system atrophy and Parkinson's disease. J Neurol. 2004;251:1317-23.

ANSWERS TO THE PRETEST

Case 1

1. This patient was unable to perform simple motor act (in this case, demonstrating the use of a toothbrush). There is a spatial error affecting the correct limb placement in space and there is finger substitution for the object. When given the actual object, he was able to automatically perform the act correctly. This **voluntary-automatic dissociation** is indicative of ideomotor apraxia.
2. The anatomical correlate of this finding is an anteriorly placed lesion in the left hemisphere, that spares the motor programs stored in the more posterior regions, especially the angular gyrus. His diffusion weighted MRI demonstrated a left hemispheric acute infarct, possibly sparing the angular gyrus and adjacent areas.

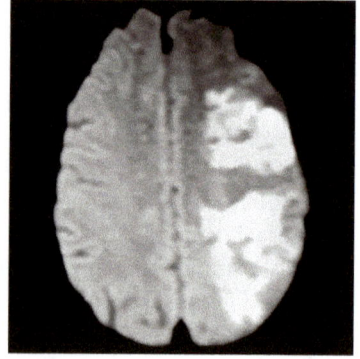

Case 2

1. It is evident from Figures 1.5C and D that there is no true left hand weakness and it is likely that the patient's disability was due to left hand apraxia. Left hand apraxia can occur in three situations:
   - Left frontal lesion: It is associated with right hand weakness. In all the figures, right hand was moving normally. Therefore, it is unlikely.
   - Left parietal lesion: Here, no weakness is expected on either side because of the intact frontal regions. But the apraxia is **always bilateral**, because the movement templates originate from left parietal areas and then project to bilateral premotor areas. In this patient, right hand praxis is preserved (Figs. 1.5A to D). Thus parietal lesion is unlikely.
   - Callosal lesion: Here also, there is no weakness of any limb. Movement templates originate in the intact left parietal lobe and project normally to left premotor area, but fail to reach right premotor area. Thus, patient will have normal right hand praxis and impaired left hand praxis to command (Figs. 1.5A and B).
   - In contrast to gestures on command, gesture imitation can occur in the right hemisphere. Therefore, the patient was able to imitate the thumbs up gesture with left hand (Fig. 1.5C)
   - Dressing praxis is lateralized to right hemisphere and is preserved in this patient (Fig. 1.5D).
2. The above features suggest that the lesion is likely to involve anterior corpus callosum that has disconnected right premotor areas from left parietal projections. Her CT scan (below) confirmed the localization.

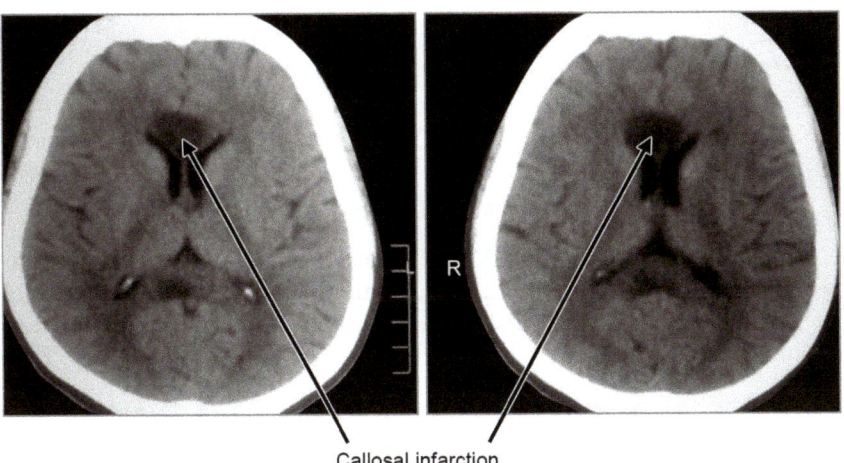

Callosal infarction

CALCULATIONS

GRK Sarma

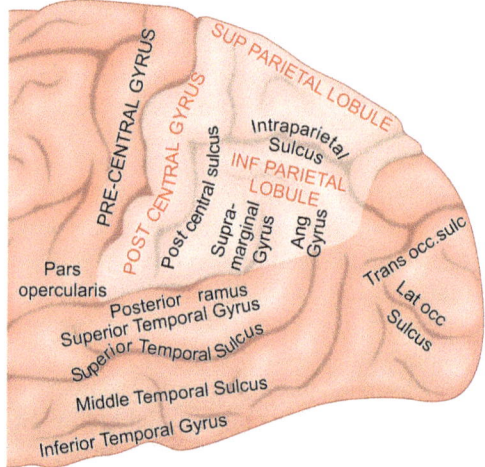

Fig. 1.7: Anatomical definition of the inferior parietal lobule.

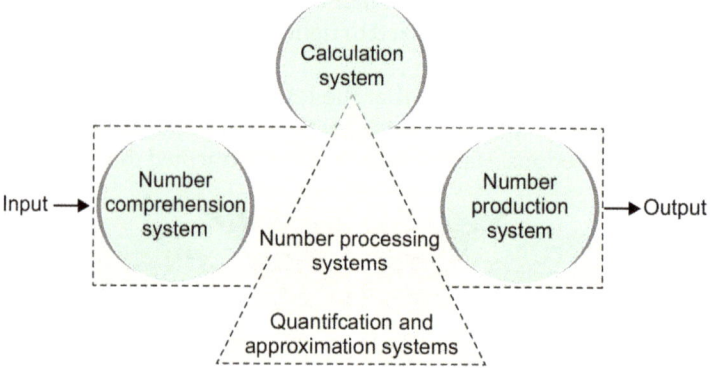

Fig. 1.8: Schematic representation of number processing and calculation.

Dehaene and Cohen (1995) put forward a schema to understand the processes involved in calculations and number processing. This model suggests that a number of lesion locations can potentially impair these functions.

CALCULATIONS AND RELATED PARIETAL LOBE FUNCTIONS (FINGER IDENTIFICATION, RIGHT-LEFT ORIENTATION)

Physiologic Basis

- Dominant inferior parietal lobule is required for calculations, right left orientation and finger identification
- Deficits in these functions along with dysgraphia constitute the Gerstmann syndrome

A. Calculation

- Proper execution of calculations requires the following:
  - Good attention and concentration
  - Intact language functions for number recognition
  - Intact visual fields and spatial attention (e.g. no hemianopia/hemineglect)
  - Intact frontal executive functions
  - Intact primary arithmetic function in the inferior parietal lobule
- Primary acalculia (due to parietal lesion): It is defined as impaired numerical concepts and impaired execution of basic operations (additions, subtractions, borrowing, carrying, etc.)
- It can be confidently diagnosed only after excluding all other deficits listed above (secondary acalculia).

Methodology

- Forward counting, backward counting
- Ask what number comes after or before a given number (e.g. before 400, after 199 and so on)
- Give two numbers and ask which is bigger or which is smaller
- Read a number and ask patient to write the word for it (e.g. give number 32, patient should write "thirty two"); show the written word and ask him to write the corresponding number (e.g. show the word "sixty nine", patient should write "69")
- Give single digit and double digit additions, subtractions
- If he does them correctly, give more complex arithmetic like multidigit additions, subtractions, multiplications, divisions, depending on his baseline capabilities. Test carry over and borrow functions
- Basic rules like $N \times 0 =?$; $N + 0 =?$; $N \times 1 =?$ have to be tested.

Interpretation

- Primary acalculia indicates left inferior parietal lobule lesion. In addition, there are reports of frontal lobe and basal ganglia lesions with primary acalculia
- Errors in tests like which is a bigger or smaller number indicate defects in numerical concepts
- Errors in "what comes after or before..." also indicate numerical concept defects
- Errors in spelling a number and writing the number to dictation indicate "transcoding defect" (i.e. conversion of visual to verbal modality and vice versa)
- Errors in actual arithmetic functions indicate defects in manipulation of numbers and application of basic arithmetic principles
- Errors of omission indicate inattention (e.g. missing to add a number in a carry-over function)
- Errors also occur in inattention to the mathematical symbols (+ and -).
- Perseveration errors manifest by sticking to same function inspite of being given another (e.g. patient may continue perform addition, even though a subtraction sum is given)

B. Right-left Disorientation

- Benton 20 point assessment scale is used by neuropsychologists for testing right left orientation
- Bedside examination can be performed by the following methods:
    - Verbal modality:
        - Ask patient to show various body regions of either side (e.g. right hand, left ear, etc.)
        - Then give more complex commands (e.g. touch your left ear with your right hand)
        - Ask him to point your (examiner's) body parts on the correct side (e.g. which is my right eye?)
        - If the patients responses are correct with verbal modality, non-verbal tests may be omitted. If verbal test is abnormal, nonverbal tests are administered to confirm true right-left disorientation (and not aphasic error)
    - Nonverbal modality: Ask patient to copy the examiner' gesture using the same body regions (e.g. touch your right ear with your left hand, patient has to reproduce the same). The same can be tested by using pictures of persons doing certain actions instead of examiner's gestures
    - Nonverbal modality: Ask patient to describe the relation of parts of a picture in terms of right and left (e.g. the child in the picture to the right or left of his mother?)
- Impairment in verbal modality may be a part of aphasia. Hence, abnormality in this modality must be verified by nonverbal tests.
- Impairment in nonverbal modality indicates true right-left disorientation.

Interpretation
- True right left disorientation is seen in left inferior parietal lobule lesions.

C. Finger Identification

- Bedside testing is done by verbal and nonverbal modalities
- If responses on verbal modality are normal, further testing may be skipped. If, they are abnormal, nonverbal modality tests are needed to confirm true finger agnosia (and not aphasic error)
- Verbal modality: Ask patient to show his thumb, index finger, little finger, pointing finger on your command
- Nonverbal modality: Show a picture of hand and ask the patient to match his own fingers to those demonstrated in the picture.

Interpretation
- True finger agnosia is a part of Gerstmann syndrome due to a lesion in the left inferior parietal lobule

THE AGNOSIAS

Madhusudanan M

PHYSIOLOGIC BASIS

- **Gnosis** essentially means "to know". It is defined as an appreciation of meaning of a stimulus
- **Agnosia:** Perception of stimuli without appreciation of its meaning. Agnosia represents a lack or loss of knowledge
- Agnosia is **modality-specific** recognition impairment that cannot be fully explained by problems in elementary sensory processing, mental deterioration, attentional disturbances, aphasic misnaming, or to unfamiliarity with the stimuli used to assess recognition abilities
- Agnosias are of **two types:** Apperceptive and associative
    - **Apperceptive agnosia:** A deficit in multimodal **perceptual processing** wherein all features of perceived stimulus cannot be synthesized so as to form a meaningful whole. The patient fails to draw, copy or match an object. In the strict sense, it is not a true agnosia. Some patients have perceptual categorization deficit, in which there is a difficulty in recognizing the objects presented in an unconventional view, for example, rotation. This deficit is seen in right parietal lesions.
    - **Associative agnosia:** A completely perceived stimulus is not recognized due to failure to access the **associated semantic store.** The patient can draw, copy or match the object, but cannot recognize it.
- **Optic aphasia:** It is a condition wherein, the patient recognizes but cannot name an object presented in visual modality, but can do so in other modalities. It represents a disconnection between visual recognition and lexicon. It is seen during recovery of associative agnosia.

Classification

Agnosia is classified according to stimulus modality:
- Visual agnosia:
    - Object agnosia
    - Color agnosia
    - Prosopagnosia (Failure of recognition of familiar faces)
    - Simultanagnosia: Unable to simultaneously appreciate multiple objects or multiple elements of an object in the same visual image
    - Topographagnosia which may be a landmark agnosia (inability to recognize familiar buildings or other landmarks) or an egocentric disorientation (inability to follow, memorize or describe route maps)
- Auditory agnosia: Inability to recognize familiar sounds. This is classified into:
    - General auditory agnosia: Impaired recognition of all types of auditory stimuli

- Agnosia for speech (verbal auditory agnosia or pure word deafness). Reading, speaking and writing are preserved
- Phonagnosia: Inability to recognize familiar voices (auditory equivalent of prosopagnosia)
- Agnosia for environmental sounds: Agnosia for non-speech environmental sounds like ticking of a clock, or a ringing bell
- Agnosia for music (amusia): Impairment in musical expression or perception

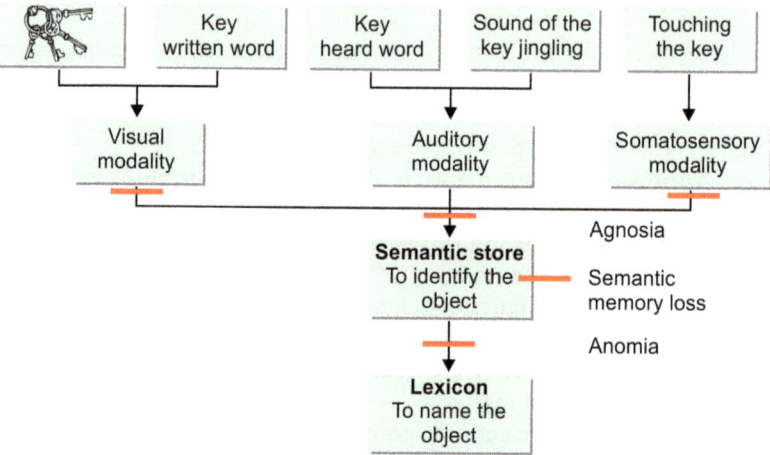

Fig. 1.9: Neuropsychological model for agnosias. A bunch of keys can be perceived by various sensory modalities. Subsequently meaning is attached to the percepts by accessing the semantic store. Connections with language centers ascribe a name to the percept. The red line indicates the lesion sites causing the various defects.

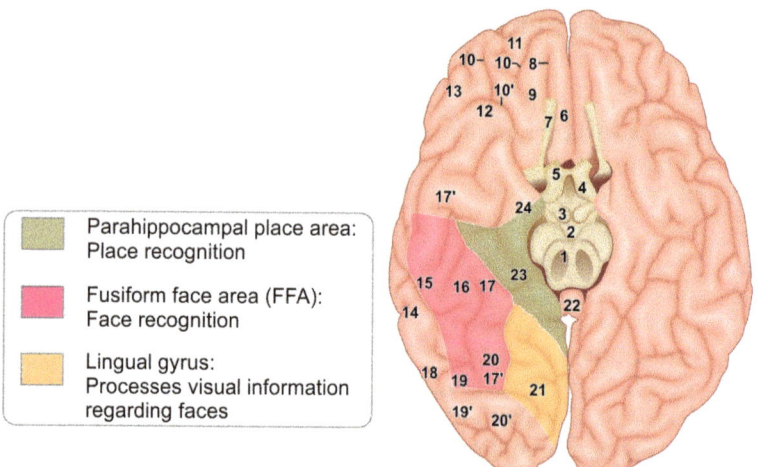

Fig. 1.10: Various category specific agnosias and their usual anatomical correlates.

- Tactile agnosia: Selective impairment of object recognition by touch despite relatively preserved primary and discriminative somesthetic perception is known as tactile agnosia.

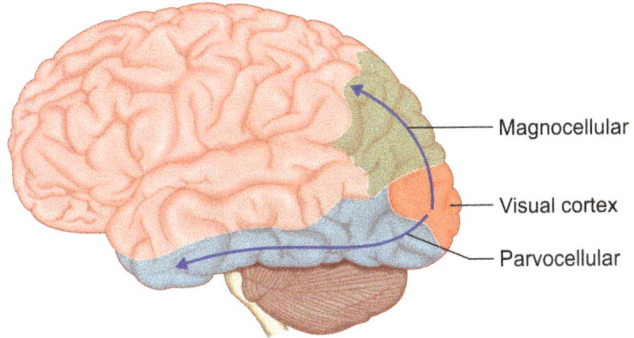

Fig. 1.11: Processing of visual information is proposed to occur along a dorsal stream to the parietal region and a ventral stream to the temporal region. The former deals with movement in space and the latter with patterns of objects and faces.

METHODOLOGY

Visual Agnosia Testing

1. Apperceptive agnosia:
   - Ask the patient to copy the simple line diagrams. Inability to reproduce these suggests defective perception (apperceptive agnosia) (Fig. 1.12)

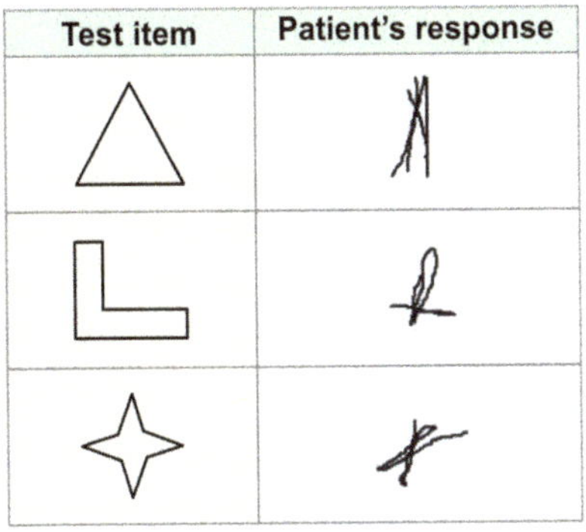

Test item	Patient's response
△	〤
L	↯
✦	⚹

Fig. 1.12: Apperceptive agnosia: Examples of defective drawing.

   - If the patient has motor impairment interfering with copying, ask him to match a test picture with multiple choices (Fig. 1.13)

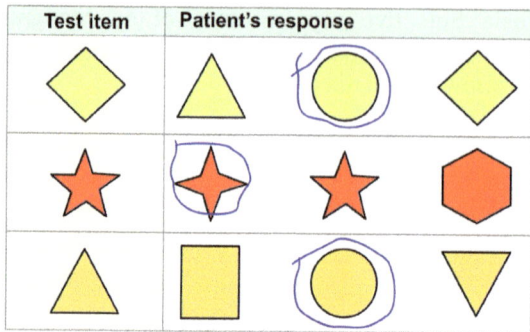

Fig. 1.13: Apperceptive agnosia: Examples of defective shape matching.

- For a more complex perception task, ask him to identify a common object presented in an unusual perspective. An example is a bucket as seen from above (Figs. 1.14A and B).

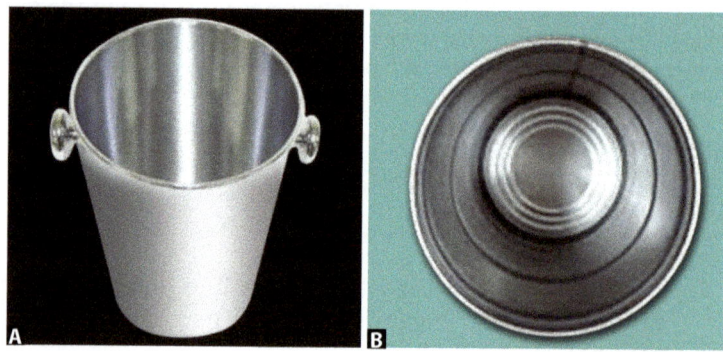

Figs. 1.14A and B: Example of perceptual categorization deficit.

2. Associative agnosia:
   - If perception is considered normal, test a associative gnosis by showing common objects like spectacles, keys, pen, etc.
   - If the patient fails to recognize these, present them in their appropriate context. For example, if he cannot recognize spectacles, show a picture of a person wearing them (Figs. 1.15A and B).
   - If the patient is able to recognize the common objects, give a more complex task like line diagrams (Fig. 1.16)

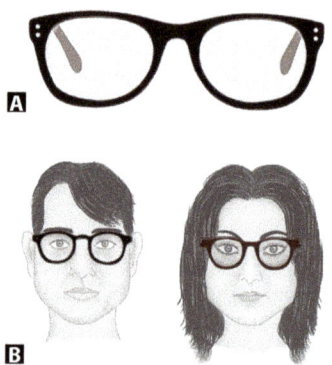

Figs 1.15A and B: Mild degrees of visual agnosia can be detected when the object is placed in its usual perspective.

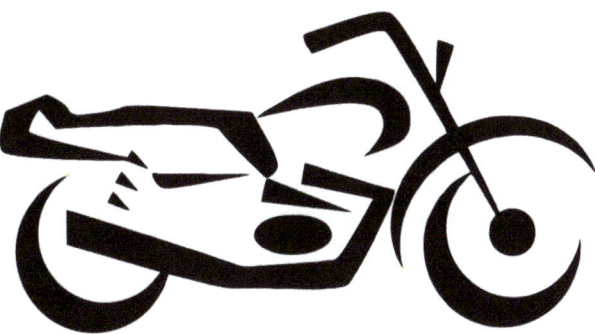

Fig. 1.16: Line diagram of motorbike.

- Show faces of familiar personalities and ask patient to identify
- Colors: Ask patient to name the colors of objects, match the test colors, and recall colors of common objects (banana, apple)
- Topographic agnosia
  - Ask patient to describe a route map in familiar area
  - Ask him to describe the lay out of his house and immediate environment
- Ask patient to close his eyes and identify sound of bunch of keys, and ticking clock.

INTERPRETATION

- **Associative visual agnosia:** The lesion is in posterior and inferior temporal and occipital regions (in the so called "what" system). The lateral occipital complex, has been found to respond in a general manner to all formed visual objects. The major cause is ischemia and degenerative conditions like posterior cortical atrophy and late Alzheimer's disease.
- **Optic aphasia:** The lesion is in left ventral temporal and occipital regions and the splenium that disconnects language areas from visual recognition areas. If the splenium is intact, visual information from right occipitotemporal region can access the language areas and there is no naming defect.
- **Prosopagnosia:** Bilateral fusiform gyrus and its adjacent inferior temporal and occipital gyri. There may be a right hemispheric dominance.
- **Color agnosia:** Dominant hemisphere lesions that involve the inferomedial aspect of the occipital and temporal lobes, and the left medial sub-splenial area.
- **Dorsal simultanagnosia:** It is characterized by a failure to see more than one "object" at a time. In this of simultanagnosia, there is an inability to sustain attention simultaneously in different locations in the visual field, causing individual objects to disappear from view or appear fragmented. There is a "shrinkage" of the attentional spotlight.
- **Ventral simultanagnosia:** It appears to be due to a slowing of visual processing speed, with difficulty in simultaneously processing the

individual elements of a complex image and may result in slow, laborious interpretation of a scene or reading by individual letters. Dorsal simultanagnosia is associated with bilateral lesions involving the posterior parietal or parieto-occipital regions as in Balint's syndrome. The ventral type is seen in left occipitotemporal lesions.
- **Landmark agnosia:** The inability to identify familiar landmarks and buildings. This follows right ventral temporo-occipital lesions. Functional imaging has revealed a "parahippocampal place area", a region adjacent to the fusiform face area.
- **Egocentric disorientation:** Right parietotemporal lesions.
- **General auditory agnosia:** Most often associated with bilateral temporal damage and can develop from cortical deafness.
- **Verbal auditory agnosia:** Typically results from bilateral temporal lesions in the superior temporal cortex or its subcortical connections. However, a unilateral left temporal lesion can also produce pure word deafness less commonly.
- **Phonagnosia:** It is seen after right parietal damage.
- **Agnosia for environmental sounds:** Bilateral auditory radiations.
- **Apperceptive amusia:** Right parietal lesions.
- **Associative amusia:** Bitemporal lesions.

CAVEATS

- Anomia may be confused with agnosia. Anomia is an inability to name when presented through any modality, whereas, agnosia is "**failure of recognition of an object despite intact perception**" and is unimodal. Anomic patients can demonstrate the use of an object, while agnostic patients cannot.
- Auditory agnosia may be mimicked by cortical deafness. The latter patients behave as if they were deaf, whereas patients with auditory agnosia are aware of sounds but have problem with sound identification.
- Wernicke's aphasia may mimic auditory agnosia. The former have impaired verbal comprehension but intact sound identification.
- Astereognosis may be confused with tactile agnosia. It is a unilateral disorder of ability to recognize basic features such as size, weight and texture of the object by palpation. In tactile agnosia, a bilateral disorder, these features are recognized, but the object recognition is impaired.
- Apraxias can interfere with tasks in which, object recognition is tested by demonstration of its use.

BIBLIOGRAPHY

1. Barton JJ. Disorders of color and object recognition: syndromes of the ventral occipitotemporal pathway. Continuum Lifelong Learning in Neurology. 2010;16: 111-27.
2. Barton JJ. Disorders of face perception and recognition. Neurologic Clin. 2003;21(2):521-48.

3. Bauer RM. The agnosias. Clinical neuropsychology: a pocket handbook for assessment. 2006.
4. Bradley's Neurology in Clinical Practice, 6th edition.
5. Brazis PW. Localization in Clinical Neurology. 6th edition.
6. Cooper SA. Higher visual function: hats, wives and disconnections. Pract Neurol. 2012;12(6):349-57.
7. De Renzi E. Disorders of visual recognition. Seminars in Neurology. 2000;20(4):479-85.
8. Greene JD. Apraxia, agnosias, and higher visual function abnormalities. J Neurol Neurosurg Psychiatr. 2005;76(Suppl 5):v25-34.
9. Lezak MD. Neuropsychological Assessment, 5th edition.
10. Mesulam MM. Principles of cognitive and behavioural neurology, 2nd edition.
11. Rizzo M. Clinical assessment of complex visual dysfunction. Seminars in Neurology. 2000;20:75-87.
12. Slevc LR, Shell AR. Auditory agnosia. Handbook of Clin Neurol. 2015;129:573-87.
13. Starr A, Rame G. Auditory neuropathy in handbook of clinical neurology, Vol 129 (3). In: Celesia GG, Hickok G, (Eds). The Human Auditory System. Elsevier; 2015.
14. The visual brain in action, 2nd edition, Milner & Goodale.

MEMORY

GRK Sarma

PRETEST

Two patients A and B with a digit span of 5 were given the following list of words to learn and recall after 60 seconds and 3 minutes. Look at the test results and comment on the memory systems that are affected and the anatomical correlates.

Word list: Banana, honesty, cow, truck

	Learning trials					Delayed recall	
	1	2	3	4	5	60 seconds	3 minutes
Patient A							
Banana	+	+	+	+	+	+	+
Honesty	-	-	+	+	+	+	+
Cow	-	-	+	+	+	+	+
Truck	+	+	+	+	+	+	+
Patient B							
Banana	+	+	+			+	+
Honesty	+	+	+			+	+
Cow	+	+	+			+	-
Truck	+	+	+			-	-

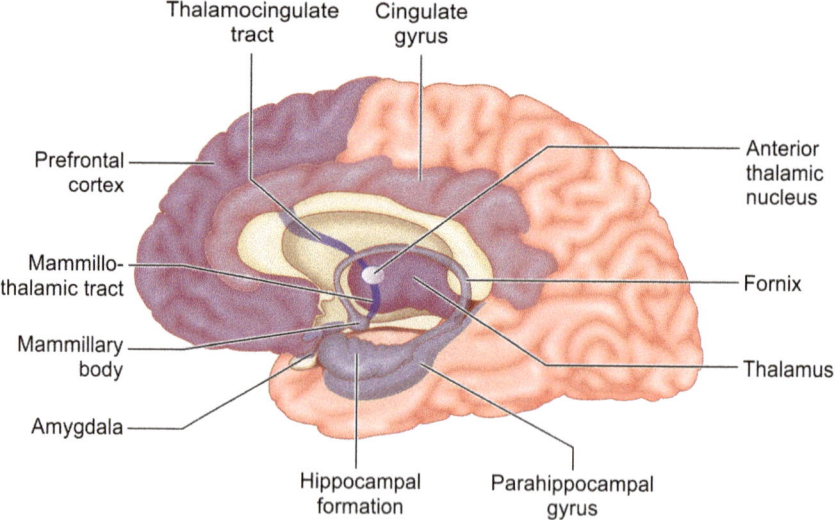

Fig. 1.17: Medial temporal lobe and its connections that are responsible for encoding short-term memory.

Assessment of Higher Mental Functions

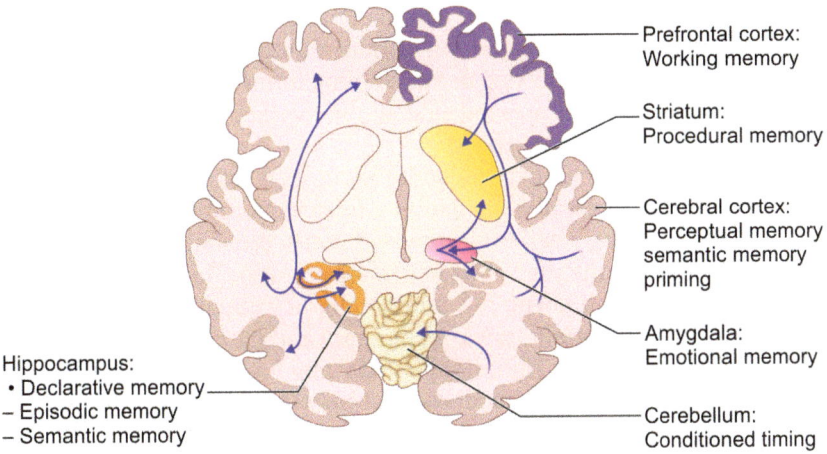

Fig. 1.18: Various brain regions responsible for different types of memory.

PHYSIOLOGIC BASIS

- Memory is defined as the ability of the brain to store and retrieve information.
- Memory is classified as follows (Flowchart 1.2):
  - Explicit memory involves conscious recall and requires integrity of various cortical regions
  - Implicit memory does not require conscious recall and does not involve medial temporal structures. Basal ganglia and cerebellum are important in this memory system
  - Immediate memory (working memory): The information that a subject can keep in conscious awareness for a brief period

Flowchart 1.2: Classification of memory.

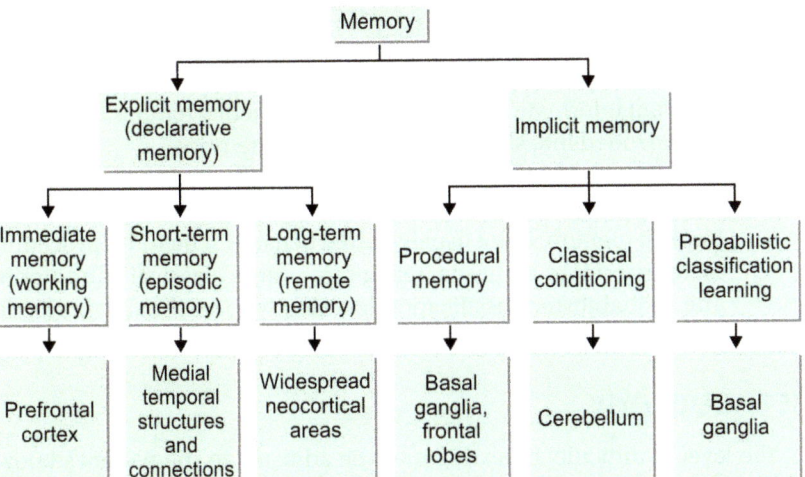

(few seconds to minutes) and manipulate it, without memorizing it (For example, remembering a phone number for dialing) prefrontal cortex is the main region sub-serving immediate memory. Verbal information activates left side and nonverbal information activates right side prefrontal cortex.

- Short-term memory (episodic memory): Involves the ability to register and recall information after several minutes or hours (e.g. remembering a series of unrelated items, remembering events that occurred in the preceding few hours or days). This is dependent on integrity of hippocampus and parahippocampal region. Perirhinal cortex is important for visual memory and parahippocampal cortex (especially on the right side) is important for spatial memory.
- Amygdala is important for recall of emotional aspects of the episodic memory, especially fear.
- Anteromedial thalamus activates medial temporal structures during memory tasks and its lesions (e.g. Wernicke-Korsakoff syndrome) can cause amnesia. However, prominent confabulations point to thalamic rather than temporal lobe lesion.
- Long-term memory (remote memory): Involves long known information regarding personal aspects as well as the external world (e.g. schooling details, famous personalities, major events in the history, etc.). Remote memory is believed to be represented in widespread neocortical networks, and is not dependent on the medial temporal structures for retrieval.
- Semantic memory is a type of long-term memory concerned with factual details outside of personal details.
- A useful concept on how memory systems work is put forward by Budson and Price. The frontal lobe can be considered as "filing clerk", deciding which information has to be filed or retrieved. The medial temporal lobes are the actual filing cabinets for recent memories. The neocortical regions are filing cabinets for remote memories.
- When presented with information, it is held and manipulated by the working memory system of the prefrontal cortex.
- Relevant information is processed by the medial temporal structures and encoded into short-term or episodic memory.
- Over longer period, the information becomes more widespread in various neocortical regions in a modality dependent way.
- Implicit memory is not usually tested bedside. It includes procedural memory (riding a bicycle, using tools, etc.), classical conditioning and probabilistic classification learning (e.g. reasonably predicting the likelihood of rain in a given situation, etc).

METHODOLOGY

- The level of difficulty of testing must be adjusted to the patient's known level of functioning and educational and professional background

- All standard MSE tools have a memory component of variable complexity.
- Neuropsychologists use the Wechsler Memory Scale-III battery that tests various aspects of memory with individual subtest scores and age relevant norms
- The following is a scheme for examining different aspects of memory in a more detailed fashion, beyond the standard tools like MMSE.
- **Working memory**
    - Forward digit span: A series of random numbers are read out at 1 per second and patient is asked to repeat the same sequence. Start with 3 to 4 digits and increase if patient succeeds. Normal digit span is 7 ± 2
    - 100-7 serial subtraction test: Ask the patient to serially subtract 7 from 100 and so on. Count the number of errors in the first 5 subtractions.
    - Ask the patient to spell "WORLD" backwards
    - If working memory (immediate recall) is impaired with >50-75% failure rate, testing the short-term and long-term memory is not fruitful
    - The digit span of the patient can be used to decide on the number of words to be given (word span) in episodic memory test (see below).
- **Episodic memory**
    - Verbal memory
        - Question about patient's breakfast, or other incidents of the day or the day before
        - Learning of 3 or more unrelated words:
            - A systematic way to determine the number of words to be given is by subtracting 1 from the digit span
            - Examiner presents the words aloud clearly at one word per second
            - Patient has to immediately repeat the words
            - If patient misses one or more words, the list is presented again until the patient repeats the list correctly three consecutive times (to ensure memory encoding)
            - Patient is distracted with serial 3s addition task and other tasks
            - After 60 seconds and again after 3 minutes, recall is tested
            - If patient fails to completely recall the test items, recognition from a list that includes test items and distracters is tested. Also, semantic cues, category cues ("it is a fruit"), phonemic cues (" br" for "brown"). Further cueing can be in the form of giving multiple choices (" is it apple/orange/banana/grapes?")
            - The number of times the list has to be presented for complete learning is a measure of the attention
            - The rate of forgetting can be measured by comparing the 60 second and 3 minute performance
            - Normal persons recall at least 3 out of 4 words after 10 minutes

- Over 80 years, this decreases to 2 out of 4 words. But, they can continue to learn if the correct responses are provided again. In dementia, this new learning is impaired
              - Story recall: A brief story is read out to the patient, followed by a set of questions based on the story
          - Nonverbal memory: Especially useful in assessment of aphasic patients
              - Hidden objects:
                  - Hide 3 to 5 common objects as the patient observes
                  - Give distracting tasks for 5 minutes
                  - Ask patient to recall the objects that are hidden and their respective locations
                  - Normal persons correctly remember 4 out of 5 objects. Remembering less than 3 objects is clearly abnormal
              - Geometric figures:
                  - Show a set of 3 simple geometric figures and ask him to copy them
                  - Give distracting tasks for 5 minutes
                  - Ask him to reproduce the 3 figures
              - Rey-Osterrieth figure: It is a complex figure with several geometric shapes and lines embedded in one. Patient has to observe the figure and reproduce as many details as possible. There are normative data for the number of components that are expected to be reproduced.
              - Family scene recall:
                  - In this, pictures of familiar family scenes are shown to the patient
                  - Patient is asked to recall the details of the picture including the people, their actions as well as locations of various objects in the picture.
- **Long-term memory**
    - Personal information: Ask about schooling, job, personal events, etc. names of children, siblings, personal phone number, address, date of birth, wedding anniversary date. There has to be means to check the correctness of the answers (presence of spouse/children)
    - General knowledge: Ask about famous personalities, events like independence day, politicians, recent prime ministers or presidents sportspersons, celebrities, capitals of states
    - Recollecting the geography of one's house or neighborhood (non-verbal and spatial memory)
    - Semantic memory: Definition of words, differences between words
- **Mini-Cog test**
    - It is a 3-minute screening test for cognitive impairment
    - It is less affected than MMSE by language, ethnicity or other factors

- In the first step, examiner reads out three words—Apple, Watch, Penny (a number of other word sets can be used, ensuring that they are from different categories). Patient is asked to repeat all the three. 3 trials are given to learn, before moving to the step 2
- In the second step, a predrawn circle is provided and patient is asked to fill in the numbers of a clock and then draw the hands of the clock to indicate the time '10 minutes past 11 O, clock' or '20 minutes past 8 O, clock'. If the task is not completed in 3 minutes, step 3 is undertaken.
- In the third step, patient is asked to recall the three words given in step 1
- Scoring: 1 point each for correct word recalled.

Interpretation
- Score 0: Cognitively impaired
- Score 1-2 with abnormal clock drawing: Cognitively impaired
- Score 1-2 with normal clock drawing: Negative for cognitive impairment
- Score 3: No cognitive impairment.

INTERPRETATION

- Isolated explicit memory impairment (with preserved attention, concentration, visuospatial skills, language, perceptual functions) is called 'cortical amnestic syndrome'. It differs from dementia, which, by definition, involves multiple domains listed above
- Impaired working memory implies a lesion involving the prefrontal cortex and its connections, especially perisylvian language areas
- **Impaired registration and recall** of new information (e.g. 3 unrelated words or pictures) is called "**anterograde amnesia**". It implies a lesion in the medial temporal lobe or its connections. Such impairment for verbal information indicates left temporal dysfunction and for non-verbal information indicates right temporal dysfunction
- **Impaired recall** of information registered within a certain interval before disease onset is called "**retrograde amnesia**". Since, the dependency of the long-term memory on medial temporal structures decreases with time (as it gets distributed to neocortical structures), the older memories are less affected than more recent memories
- Hemispheric differences in verbal and nonverbal memory hold true only in chronic lesions. In acute lesions, both types of memory may be detected even in unilateral lesions, if adequately tested
- If retrograde amnesia is noted for events that occurred more than 2 years earlier, a defect in retrieval mechanisms may be strongly suspected
- Impaired recall, in spite of cues, of verbal and nonverbal information has the same significance as impaired registration
- Impaired recall that improves with cues suggests a defect in "**retrieval system**" indicates a lesion in the **prefrontal cortex- subcortical networks.**

CAVEATS

- Depressed patients may complain of memory problems and do poorly on memory tests (pseudodementia)
- Similarly anxious patients may do poorly on these tests
- However, when tested for new learning of 4 unrelated words, psychogenic amnesic patients perform well, compared to true dementia patients
- Inattentive patients perform poorly on these tests
- Conduction aphasia can impair digit span test.

ANSWERS TO THE PRETEST

Patient A

1. Took several trials to learn 4 unrelated words indicating impaired attention/working memory system that require prefrontal cortex and its networks.
2. After 3 minutes of distracting tasks, he recalled all the four items correctly, indicating preserved short-term memory system that includes medial temporal lobe and its networks.
3. This patient had a mild metabolic encephalopathy.

Patient B

1. Has quickly learnt the 4 words, indicating preserved prefrontal cortex and its connections. After 60 seconds, he recalled 3 words and after 3 minutes, only 2 words. This suggests progressive loss of information due to unstable encoding by the medial temporal lobe and its connections.
2. This patient had Alzheimer's disease.

Assessment of Higher Mental Functions

CONSTRUCTION AND DRESSING

GRK Sarma

PICTORIAL PRETEST

A 60-year-old man was asked to copy a cube and his reproduction of the test item is shown in Figure 1.19.

1. What are the abnormalities and how do you interpret them?
2. Which further neuropsychological test is required to confirm the localization?

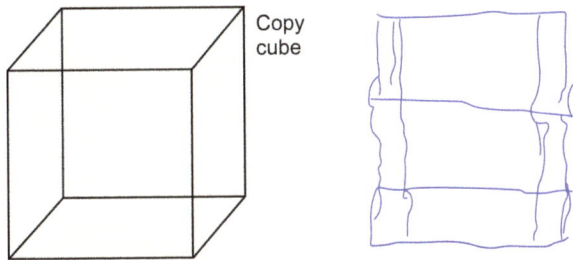

Fig. 1.19: Test for constructional tasks.

CONSTRUCTION

Physiologic Basis

- Definition: Constructional praxis is the ability to draw or construct 2 or 3 dimensional figures or shapes
- Constructional tasks require good visual-motor integration
- These tasks require an ability to perceive the several elements of an item as well as their spatial relationship, followed by an ability to execute the appropriate motor program
- Visual information from the primary visual cortex is further processed in the secondary visual cortex of the inferior parietal lobule
- The parietal lobe is the major area involved in learning and programming skilled movements
- The frontal premotor and motor cortices are involved in execution of the motor programs
- Since, extensive cortical areas are needed to perform the construction tasks, early or mild brain damage can produce deficits in these tasks
- In constructional tasks, the right hemisphere maintains the overall configuration, while the left hemisphere fills in the details.

Methodology

- Ensure at least 20/200 visual activity
- Ensure good motor power and coordination, sufficient to complete the task

- Select the appropriate task that matches the patient's expected level of capability:
  - Copying simple and complex (e.g. Rey-Osterrieth figure) geometric shapes with a pencil
  - Spontaneous drawings
  - Two-dimensional block designs
  - Stick pattern reproduction
  - Three-dimensional block constructions

  The first 2 tasks are easy to use bedside.

A. Drawing Reproduction

- A predrawn or printed design may be given or the examiner may draw them at the time of testing
- Patient is preferably given a plain white sheet, instead of a ruled one
- Ask the patient to copy a:
  - Diamond
  - Cross
  - Cube
  - Triangle within a triangle.

Observations: The following aspects of constructional task performance have to be noted:
  - Distortion of the design
  - Rotation of the figure (>90° is considered poor construction)
  - Preservation of all angles
  - Preservation of 3 dimensionality
  - Reproduction of minute details of the picture
  - Relation of parts of the picture to one another
  - Perseveration
  - Closing in phenomenon.

B. Drawing to Command

Ask the patient to draw:
- A daisy in a flower pot
- A clock with numbers and hands; ask him to place the hands of the clock so as to indicate a particular time (choose a time such that one hand points to left side and the other to the right side of the clock)
- A house in perspective.

Observations: Look for the following aspects
- Gross distortion
- Rotation
- Loss of 3 dimensionality of the house
- Symmetry of number placement in the clock
- Correct placement of the daisy in the pot.

Interpretation
- Performance on constructional tasks declines with age. Thus, subtle abnormalities should not be over-interpreted.
- Clearly abnormal deficits are:
  - Rotation more than 45° (more often in right parietal lesion)
  - Perseveration (frontal lobe lesion)
  - Fragmentation of the design (right parietal lesion)
  - Omission of parts of the design (left parietal lesion)
  - Closing in phenomenon (patient draws his picture close to the examiner's picture or even superimpose on it)
  - Substitution or addition
  - Abnormal placement of the angles
  - Incorrect integration of components of the picture
- Lesions in any quadrant can produce some impairment in constructional tasks, but severe deficits point to parietal lobe lesion
- Lesions of either parietal lobe can produce constructional impairment, but right side lesions produce more severe deficits
- If the overall picture form is disorganized, it is suggestive of right hemispheric disease
- If the overall form is relatively preserved, but the internal details are simplified, it is more suggestive of left hemispheric disease
- Severe deficits in three-dimensional cube drawing are suggestive of right hemispheric disease
- Copying of complex figures like Rey-Osterrieth figure is typically deranged in right hemispheric disease. Patients copy them in a piece meal fashion
- Missing of petals of daisy on one side suggests hemineglect on that side
- If numbers of a clock on one side are missed, it suggests hemineglect
- Closing in phenomenon is seen with a more diffuse disease process like Alzheimer's disease.

Caveats
- Impaired visual acuity (input disorders) can interfere with assessment of constructional tasks
- Motor deficits (output disorders) can also interfere with these assessments
- Lower level of education impairs performance.

DRESSING

Physiologic Basis
- Correct dressing requires proper orientation of the body parts to the garment
- Right parietal lobe is important in this function
- Either parietal lobe can cause hemispatial neglect and result in unilateral dressing deficit
- A more generalized dressing difficulty is suggestive of right parietal disease.

Methodology

- Hand over a shirt or sweater that has been turned upside down with one sleeve inside out
- Observe the smoothness of putting on the dress
- Errors include inability to re-orient the garment, to align it properly to the axis of the body and to properly introduce arms in to the sleeves.

Interpretation

- Dressing apraxia is seen with right parieto-occipital or bilateral occipitoparietal lesions
- More often, it is seen in patients with dementia or in confusional states.

ANSWER TO THE PRETEST

1. The findings in the test are:
   - There is no rotation of the Figure 1.19.
   - There is no gross distortion of the Figure 1.19.
   - Most angles are preserved
   - There is no closing in phenomenon
   - The three dimensionality of the figure is lost because of wrong placement of angles

   These features suggest a possible left parietal dysfunction.

   However, before concluding the deficits as "output defect", one has to ensure that "input function" is intact. Patient may be given 3 or 4 3-dimensional figures that include the cube and ask him to match the test picture with them. Failure to match the cubes correctly suggests perception defect. If there is no perception defect, then one can conclude that there is true construction defect.

TESTS FOR HIGHER ORDER THINKING (REASONING, ABSTRACTION, JUDGMENT, AND EXECUTIVE FUNCTIONS)

GRK Sarma

PHYSIOLOGIC BASIS

- Attention, memory and language are the basic cognitive processes
- To utilize them correctly and appropriately in a given situation, a higher level functioning is required
- These 'higher order functions' may be categorized into:
  - Fund of information/knowledge
  - Manipulation of this knowledge (problem-solving)
  - Social appropriateness and judgment
  - Abstraction
- The examination of these functions are described below.

METHODOLOGY

- **Fund of information:** The test questions must be appropriate to the educational and social background of the patient. This is especially true in India with its highly variable educational status, occupations, religious backgrounds. Some questions applicable are:
  - Name 4 Prime ministers of India
  - Capital cities of various states of the country
  - Approximate distance from patient's place to another city
  - Information about famous personalities
  - Information about famous books and authors, include religious texts.
- **Calculations:** This has been discussed in a separate section.
- **Reasoning/abstraction:** The various tests that are commonly used are:
  - Proverb interpretation: Use proverbs of increasing complexity and unfamiliarity. Look for concrete interpretation of the proverb which is common in dementia patients.
    - Do not cry over spilled milk
    - All that glitters is not gold
    - A friend in need is a friend indeed
    - An empty vessel makes loud noise
    - A drowning man will clutch a straw
  - Similarities and differences: Give a pair of items
    - Apple and orange
    - Car and aeroplane
    - Cow and orange

    Patient is asked to state the differences and similarities between the two items of a given pair.
  - Wisconsin card sorting test: Patient has to sort cards containing different shapes and colors based on examiner's instructions.

JUDGMENT, INSIGHT, AND SOCIAL APPROPRIATENESS

- Insight is the ability of a person to understand one self and the external situation
- Judgment is a process of forming opinion, making a choice considering various options, planning an action that is appropriate in the given situation
- These can be assessed by the patient's dealing ability with every day situations. For example, what do you do if a building is on fire?
- Ask the relatives for:
  - The patient's response to such situations appropriately
  - Inappropriate jocularity/remarks
  - Inappropriate familiarity with strangers
  - Inability to comprehend a joke/cartoon
  - Insight of the patient for his illness.

Interpretation

- Social judgment is impaired in frontal lesions
- Abstract thinking is more commonly impaired in posterior lesions rather than frontal lesions
- Verbal reasoning and abstraction are more disturbed in dominant hemisphere lesions (language dependent functions).

Caveats

- General intellectual impairment, poor education and social deprivation impair the performance on these tests
- Therefore, poor performance in proportion to the intellectual capacity should not be overinterpreted. Only if there is a dissociation between the two, a localizing value can be ascribed to these deficits.

MINI-MENTAL STATUS EXAMINATION

- Mini-mental status examination (MMSE) is a commonly used initial screening tool in mental status examination. It has some advantages and some limitations
- The standardized MMSE is a further improvization over the surlier version and gives clear instructions on test administration to minimize the inter-rater variability
- It is a quick (10–15 minutes) and simple way to quantify cognitive function and screen for cognitive loss
- It tests the individual's orientation, attention, calculation, recall, language and motor domains
- Each section of the test involves a related series of questions or commands.

METHODOLOGY

Tools Required

- Pencil and eraser
- White paper with command "close your eyes" clearly typed in black ink (instead of handwritten letters)
- Picture of intersecting pentagons printed in large size and black ink
- The MMSE test and scoring sheets (provided at the end of this chapter).

General Guidelines

- Seat the individual in a quiet, well-lit room without distractions
- Inform the patient that you will assess his cognitive functions and ask him to answer each question as accurately as he can
- The original version is not a timed test, but the standardized mini-mental state examination (SMMSE) has time limits to complete the tasks
- For each correct response, assign the appropriate score and add the scores at the end
- Do not indicate the errors to the patient and do not correct the mistakes
- If a patient has limitations due to a non-cognitive component (e.g. visual impairment) avoid that component and score him out of the remaining maximum score. Mention this modification on the test form
- Score the patient on his actual performance, not the potential performance
- There are no partial correct scores for "approximate answers". It is either 1 or 0.
- The individual can receive a maximum score of 30 points
- A score below 20 usually indicates cognitive impairment.

Administration of the Test

A. Three word registration:
  - Use three unrelated words
  - Read them clearly at 1 word per second. Do not repeat the words.

- Use different word sets for different assessments of the same patient
- Patient has to repeat the 3 words within 20 seconds. This is meant to reduce inter-rater and intra-rater variability. If one gives a longer time for the patient to respond, it may be mentioned so that during repeat assessment, same time is given to respond. But this latter modification has not been validated.
- The order of recalling is not important
- One point is scored for each correct answer
- If the patient has not registered all the 3 words, repeat trials are given up to a maximum of 5 to 6 trials
- Patient is informed that he will be asked later to recall these words.

B. Spelling "WORLD" backwards:
- First ask the patient to spell "WORLD" forwards
- If patient succeeds, ask him to spell it backwards
- 1 point is scored for each letter in the correct order
- For example, if he spells it " DLORW", he gets 3 points

C. Serial minus 7 (n-7) test:
- It is an alternative test to spelling "WORLD" backwards
- Ask patient to serially subtract 7 from 100 and continue the task
- Test is stopped after five consecutive subtractions
- 1 point is scored for each correct subtraction.

D. Naming:
- Show two common objects one after another, e.g. watch and pencil
- Ask the patient to name each of them
- Allow 10 seconds for each object
- Near answers get no points (e.g. clock for watch, pen for pencil).

E. Repetition:
- Ask the patient to repeat the phrase "no ifs, ands, or buts"
- About 10 seconds are given to respond
- 1 point for repeating the entire phrase correctly.

F. Third step command:
- Hold a paper in front of the patient out of his reach (so that the entire command can be finished before patient starts to respond)
- Instruct patient to "take this paper in your left (or non-dominant) hand, fold it in half once with both hands and put it on the floor"
- 1 point is scored for each of the three steps correctly performed.

G. Writing:
- Give a piece of paper and a pencil to the patient and ask him to write a complete sentence
- About 30 seconds are allowed and 1 point is scored for a sentence that makes sense
- It should have a subject, verb, and object
- Ignore the spelling mistakes.

H. Copying overlapping pentagons:
- Give a paper, pencil and eraser to the patient
- Show him the picture of overlapping pentagons
- Ask him to copy the picture (within 1 minute)
- One point is scored for correct reproduction of the picture including the four-sided figure at the overlapping region of the pentagons.

INTERPRETATION

- Maximum score: 30
- There is an inverse correlation of the score with age in normal persons:
    - 18-24 years: Score 29
    - >80 years: Score 25
- There are norms for the level of education also:
    - >9 years education: Score 29
    - 5-8 years education: Score 26
    - <4 years education: Score 22
- Score below 24-25: Definite diagnosis of dementia (high sensitivity and specificity)
- The score has direct relationship with severity of dementia:
    - 20-25: Mild dementia
    - 10-20: Moderate dementia
    - <10: Severe dementia
- The subscores on MMSE do not allow the type of dementia to be diagnosed, however, they follow a particular pattern with progression of the disease:
    - Early stage: Recall of the date, serial minus 7, recall of 3 objects
    - Moderate stage: Orientation for time and place
    - Severe stage: 3 stage commands, repetition, naming.

CAVEATS

- Mini-mental status examination may lack sensitivity in early dementias and result in false negative diagnosis (**ceiling effect**)
- In severe stages, there is **floor effect,** i.e. some tests cannot be given at all to such patients
- Attention is tested by two simple tests which can miss milder degrees of inattention
- The most important domain of memory is incompletely tested in the MMSE. Elements like personal events, general knowledge, recognition, cueing are not included
- There are no tests for judgment and abstract thinking
- When used repeatedly, learning can occur with simple instruments like MMSE. Therefore, it is better suited for initial contact evaluation.

The MMSE test and scoring sheet.

Orientation to time (1 for each correct response) Score

What is today's date?
What is the month?
What is the year?
What is the day of the week today?
What season is it?

Total: ____

Orientation to place (1 for each correct response)

Whose home is this?
What room is this?
What city are we in?
What county are we in?
What state are we in?

Total: ____

Immediate recall (1 for each correct response)

Ball
Flag
Tree

Total ____

Attention

A. Ask the individual to begin with 100 and count backwards by 7. Stop after 5 subtractions.
Score the correct subtractions (1 for each correct subtraction).

93

86

79

72

65

Total: ____

B. If patient does not attempt item A, then item B is provided
Ask the individual to spell the word "WORLD" backwards. (The score is the number of letters in correct position).

D

L

R

O

W

Total: ____

Contd...

Contd...

Delayed verbal recall

Ask the patient to recall the 3 words you previously asked him/her to remember. 1 point for each correct answer

Ball

Flag

Tree

Total: _____

Naming

Show a wrist watch and ask him/her what it is. Repeat for pencil.
(1 point for each correct response)

Watch

Pencil

Total: _____

Repetition

Ask the individual to repeat the following (1 point):
"No if, ands, or buts"

Total: _____

3-Stage command

Give the individual a plain piece of paper and say,
"Take the paper in your hand, fold it in half, and put it on the floor."
(1 point for each correct step)

Takes

Folds

Puts

Total: _____

Reading (1 Point)

Hold up the card reading: "Close your eyes" so the individual can see it clearly. Ask him/her to read it and do what it says.

Score correctly only if the individual actually closes his/her eyes.

Total: _____

Writing (1 Point)

Give the individual a piece of paper and ask him/her to write a sentence. It is to be written spontaneously. It must contain a subject and verb and be sensible.

Total: _____

Copying

Give the individual a piece of paper and ask him/her to copy a design of two intersecting shapes. One point is awarded for correctly copying the shapes. All angles on both figures must be present, and the figures must have one overlapping angle.

Total : _____

TOTAL SCORE: _____

BIBLIOGRAPHY

1. Borson S, Scanlan JM, Chen P, et al. The Mini-Cog as a screen for dementia: validation in a population-based sample. J Am Geriatr Soc. 2003;51(10):1451-4.
2. Budson AE, Price BH. Memory dysfunction. N Engl J Med. 2005;352:692-9.
3. Brazis PW, Masdeu JC, Biller J. The localization of lesions affecting the cerebral hemispheres, In: Localization in clinical neurology, 5th edition. Lippincott Williams & Wilkins; 2007.
4. Dehaene S, Cohen L. Towards an anatomical and functional model of number processing. Mathematical Cognition. 1995;1:83-120.
5. Gitelman DR. Acalculia: a disorder of numerical cognition. In: Esposito MD (Ed). Neurological Foundations Of Cognitive Neuroscience: a bradford book, Cambridge: The MIT Press; 2003.
6. Kirshner HS. Approaches to intellectual and memory impairment. In: Bradley WG, Daroff RB, Fenichel GM, Jankovic J (Eds). Neurology in clinical practice. Butterworth Heinemann publications; 2008.
7. Markowitsch HJ. Memory and amnesia. In: Mesulam M. Principles of behavioral and cognitive neurology, 2nd edition. Oxford press; 2000.
8. Mesulam M. Principles of behavioral and cognitive neurology, 2nd edition. Oxford press; 2000.
9. Molloy DW, Alemayehu E, Roberts R. Reliability of a standardised Mini-Mental State Examination compared with the traditional Mini-Mental State Examination. American Journal of Psychiatry. 1991;148(1):102-5.
10. Molloy DW, Standish TI. A guide to the standardized mini-mental state examination. International Psychogeriatrics.1997; 9 (1): 87-94.
11. Nehl C, Paulsen JS. Behavior and personality disturbances. In: Bradley WG, Daroff RB, Fenichel GM, Jankovic J (Eds). Neurology in clinical practice. Butterworth Heinemann publications, 5th edition, 2007.
12. Simard M. The mini-mental status examination: strengths and weaknesses of a clinical instrument. Canadian Alzheimer's Disease Review. 1998; 10-2.
13. Spencer MP, Folstein MF. The Mini-Mental State Examination. In: Keller PA, Ritt LG (Eds). Innovations in clinical practice: a source book, Vol 4. Sarasota, FL: Professional Resource Exchange, Inc., 1985.p.307-8.
14. Strub RL, Black FW. The mental status examination in neurology. Jaypee Brothers Medical publishers (p) ltd. 2003.
15. Weintraub S. Neuropsychological assessment of mental state. In: Mesulam M. Principles of behavioral and cognitive neurology, 2nd edition. Oxford press; 2000.

For references related to language and praxis, please see the respective chapters.

Summary of MSE of a Dementia Patient
(To be modified on individual case basis)

A. **Mood, motivation, behavioral changes**
B. **Attention, orientation, working memory and other executive functions**
   - Orientation to:
     - Time (day, date, time, month, season, year)
     - Place (country, state, city, hospital name, floor)
     - Person (relatives, friends, caregivers)
   - Digit span: Forward and backward
   - Name the months forward and backward
   - Recite alphabets in reverse order
   - Fist-palm-edge test, Luria alternating sequence test
   - Trail making test
   - Stroop procedure
   - 'A' cancellation test
   - FAS list generation
   - Semantic list generation
C. **Language**
   - Spontaneous speech
   - Naming various categories (objects, colors, animals, body parts)
   - Auditory comprehension: One step commands, Two step commands, Yes or no questions
   - Repetition: One word, and sentence
   - Reading:
     - Simple letters, words
     - Obeying written commands
     - Reading comprehension
   - Writing: Few sentences spontaneously and to dictation
D. **Praxis**
   - Eyes: Close your eyes
   - Buccofacial: Blow a candle, Sniff a flower, suck through a straw, protrude your tongue, lick your lips
   - Limbs:
     - Transitive: Comb, toothbrush, key, kick a football
     - Intransitive: Salute, wave bye, snap fingers, make a fist
   - Ideational:
     - Light a candle with a matchbox
     - Write and post a letter
   - Limb kinetic: Turn over a coin on fingertips/pick up a needle from the ground
   - Constructional: Draw a daisy, 3-dimensional figure (cube) clock with a specified time, copy a complex figure
   - Dressing: Wear a shirt that is turned inside out
E. **Calculations**
   - Forward counting, backward counting
   - What number comes after or before a given number (e.g. before 400, after 199 and so on)
   - Give two numbers and ask which is bigger or which is smaller
   - Read a number and ask patient to write the word for it
   - Show the written word and ask him to write the corresponding number
   - Give single digit and double digit additions, subtractions
   - If he does them correctly, give more complex arithmetic that tests the carry over and borrow functions
   - Basic rules like $N \times 0 =?$; $N + 0 =?$; $N \times 1 =?$ have to be tested.

Contd...

Contd…

F. Right left orientation
- Simple commands (e.g. right hand, left ear, etc.)
- Complex commands (e.g. touch your left ear with your right hand)
- Pointing the examiner's body parts on the correct side
- Nonverbal modality (if patient has aphasia): Copy the gestures of examiner or persons in a picture using the correct sided body part

G. Finger identification
- Ask to show various fingers while you name them
- Ask patient to match his fingers with those shown on a hand picture card.

H. Memory
- **Working memory**
  - Forward digit span, 100-7 serial subtraction test
  - Ask the patient to spell "WORLD" backwards
- **Episodic memory**
  1. Verbal memory:
     - Question about incidents of the day or the day before
     - Learning of 3 or more unrelated words (word span = digit span -1)
     - Story recall
  2. Nonverbal memory
     - Hidden objects
     - Geometric figures reproduction after distraction
     - Rey-Osterrieth figure
     - Family scene recall
- **Long-term memory**
  - Personal information
  - General knowledge
  - Geography of one's house or neighborhood
  - Semantic memory: Definition of words, differences between words

I. Construction
- Ask the patient to copy a diamond, cross, cube, triangle within a triangle
- Ask the patient to draw: A daisy in a flower pot, A clock with numbers and hands, A house in perspective

J. Higher order functions
- Fund of information (general knowledge questions)
- Proverb interpretation
- Similarities and differences
- Judgment: In a day-to-day situation (hypothetical or real).

Tool kit checklist

The following list includes some important test items required for mental status examination:
- Working tools:
  - Pencil
  - Eraser
  - Plain (unruled) white papers
- Memory:
  - Pictures of common domestic and wild animals
  - Pictures of famous personalities, politicians, sports persons
  - List of words containing test words and distraction words.
  - Pictures of simple geometric figures
  - Picture containing a family scene
  - A brief story and questions
  - Objects to hide (key, watch, pen, coin, comb)

Contd…

Contd...

- Construction:
    - Pictures of diamond, cross, cube, triangle within a triangle
    - Rey-Osterrieth figure
    - Picture of house, daisy, clock outline
    - Intersecting pentagons
- Executive functions and higher order thinking:
    - Luria test pattern of squares and triangles
    - Trail test pattern
    - Stroop test items (spelling of various colors printed in distracting colors)
    - Common proverbs with increasing difficulty level
- Language:
    - Command card ("close your eyes").

CHAPTER 2

Examination of a Patient in Coma

Raghunandan Nadig, GRK Sarma

PICTORIAL PRETEST

This 63-year-old man was brought in coma of acute onset. His spontaneous eye positions over a 2-minute observation are shown in Figures 2.1A and B.

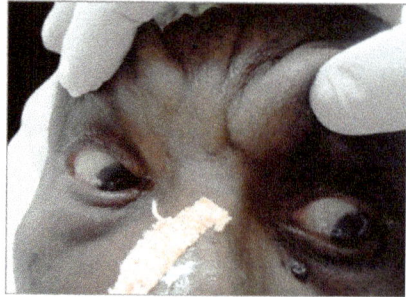

Fig. 2.1A: Spontaneous eye position (left ward).

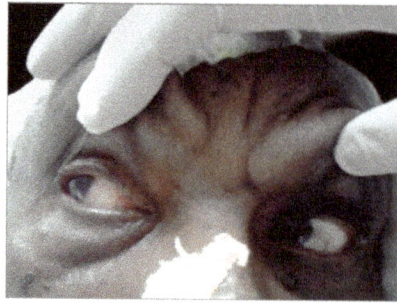

Fig. 2.1B: Spontaneous eye position (right ward).

Questions

1. What is the eye movement abnormality?
2. What is the significance of this observation?

(Answers are discussed at the end of the chapter)

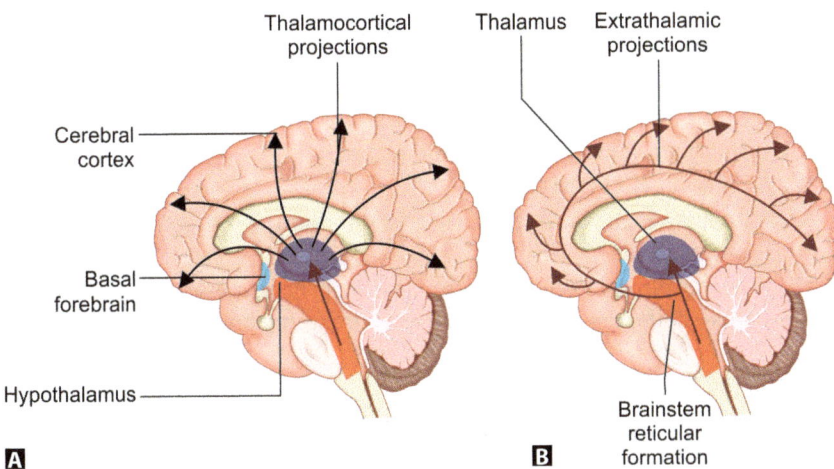

Figs. 2.2A and B: Lateral view of the brain showing the components of the consciousness system. Note that neurons of the brainstem reticular formation may control activity of the cerebral cortex both through a relay in the thalamus and by direct projections to the cerebral cortex (extrathalamic pathways).

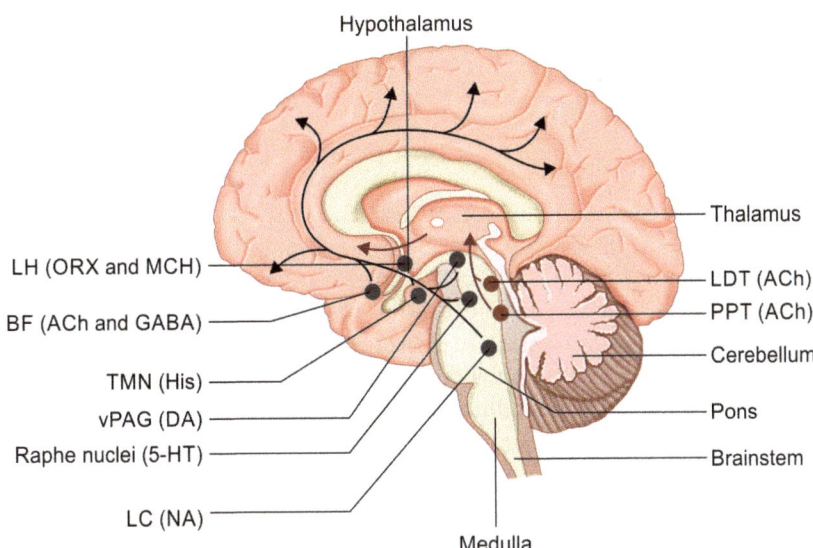

Fig. 2.3: Neurotransmitters involved in maintaining consciousness.
(Ach: acetylcholine; BF: basal forebrain; DA: dopamine; GABA: gamma aminobutyric acid; 5-HT: 5 hydroxy tryptophan; His: Histamine; LC: locus coeruleus; LDT: laterodorsal tegmental nucleus; LH: lateral hypothalamus; MCH: melanin concentrating hormone; NA: norepinephrine; ORX: OREXIN; PPT: pedunculopontine tegmentum; v PAG: periaqueductal gray matter; TMN: tuberomammillary nucleus)

INTRODUCTION

- The essence of clinical evaluation of coma is to answer **4 questions:**
  1. **Is it coma (or its mimic)?**
  2. **If it is coma, is it metabolic or structural?**
  3. **If it is structural, where is the lesion?**
  4. **How severe is the insult?**
- This chapter is devoted to present a systematic approach to answering these 4 questions
- It must be remembered that the first step in the management of the comatose patient is "A, B,C", i.e. airway, breathing and circulation.

DEFINITIONS

- Consciousness is the state of full awareness of the self and one's relationship to the environment
- Coma is best defined as a completely unaware state where a patient is unresponsive to both external stimuli as well as internal stimuli
- There are two components of conscious behaviors:
  1. Arousal—the appearance of wakefulness (a function of the ARAS)
  2. Content—the sum of cognitive and affective function (a cortical function)
- Content depends on arousal but normal arousal does not guarantee normal content
- Coma implies dysfunction of ARAS or both hemicortices.

PHYSIOLOGICAL BASIS

Arousal

- It is localized to ascending reticular activating system (ARAS) situated in the 'core of the brainstem'; which receives input from numerous somatic afferents and projects to midline thalamic nuclei (which are in a circuit with cortical structures) and the limbic system (Figs. 2.2A and B).
- ARAS acts as a gating system, increasing or decreasing thalamic inhibitory influence on the cortex and alters the effect of ascending sensory stimuli and also alters the descending cortical stimulation (Fig. 2.3).
- Function of ARAS—thalamic-cortical system depends on:
  a. Anatomic integrity of structures
  b. Metabolic integrity (circulatory integrity)
  c. Communicative integrity (neurotransmitter function).
- Lesions that involve the midbrain and pontine reticular formation impair the basic arousal mechanism and causes true coma (e.g. uncal herniation, infarct, hemorrhage, etc.)

- Lesions that involve the ARAS at higher levels in thalamus or hypothalamus result in coma-like states due to inadequate cortical activation, but not true coma. These states are characterized by an apparent visual alertness but a lack of speech and movement.

Content

It is localized to both hemispheres and their interconnections (circuits) with different lobes of brain and also with basal ganglia.

EXAMINATION OF THE COMATOSE PATIENT

The clinical assessment of the comatose patient consists of:
- History (from relatives, friends, or attendants)
- General physical examination
- Neurologic examination.

History: The key aspects in history taking are:
- Onset of coma (abrupt, gradual)
- Recent complaints (e.g. headache, fever, seizures, depression, focal weakness, vertigo)
- Recent injury
- Previous medical illnesses (e.g. diabetes, renal failure, heart disease)
- Previous psychiatric history
- Access to drugs (sedatives, psychotropic drugs).

General Physical Examination

- Vital signs—pulse, respiration, blood pressure
- Evidence of trauma
- Evidence of acute or chronic systemic illness like chronic liver disease, chronic renal failure
- Evidence of drug ingestion (needle marks, alcohol on breath)
- Nuchal rigidity (assuming that cervical trauma has been excluded).

Neurological Examination

The neurological examination focuses on assessment of integrity of **three systems** to answer the **primary questions:**
1. **ARAS** and the cortical networks: Level of consciousness—to assess the severity of the insult
2. **Brainstem** functions: To localize the level of lesion
    - Respiratory pattern and circulatory changes

- Cranial nerve examination:
  - Eye opening
  - Optic fundi
  - Pupillary reactions
  - Corneal responses
  - Spontaneous eye movements
  - Oculocephalic responses (assuming cervical trauma has been excluded)
  - Oculovestibular responses.
3. **Motor** system: To localize the level of lesion.

Further discussion elaborates on these three systems and the whole discussion is summarized to help a quick localization is discussed in Figure 2.8.

LEVEL OF CONSCIOUSNESS

Methodology

- **Stimuli:** Increasing intensity are given bilaterally:
  - Visual
  - Auditory
  - Somatosensory (touch, pain)
- **Responses may be graded qualitatively and quantitatively:**
  - Eye opening
  - Speech
  - Motor movements
- **Qualitative grading:**
  - Alert—normal awake and responsive state
  - Lethargic—easily aroused with mild stimulation, can maintain arousal
  - Somnolent—easily aroused by voice or touch; awakens and follows commands; requires stimulation to maintain arousal
  - Obtunded/stuporous—arousable only with repeated and painful stimuli; verbal output is unintelligible or nil; some purposeful movement to noxious stimuli
  - Comatose—no arousal despite vigorous stimulation, no purposeful movement—only posturing, brainstem reflexes often absent
- **Quantitative grading:** It is usually done using the **Glasgow coma score (GCS)** (Table 2.1)
- The newer Full Outline of UnResponsiveness (FOUR) score provides a replacement for all patients with fluctuating levels of consciousness and is gradually gaining wide acceptance.

Table 2.1: Glasgow coma score.

Eye opening	Verbal response	Motor response
4 = Spontaneous	5 = Normal conversation	6 = Normal
3 = To voice	4 = Disoriented conversation	5 = Localizes to pain
2 = To pain	3 = Words, but not coherent	4 = Withdraws to pain
1 = None	2 = No words only sounds	3 = Decorticate posture
	1 = None	2 = Decerebrate
		1 = None
		Total = E + V + M

Record 'D' if patient is dysphasic and 'T' if he has tracheostomy tube in situ.

BREATHING

- There are number of characteristic patterns of breathing that may be seen in patients in stupor or coma depending on the level of damage to the neural axis (Figs. 2.4A to E).
- These are best recorded by chest and abdomen pneumography, but bedside clinical examination can provide good information, when a few minutes are spared to observe them.

1. Cheyne-Stokes respiration (Fig. 2.4A)
   - This type of respiration consists of brief periods of hyperpnea alternating regularly with even shorter periods of apnea. After the apneic phase, the amplitude of respiratory movements increases gradually to a peak and then slowly wanes to apnea
   - This occurs due to bilateral widespread cortical lesions or associated with bilateral thalamic dysfunction and has also been described with lesions of the descending pathways anywhere from the cerebral hemispheres to the level of the upper pons
   - Metabolic disturbances, such as uremia, diffuse anoxia, and heart failure, often underlie this breathing disorder
   - In patients with supratentorial mass lesions, this pattern of respiration may indicate incipient transtentorial herniation
2. Hypothalamic–midbrain damage (Fig. 2.4B)
   - Central reflex hyperpnea is a condition characterized by rapid, regular hyperventilation that persists in the face of alkalosis, elevated PO_2, low PCO_2, and in the absence of any pulmonary or airway disorder.
3. Lower pontine tegmentum damage or dysfunction (Fig. 2.4C)
   - Apneustic breathing: There are sustained inspiratory cramps with a prolonged pause at full inspiration or alternating brief end-inspiratory and end-expiratory pauses.
4. Medullary dysfunction (Fig. 2.4E)
   - Ataxic breathing is characterized by a completely irregular respiratory cycle of variable frequency and tidal volume alternating with periods of apnea (Fig. 2.5D)
   - Slow regular breathing
   - Loss of autonomic breathing with preserved voluntary control
   - Gasping.

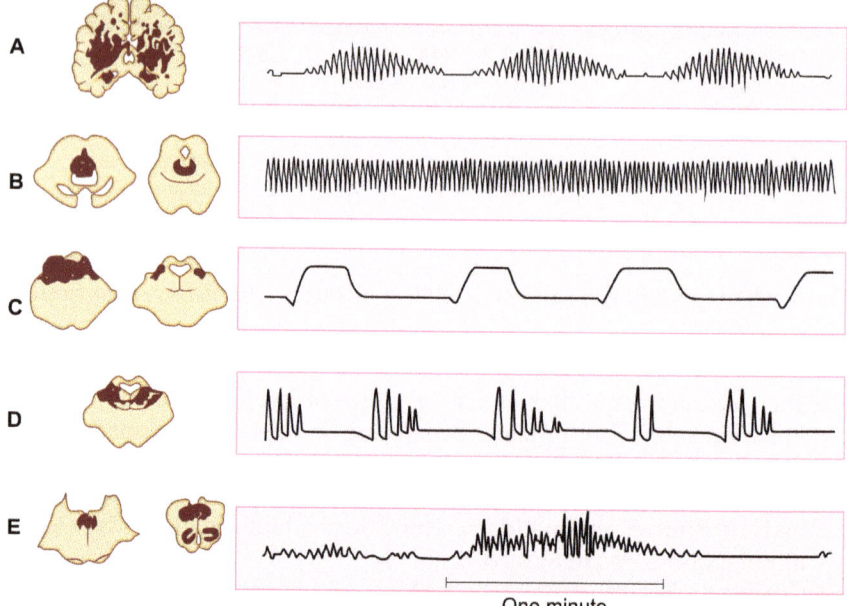

Figs. 2.4A to E: Abnormal respiratory patterns associated with pathologic lesions (shaded areas) at various levels of the brain. (A) Cheyne–Stokes respiration—diffuse forebrain damage; (B) Central neurogenic hyperventilation—lesions of low midbrain ventral to aqueduct of Sylvius and of upper pons ventral to the fourth ventricle; (C) Apneusis—dorsolateral tegmental lesion of middle and caudal pons; (D) Cluster breathing—lower pontine tegmental lesion; (E) Ataxic breathing— lesion of the reticular formation of the dorsomedial part of the medulla.

CIRCULATION

- Damage to the descending sympathetic pathways that support blood pressure may result in a fall to levels seen after spinal transaction (mean arterial pressure about 60 to 70 mm Hg)
- Persistent hypotension below these levels in a comatose patient is almost never caused by an acute neurologic injury
- Lesions that result in stimulation of the sympathoexcitatory system (insular region) may cause an increase in blood pressure
- Direct pressure to the floor of the medulla can activate the Cushing reflex, an increase in blood pressure and a decrease in heart rate.

Cranial Nerve Examination

- Cranial nerve examination helps in systematic assessment of brainstem function
- This is performed in a comatose patient by assessing following reflexes, each one targeted at different levels of brainstem (Fig. 2.5).

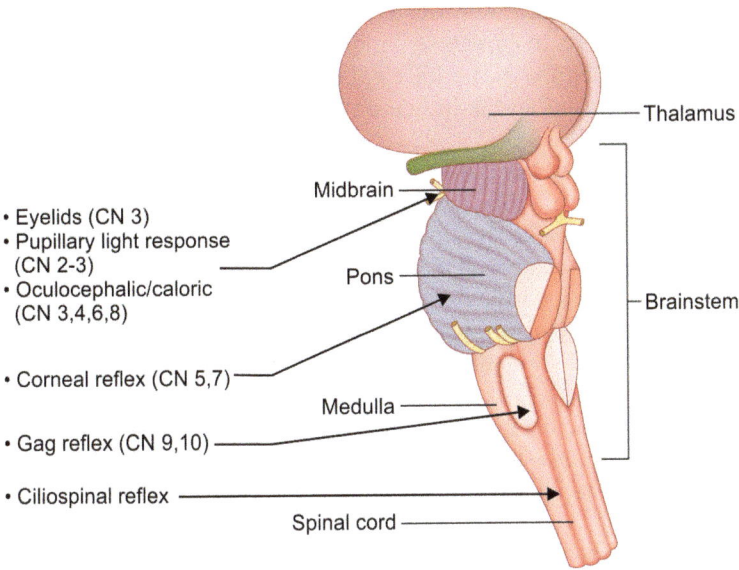

Fig. 2.5: Levels of brainstem and the corresponding reflexes.
(CN: cranial nerve)

Eyelids

- In the comatose patient, opening of the eyelids by an examiner is followed by slow re-closure
- In pseudocoma there is forced resistance to eyelid opening and active closure
- Rarely, the eyelids may be open in coma ('eyes-open coma'); because of a failure of levator inhibition associated with lesions in the pontomesencephalic region.

Fundus Examination

This is described in detail in Chapter 3: II Cranial Nerve.

Pupil Examination

- Observe the pupils in ambient light, if room lights are bright and pupils are small, dimming the light may make it easier to see the pupillary responses.
- They should be equal in size and about the same size as those of normal individuals in the same light (8–18% of normal individuals have anisocoria greater than 0.4 mm)
- Unequal pupils can result from sympathetic paralysis making the pupil smaller or parasympathetic paralysis making the pupil larger
- If one suspects sympathetic paralysis, dim the lights in the room, allowing the normal pupil to dilate and thus bringing out the pupillary inequality
- View the pupil through the bright light of an ophthalmoscope using a plus 20 lens or through the lens of an otoscope to better appreciate the pupillary reflex.

The method of examination and interpretation of pupils has been described elsewhere. In comatose patient, based on the pupil response, one can localize the lesion in the neural axis (Fig. 2.6). Abnormalities of this reflex, particularly when unilateral, indicate structural lesions of the midbrain or oculomotor nerve.
- Normal pupillary reaction to light in a comatose patient is strongly suggestive of a metabolic rather than structural cause of the coma
- Bilateral diencephalic dysfunction (metabolic coma) is accompanied by small pupils that react well to light
- Unilateral hypothalamic damage induces miosis and anhidrosis on the side of the body ipsilateral to the lesion
- Midbrain lesions causing coma usually produce distinct pupillary abnormalities:
    1. Tectal or pretectal lesions affecting the posterior commissure abolish the light reflex, but the pupils, which are midsized or slightly large, may show spontaneous oscillations in size (hippus)

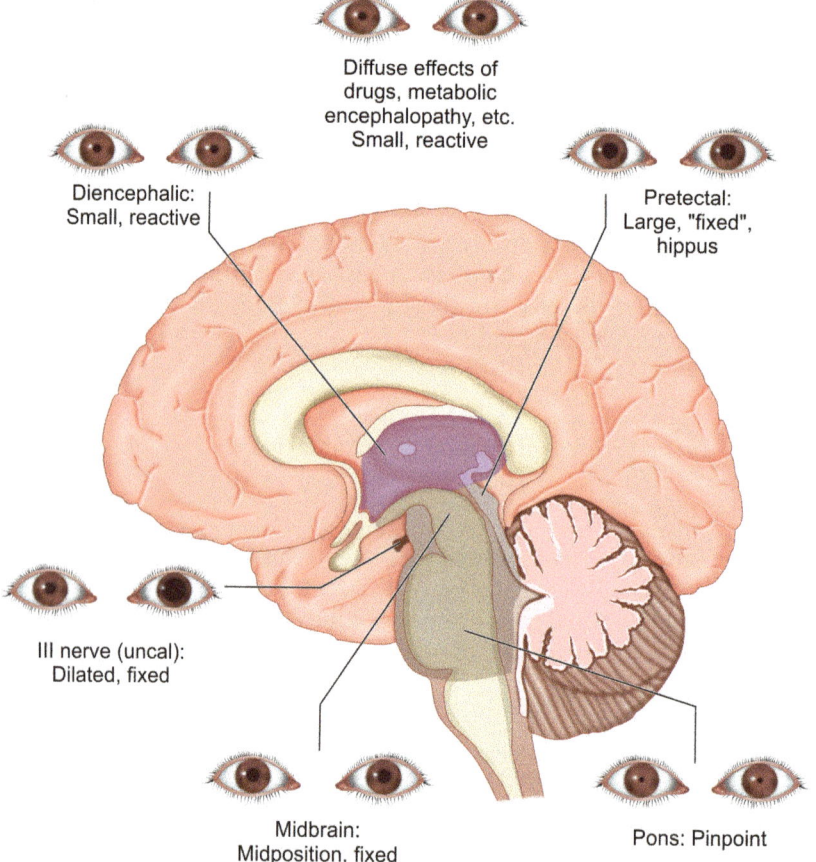

Fig. 2.6: Pupillary abnormalities in lesions at various sites.

2. Tegmental lesions, which involve the third nerve nucleus, may cause irregular constriction of the sphincter of the iris, with a resultant pear-shaped pupil or displacement of the pupil to one side. The pupils, often unequal, tend to be midsized and lack light or ciliospinal responses
- Pontine tegmental lesions cause small pupils due to interruption of the descending sympathetic pathways. Pinpoint pupils, which may be seen to constrict to light when observed with a magnifying glass, may occur with pontine hemorrhage, and are due to a combination of sympathetic damage and parasympathetic irritation.
- Lateral pontine, lateral medullary, and ventrolateral cervical cord lesions produce an ipsilateral Horner syndrome.
- Oculomotor nerve compression and elongation by herniation of the uncus of the temporal lobe affect pupillary function earlier.
- Possible explanations for pupillary dilation on the side of a mass lesion include compression of the third cranial nerve by uncal herniation beneath the tentorial edge. The light reflex is sluggish or absent and the pupil becomes widely dilated owing to sparing of the sympathetic pathways (Hutchinson's pupil).

Ciliospinal Reflex

- About 1-2 mm pupillary dilatation evoked by noxious cutaneous stimulation, pinching the nape of the neck and observing the pupil
- More prominent in sleep or coma than during wakefulness
- Tests integrity of sympathetic pathways in comatose patients
- Not particularly useful in evaluating brainstem function
- A normal ciliospinal response ensures integrity of these circuits from the lower brainstem to the spinal cord, thus usually placing the lesion in the rostral pons or higher.

Corneal Reflex

- Tests the integrity of the dorsal midbrain (Bell's phenomenon) and pons (eye closure)
- The corneal reflex has a higher threshold in comatose patients
- It must be elicited by a gentle and aseptic stimulus to avoid the risk of an infected corneal ulceration or impaired eye closure
- Afferent: Trigeminal nerve
- Efferent: Third nerve (Bell's phenomenon) and facial nerve (eye closure).

Spontaneous Eye Movements

- Note resting position of eye:
  - Midline position is seen in metabolic coma or brain death
  - Deviation suggests frontal/pontine damage

- Roving eye movements:
  - Description: Slow random predominantly horizontal conjugate eye movements (though there may be a degree of exophoria) similar to those seen in deep sleep.
  - Likely cause: Metabolic encephalopathy (may be absent in deep coma), bilateral supranuclear lesions
- Ocular bobbing:
  - Description: Rapid, conjugate, downward movement; slow return to primary position
  - Likely cause: Pontine strokes; other structural, metabolic, or toxic disorders
- Ocular dipping:
  - Description: Slow downward movement; rapid return to primary position
  - Likely cause: Unreliable for localization; follows hypoxic–ischemic insult or metabolic disorder
- Reverse ocular bobbing:
  - Description: Rapid upward movement; slow return to primary position
  - Likely cause: Unreliable for localization; may occur with metabolic disorders
- Reverse ocular dipping:
  - Description: Slow upward movement; rapid return to primary position
  - Likely cause: Unreliable for localization; pontine infarction and with acquired immunodeficiency syndrome (AIDS)
- Ping-Pong gaze:
  - Description: Horizontal conjugate deviation of the eyes, alternating every few seconds
  - Likely cause: Metabolic encephalopathy, bilateral cerebral hemispheric dysfunction; toxic ingestion
- Periodic alternating gaze deviation:
  - Description: Horizontal conjugate deviation of the eyes, alternating every 2 minutes
  - Likely cause: Hepatic encephalopathy; disorders causing periodic alternating nystagmus and unconsciousness or vegetative state
- Vertical myoclonus:
  - Description: Vertical pendular oscillations (2–3 Hz)
  - Likely cause: Pontine strokes
- Horizontal myoclonus:
  - Description: Rapid horizontal pendular oscillations; the eyes appear to be shaking
  - Likely cause: Serotonin toxicity.

Reflex Eye Movements

- Oculocephalic reflex, elicited by the doll's eye maneuver
- The oculovestibular reflex, elicited by instillation of cold or warm water into the external auditory canal. These are discussed in the section on VIII cranial nerve.

Oculocephalic reflex

- Afferent: Eighth nerve
- Efferent: Cranial nerve 3,4,6 via medical longitudinal fasiculus (MLF) and paramedian pontine reticular formation (PPRF)
- Oculocephalics may also involve proprioceptive afferents from the neck
- It is important first to rule out the possibility of a fracture or dislocation of the cervical spine
- The head is rotated first in a lateral direction to either side while holding the eyelids open. This can be done by grasping the head on either side with both hands and using the thumbs to reach across to the eyelids and hold them open
- The head movements should be brisk, and when the head position is held at each extreme for a few seconds, the eyes should gradually come back to midposition (Figs. 2.7A and B)
- The eye movements should be smooth and conjugate
- The head is then rotated in a vertical plane and the eyes are observed for vertical conjugate movement. During downward head movement, the eyelids may also open (the doll's head phenomenon)

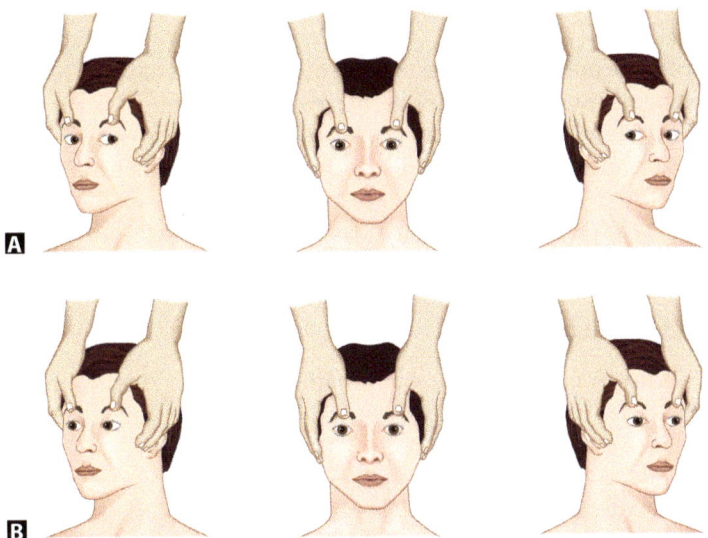

Figs. 2.7A and B: Testing the oculocephalic reflex: (A) Normal reaction—eyes move from side to side when head is turned; (B) Abnormal reaction—eyes remain in fixed position in skull when head is turned.

- The normal response generated by the vestibular input to the ocular motor system is for the eyes to rotate counter to the direction the examiner's movement
- It is a normal response to head rotation. Its absence in cases of coma patient is suggestive of involvement of the MLF and, therefore, a lesion of the brainstem.

The Caloric Vestibulo-Ocular Reflex

This is discussed in Chapter 3: VIII Cranial Nerve.

MOTOR RESPONSE TO STIMULUS

Neuroanatomy

- Rubrospinal tracts beginning in midbrain project to ventral horn cells of contralateral flexors of upper extremities
- Pontine reticulospinal tracts and medullary vestibulospinal tracts (both excitatory) project to ventral horn cells of extensors of extremities
- Corticospinal tract projects to extremities to control fine motor movements, and varying influences of corticospinal and extrapyramidal tracts result in normal tone.

Observation of the movements and of the tone and reflexes of the limbs supplies information that has a less localizing value than similar findings in alert patients.
- **Decorticate posturing**, i.e. flexion of upper extremities, extension of lower extremities: the lesion is above the red nucleus and cortical influence is impaired
- **Decerebrate posturing**, i.e. extension of all four extremities: The lesion is below the red nucleus and/above the vestibular nuclei
- Lesions below the vestibular nuclei may result in absent movement of the extremities because of disruption of projections from vestibular and pontine reticular nuclei that provide extensor tone; the medullary reticulospinal tract remains intact and is inhibitory to motor neurons controlling extensors of the extremities.

Differential Diagnoses

It is important to conclude the examination by answering the following questions:
1. Is it coma or a coma-mimic? (Table 2.2)
2. If it is coma, is it metabolic or structural? (Table 2.3)
3. If it is structural, where is the level of the lesion? (Fig. 2.8)

Table 2.2: Differences between coma and its mimics.

State	Lesion	Level of consciousness	Eye responses	Speech	Limb tone	Voluntary movements	Reflexes
Akinetic mutism (Apathetic type)	Midbrain reticular system, sparing corticospinal and corticobulbar tracts	Lethargic	Open on stimulation with good eye contact; may have ophthalmoplegia, pupillary abnormalities	On stimulation can produce normal short phrases	Normal or increased	Mostly limited, but on stimulation, can produce purposeful limb movements	Normal or increased
Locked-in syndrome	Pontine tegmentum involving corticospinal, coricobulbar tracts, sparing ARAS (exact opposite of akinetic mutism)	Awake, alert	Vertical, and sometimes horizontal, eye movements preserved, and are the only means of communication	None	Increased	None (other than eye movements)	Increased
Coma vigil (some consider this a type of akinetic mutism)	Bilateral orbital/ mesial frontal lobes, cingulated cortex, anterior hypothalamus, septal area	Awake most of the day and night (appear vigilant), may have rage during arousal state	Open mostly, no ophthalmoplegia (gaze defects may occur), pupils normal	On stimulation, can produce normal phrases	Increased in legs	Little, but can produce purposeful arm movements. Paraparesis in medial frontal lesions	Frontal release reflexes, lower limb hyperreflexia
Persistent vegetative state	Diffuse cortical damage as in hypoxia, hypoglycemia, severe trauma	Awake, no interaction with environment	Open, scan the environment, no eye contact	None (grunts occasionally)	Increased in all limbs	Double hemiplegia, often in flexion (decorticate posture)	Increased in all limbs; pathological reflexes present
Psychogenic unresponsiveness	No organic brain lesion	Appears in coma, but inconsistent	Eyes open or closed. If closed, resists passive opening, pupils constrict on passive opening they dilate in true coma, if passively opened, they close quickly (in true coma, there is gradual closure); no roving movements	None or minimal	Variable, inconsistent	Variable, inconsistent	Normal
Catatonia	Psychiatric disorders (affective disorders usual) [electroencephalography (EEG): low voltage fast activity instead of slowing)] Also seen in metabolic or drug-induced states	Awake, unresponsive	Open, unblinking, pupils dilated but reactive	None	Increased	None or minimal, waxy flexibility may be seen	Variable

Table 2.3: Differences between metabolic and structural causes of coma.

Clinical features	Structural	Metabolic/toxic
State of consciousness	Same level of arousal or progressively deteriorate	Alterations in arousal, waxing and waning of the behavioral state
Deep and increased respiratory rate	Uncommon	Common
Funduscopic examination. Subhyaloid hemorrhage or papilledema	Common	Uncommon except in malignant hypertension and hypercalcemia
Pupil size	Constricted/dilated	Symmetrical, small pupils with preserved reactivity
Pupil reactivity	Abnormal early in the course	Normal reaction, usually is spared, even when other brainstem reflexes are absent
Ocular motility	Asymmetry in oculomotor function	Symmetrical
Spontaneous eye movements	Bobbing, dipping	Roving eye movements
Reflex eye movements	Abnormal	Intact except rarely in phenobarbital or phenytoin intoxication or deep metabolic coma
Abnormal movements	Uncommon	Tremor, myoclonic are common
Muscle tone	Asymmetrical, may be increased, normal, or decreased	Symmetrical and normal or decreased

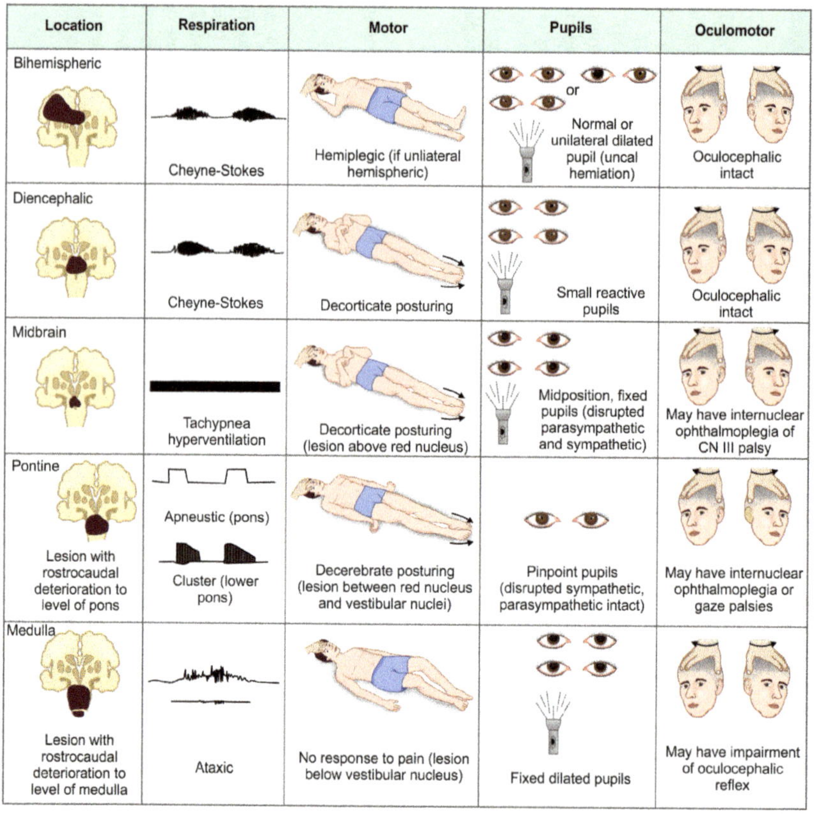

Location	Respiration	Motor	Pupils	Oculomotor
Bihemispheric	Cheyne-Stokes	Hemiplegic (if unilateral hemispheric)	Normal or unilateral dilated pupil (uncal herniation)	Oculocephalic intact
Diencephalic	Cheyne-Stokes	Decorticate posturing	Small reactive pupils	Oculocephalic intact
Midbrain	Tachypnea hyperventilation	Decorticate posturing (lesion above red nucleus)	Midposition, fixed pupils (disrupted parasympathetic and sympathetic)	May have internuclear ophthalmoplegia of CN III palsy
Pontine — Lesion with rostrocaudal deterioration to level of pons	Apneustic (pons) / Cluster (lower pons)	Decerebrate posturing (lesion between red nucleus and vestibular nuclei)	Pinpoint pupils (disrupted sympathetic, parasympathetic intact)	May have internuclear ophthalmoplegia or gaze palsies
Medulla — Lesion with rostrocaudal deterioration to level of medulla	Ataxic	No response to pain (lesion below vestibular nucleus)	Fixed dilated pupils	May have impairment of oculocephalic reflex

Fig. 2.8: Localization of lesion in structural coma.

ANSWERS TO THE PRETEST

1. The patient has 'periodic alternating gaze deviation (PAGD)'. His eyes initially were deviated to left side. After nearly 1and ½ minutes, they were deviated to the right. This cycling continued. 24 hours later, PAGD disappeared. Patient succumbed to his illness few hours later (due to large intracerebral hemorrhage with intraventricular extension).
2. In a comatose patient, presence of PAGD suggests large bilateral hemispheric lesions (usually ischemic), with intact brainstem function. The brainstem gaze centers are hypothesized to have become independent of cortical inhibition. Disappearance of PAGD in such patients who continue to be in coma may indicate that brainstem dysfunction is setting in and indicate grave prognosis as in this patient.

BIBLIOGRAPHY

1. Berger Jr. Stupor and coma. In: Bradley WG, et al. (Eds). Neurology in clinical practice, 5th edition; 2008.
2. Bordini AL, Luiz TF, Fernandes M, et al. Coma scales: a historical review. Arq Neuropsiquiatr. 2010;68(6):930-7.
3. BraZls PW. Localization in clinical neurology, 6th edition. LWW; 2011.
4. Cartlidge N. States related to or confused with coma. J Neurol Neurosurg Psychiatry. 2001;71:i18-9.
5. Greer DM. Clinical evaluation of coma and brain death: Neurocritical Care Society Practice Update; 2013.
6. Misra M, Lenka BD, Raths S. Ping Pong gaze (periodic alternating gaze): A case report. Ind J Ophthalmol. 1994;42(4):212-3.
7. Plum F, Posner JB. The diagnosis of stupor and coma, 3rd edition. Oxford University Press: New York; 2007.
8. Young GB, Wijdicks EFM (Eds). Handbook of clinical neurology, Vol. 90 (3rd series), Disorders of consciousness; 2008.

CHAPTER 3

Cranial Nerves

THE OLFACTORY NERVE (I N)

GRK Sarma

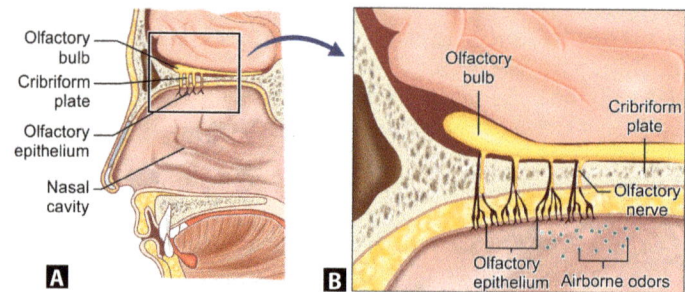

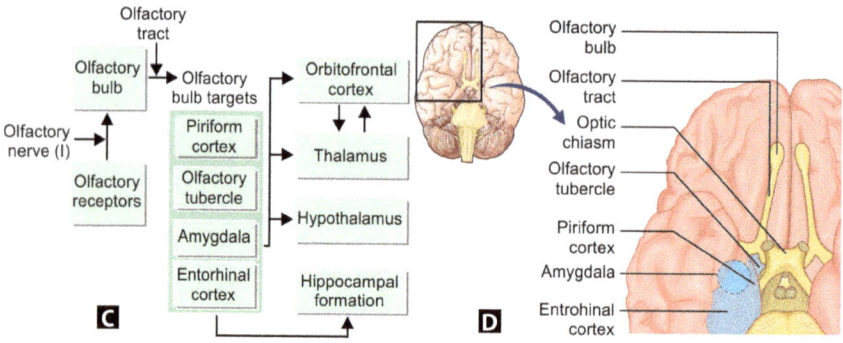

Figs. 3.1A to D: The olfactory nerve and pathways.

PHYSIOLOGIC BASIS (FIGS. 3.1A TO D)

- Olfaction is a **selective** chemosensory function of the **olfactory nerve**, wherein, the stimulus is a volatile chemical substance
- In contrast, pungent odors stimulate the free nerve endings of the **trigeminal nerve** in **nonselective** manner

- The olfactory receptors are located in the **roof** of the nasal cavity in the lateral wall and the septum, just below the **cribriform plate**. They are bipolar cells whose distal processes extended into the mucosal layer
- Their proximal processes pass through the cribriform plate to reach the olfactory bulb and synapse with the interneurons and mitral cells (output neurons)
- The central processes of output neurons contribute to the olfactory tract and terminate in the **olfactory cortex** (piriform cortex, anterior olfactory nucleus, olfactory tubercle, amygdala and entorhinal cortex)
- Olfaction is not processed in thalamus, unlike other sensations
- The olfactory pathways decussate in the anterior commissure to ensure **bilateral representation of smell**
- In addition, **insula and cingulate** cortex also are activated by stimuli that stimulate both olfactory and trigeminal system together (pungent odors)
- To simplify the olfactory function, it may be stated as follows:
    - Smell perception = Peripheral function
    - Smell identification = Central cortical function
    - Intact smell perception = Intact continuity of olfactory pathways
    - Intact smell recognition = Intact cortical function.

DEFINITIONS
- Hyposmia: Diminished smell perception
- Anosmia: Complete loss of smell perception
- Parosmia (perversion of smell): Seen after head trauma/depression
- Olfactory hallucinations: Seen in partial seizures/migraine
- Hyperosmia (heightened smell perception): Seen in migraine, hyperemesis gravidarum.

METHODOLOGY
- The objective of examination of smell is to localize the deficits to:
    - **Conductive** deficits (local nasal conditions that interfere with the interaction of the stimulus with the olfactory receptors), e.g. rhinitis
    - **Peripheral** sensorineural deficits (conditions that interrupt the olfactory pathways), e.g. orbital frontal tumors
    - **Central** neurogenic deficits (conditions that interfere with higher order processing of smell), e.g. Parkinson's disease.
- The objective is achieved by **3 sets of tests**:
    1. Conductive deficits: Thorough history and **local examination** of the nasal passages
    2. Peripheral sensorineural deficits: **Smell perception** tests
    3. Central neurogenic deficits: **Smell recognition** tests.

HISTORY
Some useful historical points are:
- Head trauma

- Recent upper respiratory infection
- Drugs (especially cytotoxic drugs)
- Intranasal substance use (cocaine, glue sniffing, etc.)
- Smoking, alcohol
- Radiation therapy
- Cognitive decline
- Parkinson's symptoms.

EXAMINATION TECHNIQUE

- Ensure that nostrils are patent and there is no active rhinitis or sinusitis
- Keep familiar test substances ready (soap, cloves, cinnamon, toothpaste, coffee powder)
- Avoid pungent or irritant substances like ammonia. The exception is when malingering is suspected. If the patient claims that he cannot perceive ammonia too, malingering is likely
- Test one nostril at a time, occluding the other
- Examine the possible abnormal side first
- Ask patient to close his eyes
- Bring the test substance close to the nostril
- Ask the patient to sniff deeply
- Patient has to report if he can smell something. If he can smell, he has to identify the substance
- Repeat the test on the other nostril
- Commercial quantitative smell tests kits are available like the Smell Identification Test (SIT).

INTERPRETATION

- If the patient cannot smell the test substance at all, he has anosmia. Odor perception indicates intact olfactory pathways
- Anosmia indicates a lesion distal to the olfactory decussation. More proximal lesion does not cause anosmia because of bilateral innervation
- If he can smell the substance but cannot identify it, he has olfactory agnosia, not anosmia. Identification of the odor indicates intact cortical function
- If a patient reports exaggerated sense of smell, it is called hyperosmia. It is seen in migraine and in psychiatric diseases.
- If a patient reports distorted smell, it is called parosmia and is seen in local nasal diseases and in psychiatric conditions.
- If the patient reports complete inability to perceive even pungent odors, it suggests possible conversion disorder (see below for explanation).
- Unilateral anosmia indicates ipsilateral lesion in the olfactory pathway. Most common cause is frontal lobe tumor or meningioma of olfactory groove/sphenoidal wing.

- Bilateral anosmia indicates bilateral orbitofrontal lesion (e.g. meningioma) or a toxic/metabolic/nutritional/systemic/degenerative disease.
- Anosmia in a patient with Parkinsonism is a valuable clue. Its absence suggests atypical parkinsonism, while its presence favors idiopathic Parkinson's disease.
- Anosmia in a patient with dementia suggests Lewy body disease or Alzheimer's disease.
- Disturbance of smell has been linked to vitamin deficiency (B_{12}, B_6, A) and zinc deficiency.

CAVEATS

- Avoid pungent or irritant substances like ammonia. These substances are perceived even in patients with olfactory nerve disease because they stimulate trigeminal nerve endings.
- If the patient does not sniff while testing, the test substance may not reach the olfactory epithelium located high up in the roof of nasal cavity. This may erroneously be interpreted as anosmia.
- Anosmia is common with advancing age due to ossification of foramina of cribriform plate. 75% of those above 80 years have anosmia. Therefore, all anosmias should not be interpreted as pathological.
- In patients with malingering, differentiating from true anosmia is difficult, because tests of smell are subject-dependent. This can be overcome by giving substances with different degree of pungentness like ammonia. Malingering patients report absolute loss to all substances, while true anosmia patients report "irritation" sense with pungent substances (this latter depends on trigeminal free endings and not the olfactory nerves).
- Perception of taste and smell are inter-related. Dysfunction of one is often perceived as dysfunction of another. Hence, it is important to clearly identify which system is impaired.

BIBLIOGRAPHY

1. Brazis PW, Masdeu JC, Biller J. Localization in clinical neurology, 6th edition. Wolters Kluver/Lippincott Williams & Wilkins; 2011.
2. Campbell WW. DeJong's The Neurologic Examination, 7th edition. Wolters Kluwer/Lippincott Williams & Wilkins publication.
3. Doty RL. The olfactory system and its disorders. Semin Neurol. 2009;29:74-81.
4. Feldman JI, Wright HN, Leopold DA. The initial evaluation of dysosmia. Am J Otolaryngol. 1986;7:431.
5. Finelli PF, Mair RG. Disturbances of smell and taste. In: Bradley WG et al. (Eds). Neurology in clinical practice. 5th edition. Butterworth Heinemann publications; 2008.
6. Hawkes C. Olfaction in neurodegenerative disorders. Mov Disord. 2003;18:364-72.
7. Schiffman SS. Taste and smell losses in normal ageing and disease. JAMA.1997;278:1357-62.

THE OPTIC NERVE (II N)

Seshu Babu G

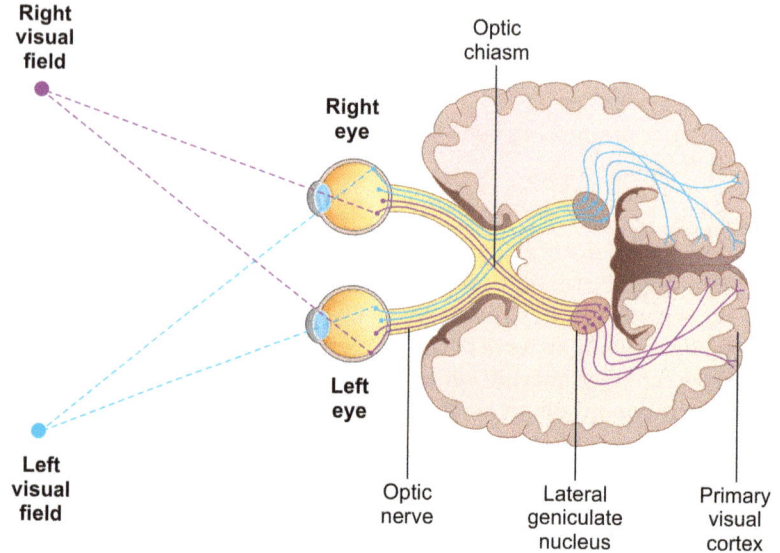

Fig. 3.2: The visual pathways.

PHYSIOLOGIC BASIS (FIG. 3.2)

Retina and Optic Nerve

- The retina is the only part of the nervous system that can be visualized directly
- The ganglion cells are located in the innermost retinal layer.
- Axons of the ganglion cells that enter the temporal aspect of the disc are called the papillomacular bundle. They carry the central visual fibers from the macula
- Axons from the nasal retina enter the nasal aspect of the disc.
- Axons from the temporal retina travel around the papillomacular bundle to enter the disc on its superior and inferior aspect.
- The nasal retina is stimulated by the temporal visual field and vice versa.
- Similarly, the inferior retina is stimulated by superior aspect of the visual field and vice versa.
- The retinotopic organization is preserved up to the visual cortex level.
- The visual field loss pattern gives a clue to the lesion at various prechiasmatic levels:
    - Field defect **not respecting any meridian**: Typical of retinal disorders
    - Field defect **respecting horizontal meridian**: Optic nerve disease (nerve bundles are segregated into superior and inferior arcuate bundles)

- Field defect **respecting vertical meridian**: Chiasmal or retrochiasmal lesion (because of segregation of the fibers in-to nasal and temporal bundles)
- Other field defects typical of optic nerve disease are: central scotoma, centrocecal scotoma, altitudinal defects, arcuate defects.

Optic Chiasm

- The two optic nerves join to form the optic chiasm just above the sella and below the hypothalamus and 3rd ventricle
- Thus sellar lesions cause superior field defects and 3rd ventricular lesions cause inferior field defects
- The temporal fibers of each optic nerve continue in the chiasm ipsilaterally, while the nasal fibers cross to opposite side
- The lower most nasal fibers, while crossing, travel close to the opposite optic nerve or may even loop into it for a short distance (Willebrand's knee). This explains the **junctional scotoma** (in which, an **anterior chiasmal** lesion produces ipsilateral central scotoma and contralateral superior temporal field defect) (Figs 3.3A and B)
- **Chiasmal body** lesions, in contrast, typically cause **bitemporal hemianopia** by involvement of bilateral nasal retinal fibers.

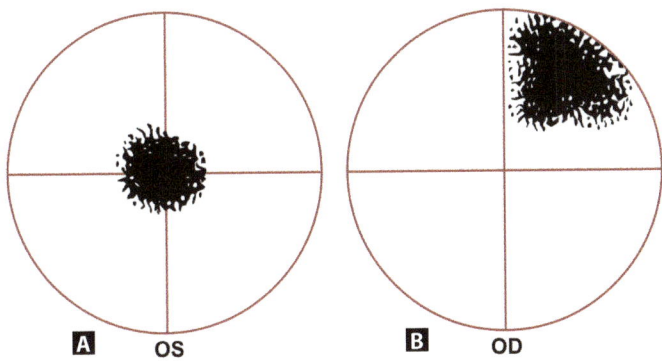

Figs. 3.3A and B: Junctional scotoma.

Retrochiasmal Pathways

- The optic tracts travel below the 3rd ventricle to reach the lateral geniculate bodies
- Most fibers synapse in the lateral geniculate body (LGB) of the thalamus
- Fibers that serve the pupillary light reflex do not reach the LGB, but branch off to synapse in the pretectal region of the midbrain
- Fibers from the LGB form the optic radiations. These radiations consist of superior and inferior fibers
- The superior optic radiations (parietal fibers) carry the information from the inferior fields and the inferior (temporal) optic radiations carry the information from the superior field

- The superior and inferior optic radiations project to the superior and inferior banks of the calcarine cortex respectively
- The macular vision is represented in the occipital pole, occupying a large area of this region. The fovea is represented in the tip of the occipital pole
- The occipital pole has dual blood supply from the middle and the posterior cerebral arteries. This explains macular sparing in the posterior circulation strokes.
- The visual association areas perform the following functions:
    - Occipito-temporal region: Object recognition
    - Mesial occipitotemporal region: Face recognition
    - Lingual and fusiform gyri: Color perception
    - Parietal lobe: Spatial orientation
- The visual field defects at various levels of retrochiasmatic pathway are as follows:
    - Optic tracts: incongruous contralateral homonymous hemianopia with RAPD
    - Lateral geniculate body: Incongruous contralateral homonymous hemianopia, no RAPD; also possible are congruous sectoranopia
    - Optic radiations: Homonymous hemianopia affecting either superior or inferior fields predominantly
    - Occipital cortex: Congruous, macular sparing homonymous hemianopia. Also possible are superior or inferior predominant field defects (if one bank of the visual cortex is involved). Sometimes, bilateral constriction of visual fields (tube vision) can occur with bilateral occipital lesions.

METHODOLOGY

The examination of the optic nerve consists of:
- Assessment of central vision (both distant and near vision)
- Assessment of color vision
- Perimetry
- Fundoscopy
- Pupillary reflexes

Central Vision

Principles

- Measuring visual acuity is by a psychophysical procedure relating the physical characteristics of a stimulus to a patient's perception and responses
- Visual acuity is a measure of the spatial resolution of the visual processing system, tested by requiring identification of optotypes, i.e. black symbols against a white background (for maximum contrast), on a printed chart from a set viewing distance
- Standard viewing conditions are correct luminance of the eye chart, correct viewing distance and enough time for responding

- Many patients do not cooperate. Providing adequate time and coaxing patients tend to yield more accurate results
- Visual acuity is measured with and without the patient's own glasses
- If patients do not have their glasses, a pinhole is used
- If pinhole is unavailable, one can be made at the bedside by poking holes through a piece of cardboard using an 18-gauge needle and varying the diameter of each hole slightly
- Patients choose the hole that corrects vision the most. If acuity corrects with pinhole refraction, the problem is a refractive error
- Pinhole refraction is a rapid, efficient way to diagnose refractive errors, which are the most common cause of blurred vision.

Steps of visual acuity testing
1. Stand/seat the patient at 6 meters from the Snellen chart Fig. 3.4.
2. If the patient normally uses distance glasses, ensure they wear them for the assessment.
3. Ask the patient to cover one eye and read to the lowest line they can manage
4. Visual acuity is recorded as chart distance *(numerator)* over number of lowest line read *(denominator)*. *This ratio can also be understood as the distance at which the patient reads a particular line (numerator) as against the distance at which a normal person would read the same line (denominator).*
5. Record the lowest line the patient was able to read *(e.g. 6/6)*.
6. If patient reads the 6/6 line, but gets 2 letters incorrect, you would record as 6/6 (-2).
7. If patient gets more than 2 letters wrong, then the previous line should be recorded as their acuity.
8. You can have the patient read through a pinhole to see if this improves vision.
9. If vision is improved with a pinhole, it suggests there is a refractive element to their poor vision.
10. Repeat above steps with the other eye.
11. Both distance and near acuities should be measured as greater reduction in near than distance visual acuity is suggestive of macular dysfunction.
12. Near vision is checked by asking patients to read a standard near card or newsprint at 14 in (35 cm); patients > 40 year who require corrective lenses (reading glasses) should wear them during near vision testing.

Recording the acuity by Snellen notation
- A Snellen notation of 6/12 (20/40) indicates that the smallest letter that can be read by someone with normal vision at 12 m (40 ft) has to be brought to 6 m (20 ft) before it is recognized by the patient
- Vision is recorded as the smallest letter patients read correctly, even if patients feel that the letter is blurry or they have to guess
- If the patient cannot read the top line of the Snellen chart at 20 ft (6 m), acuity is tested at 10 ft (3 m)
- If nothing can be read from a chart even at the closest distance, the examiner holds up different numbers of fingers to see whether the patient can accurately count them

- If not, the examiner tests whether the patient can perceive hand motion
- If not, a light is flashed into the eye to see whether light is perceived.

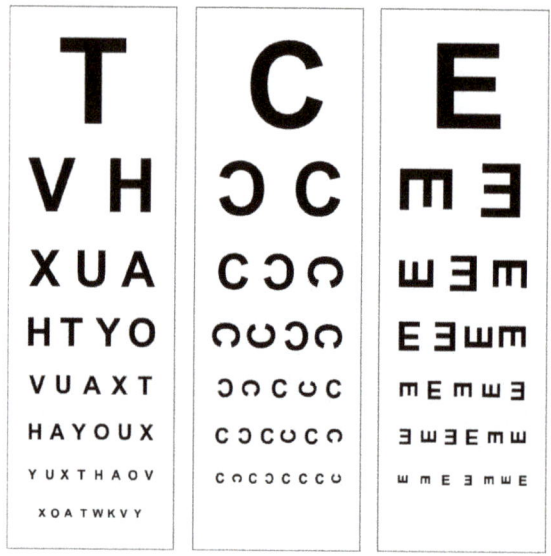

Fig. 3.4: Snellen's charts for literate and illiterate persons.

Contrast sensitivity charts, using either letters [Pelli-Robson charts (Fig. 3.5)] or sinusoidal gratings (Vistech chart), provide more comprehensive assessment of spatial resolution. Impaired contrast sensitivity (along with impaired color vision) is highly **characteristic of optic neuritis.**

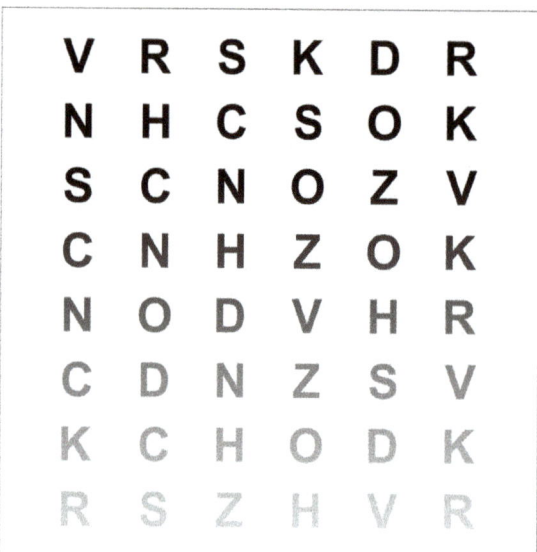

Fig. 3.5: Pelli-Robson contrast sensitivity chart.

Color Vision

Principles

- Color vision defects occur in two situations:
  1. **Macular** disease: Here both color vision and **visual acuity** are impaired.
  2. **Optic nerve** disease: Here, color vision impairment may often be **disproportionate** to the visual acuity impairment. In some cases, both are equally affected.
- *Kollner's rule* states that red/green dyschromatopsia indicates optic nerve or posterior visual pathway disease and blue/yellow dyschromatopsia indicates retinal disease
- There are a number of conditions that contradict this rule, particularly glaucoma, autosomal dominant optic atrophy, chronic papilledema, and even acute demyelinating optic neuropathy
- In clinical practice, the Ishihara pseudoisochromatic color plates, originally designed to detect inherited red-green color vision defects with little ability to test for blue-yellow dyschromatopsia, are most commonly used because of their speed and simplicity. To a color deficient patient, all the dots in one or more plates appear same or similar (isochromatic). In a normal person, some dots appear dissimilar from other dots and appear as a number or a pattern (pseudoisochromatic).

Methodology

Ishihara Color Test (Figs. 3.6A and B): Consists of a set of 24 plates.

Plates 1–17 each contain a number, plates 18–24 contain one or two wiggly lines. To pass each test one must identify the correct number, or correctly trace the wiggly lines.

1. Plate 1 and 24 are control tests – people with normal vision and all forms of color blindness should be able to distinguish these.
2. Keep the plates approximately 75 cm from the patient, with each circle set at eye level.
3. Preferably have mild **natural light** and no glare on the screen. **Interior lights and glare can alter the color of the pictures.**
4. Ask the patient to identify the hidden number or line within 5 seconds.
5. Continue to the next Ishihara test, complete all the charts to help gauge the color blindness severity.

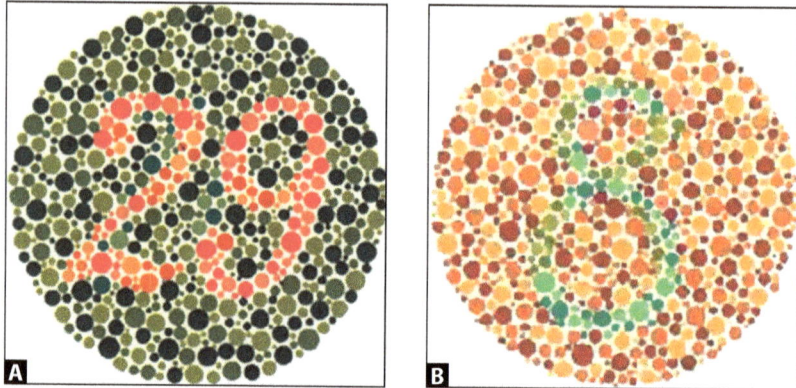

Figs. 3.6A and B: Ishihara color charts.

Interpretation

1. If the patient cannot see some or all of the hidden numbers or lines, it indicates color blindness.
2. Most congenital color blindness is red-green.
3. Blue-yellow color blindness suggests acquired disease (e.g., caused by glaucoma or optic nerve disease).

Visual Field Assessment

Pictorial Pretest

A 35-year-old male presented with painless progressive visual loss of his left eye. His perimetry is shown as follows:

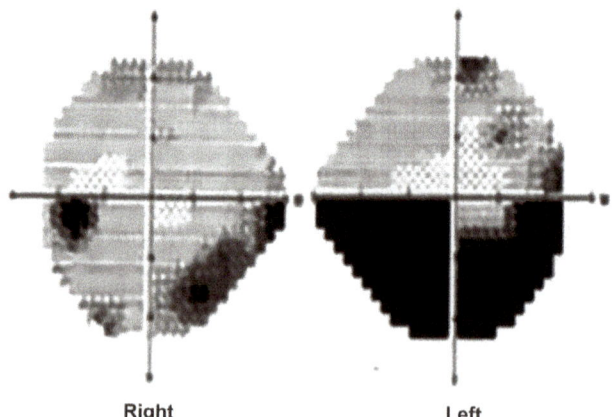

Questions

1. What does the perimetry show?
2. Where is the likely lesion based on the perimetry result?
3. What is the likely cause of his visual loss?

- Visual field assessment is crucial for the diagnosis and monitoring of optic neuropathies
- Certain visual field defects are associated with, but not specific to, various optic neuropathies
- The methods of visual field testing are:
    1. **Confrontation method** is a semiquantitative, kinetic or static (red desaturation) test. It is the most easily and readily performed test. A full field test is best performed with small (5 mm) red target. At suprathreshold, there is a interexaminer variability.
    2. **Amsler grid** testing is a semiquantitative, static test. It is easy to perform and tests central 10° of field. It is portable.
    3. **Tangent screen** is a semiquantitative kinetic or static method using colored targets.and easy to perform and tests central 30° of field of vision. It is suitable for detection of subtle central scotomas and non-organic visual loss. It is a suprathreshold test and interexaminer variability limits it use.
    4. **Goldmann perimetry** is a suprathreshold or threshold, kinetic or static test and requires experienced examiner.
    5. **Computerized static (or kinetic) test (Humphrey's visual field analyzer)** is a quantitative test, difficult to perform perimetry. It tests central (30, 24 or 10) or full field and is a very sensitive test with reproducible results. Threshold (full threshold/SITA) with fixation monitoring blind spot, gaze-tracking, testing central 30-2, 24-2, 10-2 fields and generating report with reliability indices, fixation losses, false positives, false negatives is an advantage over the rest of the methods. Standard target size (III) and other sizes are available. Colored stimuli can also be used. Absolute retinal thresholds (numerical and gray scale) including foveal sensitivity. Comparison with age-matched controls, and indices like total and pattern deviation (numerical and probability), overall performance indices mean deviation, pattern standard deviation, corrected pattern standard deviation help in differentiating normal from abnormal.

In this chapter, computerized visual field testing and bedside confrontation testing are described.

Static Perimetry

- The most common type of modern visual field testing employs a device with fixed light sources, either stationary pinpoint light sources or projected dots within a large white bowl
- Popular devices include the Octopus or the Humphrey-Zeiss field analyzer
- These tests are automated and run by the onboard computer, thus minimizing the time spent by a technician running the test
- Patient is required to fix on a central target
- He has to push a button each time a light source is illuminated randomly. This stimulus-response data is captured by the computer and analyzed for various parameters

- The visual field report generated by visual field devices includes a lot of information, for interpreting the results (Fig. 3.7):

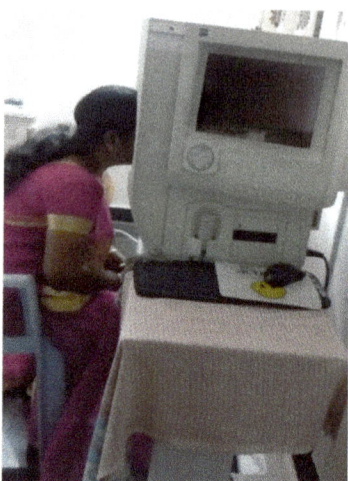

Fig. 3.7: Humphrey visual field test.

Interpretation

1. Fixation errors: The number of times the patient looks away from the central target. This is a key indicator of patient cooperation or fatigue.
2. False positives: The number of times the patient pushes the button when, in reality, a light source is not illuminated.
3. False negatives: The number of times the patient fails to push the button when, in reality, there is a light source illuminated. These spots can be repeat tested by the onboard computer at exactly the same spot to best understand the patient's ability to produce an accurate field test.
4. Points tested: Indicates the total number of separately illuminated testing points, and therefore data points presented to the patient for testing. Reliable patients can produce a very useful field with a limited number of test points.
5. Reliability index: The overall reliability of the patient's testing for each eye. Poor reliability may indicate patient fatigue, insufficient understanding of the test, or poor vision for other reasons such as cataracts. Visual field tests can also be used to ferret out malingerers.
6. Standard deviation: The difference in peripheral field acuity when compared to a normative data base, or simply put, a large group of similar normal patients. This tells the doctor whether or not a particular part of the peripheral field is normal, depressed, or absent.
7. Visual field map: The final basic report indicating the patient's visual field anywhere from the central 10° all the way out to the farthest reaches of the field at 90°. Altered patterns in the field map from reliable patient testing are often extremely useful in the diagnosis of ocular or neurological disorders (Fig. 3.8).

Cranial Nerves

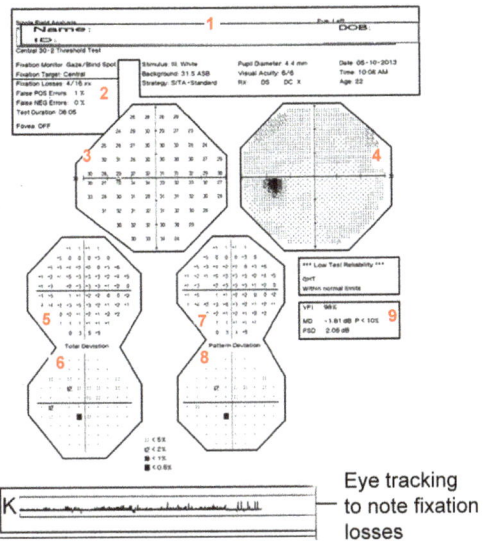

Fig. 3.8: Visual field map and interpretation.

Field analysis: Areas to be analyzed in the perimetry report.
1. Patient details
2. Reliability indices
3. Raw data
4. Grey scale
5 and 7. Total and pattern deviation numerical plot
6 and 8. Total and pattern deviation probability plot
9. Global indices.

Types of Visual Field Defects on Humphrey's Method

Focal
a. Central scotoma:

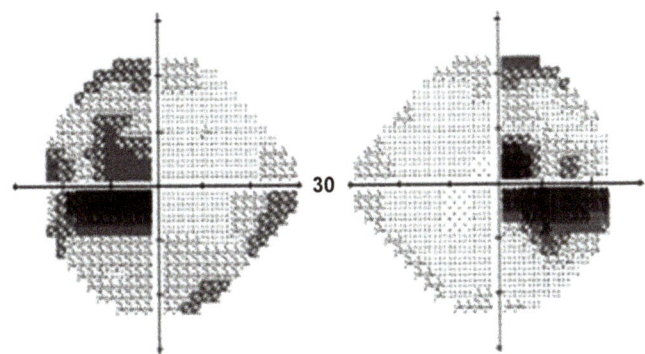

- Demyelinating optic neuropathy (centered on fixation with sloping border on Goldmann perimetry, diffuse/global loss on Humphrey 30-2)
- Toxic/nutritional optic neuropathy (small, best detected with red target)
- Leber's hereditary optic neuropathy (large, dense, steep-sided)
- Compressive optic neuropathy

b. Enlarged blind spot:

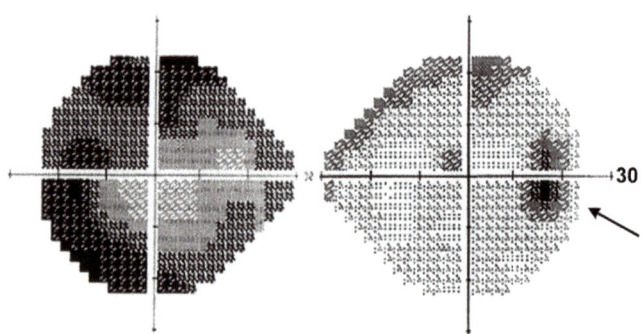

- Papilledema
- Congenital optic disc anomalies

c. Constriction (Respecting horizontal meridian altitudinal, arcuate, nasal step, or inferonasal):

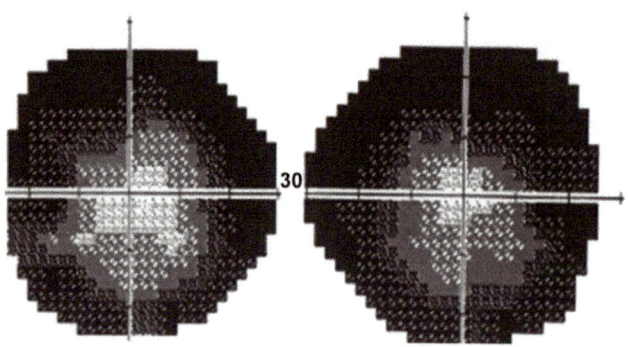

- Anterior ischemic optic neuropathy (inferior altitudinal)
- Papilledema
- Glaucoma
- Optic nerve head drusen

d. Upper temporal field loss not respecting vertical meridian:
   - Tilted optic discs

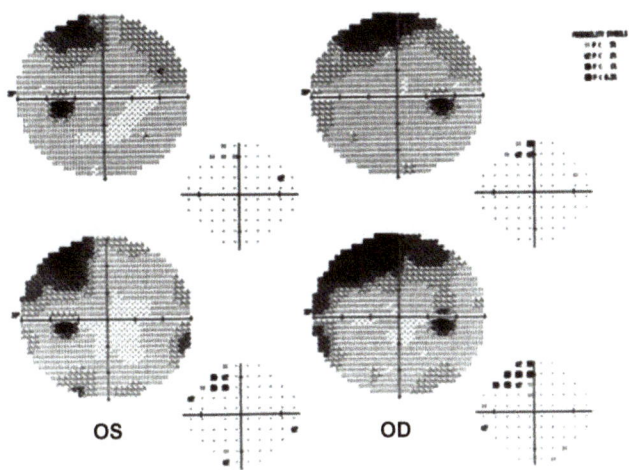

Fig. 3.9: Upper temporal field loss not respecting vertical meridian.

e. Nasal field loss respecting vertical meridian:
   - Intracranial optic nerve compression
   - Primary empty sella syndrome
f. 'Junctional scotoma' (central scotoma with contralateral superotemporal depression) prechiasmatic optic nerve
g. Diffuse:
   - Generalized depression
   - Generalized constriction

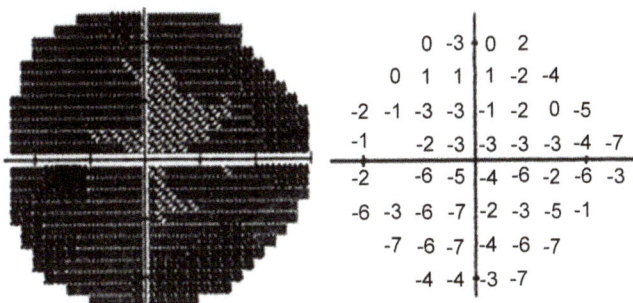

Fig. 3.10: Generalized depression.

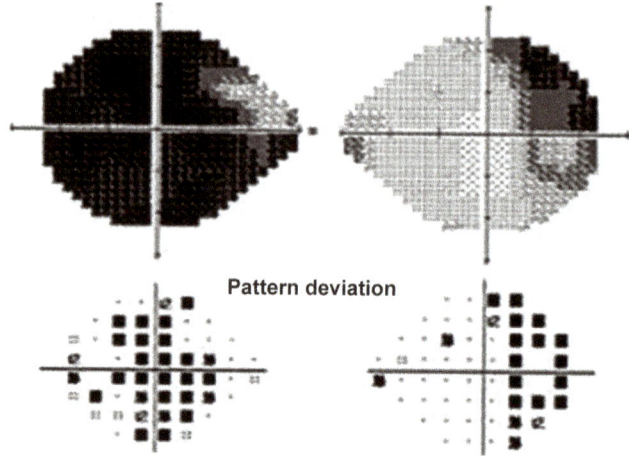

Fig. 3.11: Generalized constriction.

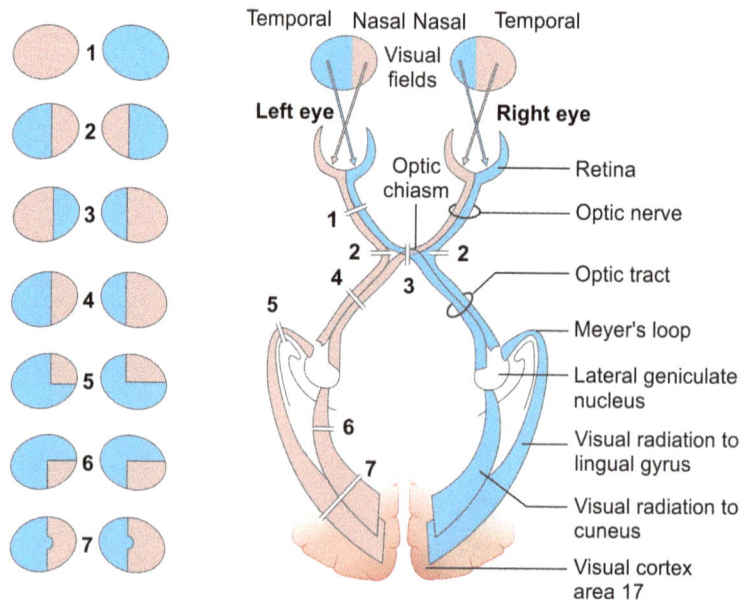

Fig. 3.12: Schematic diagram to show various expected visual field defects with lesions at various levels along the visual pathway.

Visual Field Testing by Confrontation Method

Steps of examination
1. Sit directly opposite the patient, at a distance of around 1 meter
2. Ask patient to cover one eye with his hand
3. If the patient covers their right eye, you should cover your left eye (*just mirror the patient*)

4. Ask patient to focus on your face and not move their head or eyes during the assessment, you should do the same and focus your gaze on the patient's face.
5. Ask the patient to tell you when they can see your fingertip wiggling.
6. Position your fingertip at the border of one of the quadrants of your visual field.
7. Slowly bring your fingertip inwards, toward the center of your visual field until the patient sees it.
8. If you are able to see your fingertip, but the patient cannot, this would suggest a reduced visual field.
9. Repeat this process for each quadrant, then repeat the entire process for the other eye.
10. Document your findings.

ANSWERS TO THE PRETEST

1. The perimetry shows unilateral **inferior altitudinal** field defect **respecting the horizontal meridian.** Field deficits respecting horizontal meridian are typical of optic nerve lesions.
2. This indicates a prechiasmatic lesion impinging the optic nerve on its superior aspect.
3. An injury to the optic nerve anywhere along its pathway by an extrinsic lesion is termed compressive optic neuropathy (CON). The optic nerve is most vulnerable to injury by a compressive force where it is adjacent to bone or in a confined space (e.g. orbital apex, optic canal). The clinical hallmark of compressive optic neuropathy is slowly progressive vision loss. Characteristic findings on clinical examination include reduced visual acuity, dyschromatopsia, a relative afferent pupillary defect, visual field defect, and optic atrophy (or edema). The MRI confirmed the compressive lesion (red arrow) (Fig. 3.13).

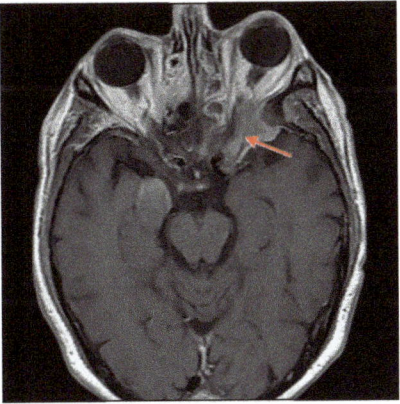

Fig. 3.13: Compressive lesion involving left optic nerve.

Optic Disc Examination

Pictorial Pretest

A 22-year-old girl presented with unsteadiness of gait for 4 years. She was born of nonconsanguineous parentage and her birth, development, schooling have been normal. No other family members had neurological illness. On examination, she had bilateral cerebellar signs and brisk reflexes. Her MRI showed severe cerebellar atrophy. Her fundus examination revealed the following:

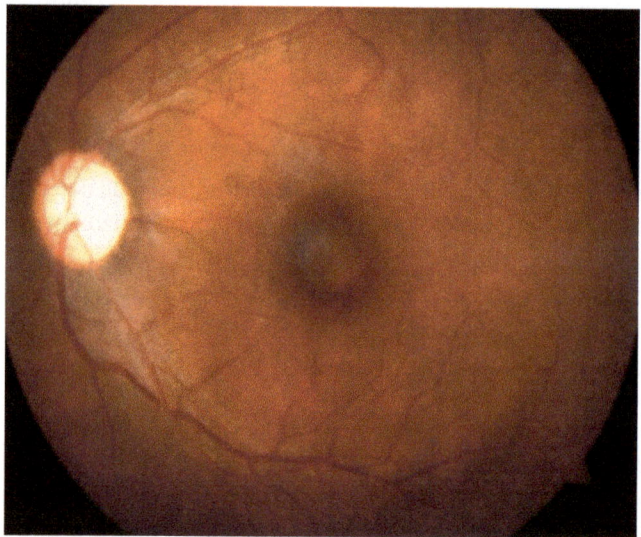

Questions

1. What are the findings on the ophthalmoscopic examination?
2. What is the ophthalmoscopic diagnosis?
3. What is the neurological diagnosis, given the combination of her clinical and ophthalmoscopic findings?

Principles

- Direct ophthalmoscopy using a hand held ophthalmoscope provides an upright, magnified (approximately 15 X), monoscopic view of the optic nerve head.
- Ideally, the aperture should approximate the size of the pupil to allow sufficient light to enter eye to provide enough illumination of the fundus.
- The selection of an aperture larger than the pupil introduces more light than can enter the eye and creates secondary problems such as glare and constriction of the pupil.

- Additionally, the use of the red-free light can help identify hemorrhages such as optic nerve head (Drance) hemorrhages.

Observations Relevant in Ophthalmoscopy

The following parameters have to be noted while performing ophthalmoscopic examination:
- Shape: Normal disc is almost circular
- Size: Normal disc is 1.5 mm in diameter. In aplasia and hypoplasia it is smaller
- Margin: Normal disc margin is sharp. Margins are blurred in various optic nerve diseases (optic neuritis, papilledema, atrophy, drusen of disc, myelinated fibers, etc.)
- Cup-disc ratio:
    - The cup is a normal depression within the center of the disc due to backward bowing of lamina cibrosa
    - It is 1/3 of the size of disc
    - Its lateral floor slopes towards center
    - It is paler than disc
    - It is also identified by the areas where vessels appear to be kinking in addition to that of pallor as the former would more accurate in identifying the cup
    - Measurements of the vertical and horizontal cup-to-disc ratios should be determined.
- Cup depth/elevation:
    - Measured by the change in diopters (by adding minus lenses for depth and plus lenses for elevation) needed to shift the focus of the scope from the retina to the bottom of the cup
    - Three diopters of change in depth equivalent to 1 mm excavation or elevation
    - In glaucoma, myopia and coloboma of disc, cup appears deep
    - In optic neuritis, papilledema, drusen of disc appears, elevated
- Disc color:
    - The nerve fibers are unmyelinated up to the retrolaminar portion of the optic nerve. The nerve fibers over the disc are transparent and pink color is due to the capillaries.
    - Normal disc looks pink due to the small capillaries over the surface of disc. Its true color is white as it is a nerve.
    - If the number of capillaries is more (normally 10–15), it appears as hyperemic and if less capillaries, it appears pale.
    - The pallor associated with glaucomatous changes in the cup is due to the thinning of the neuroretinal rim.
- Retina:
    - Normal red/orange color
    - Macula is dark and is approximately 2 disc diameters away from disc and 1.5° below horizontal raphae

- Vessels: Arterial/venous ratio 2 to 3; the arteries appear a bright red, the veins a slightly purplish color.

Methodology

- The ophthalmoscope (Fig. 3.14) has different size apertures, filters and slit
- A micro spot aperture allows quick visual entry in small and undilated pupils
- A large aperture is the standard aperture, used in dilated fundus examination.

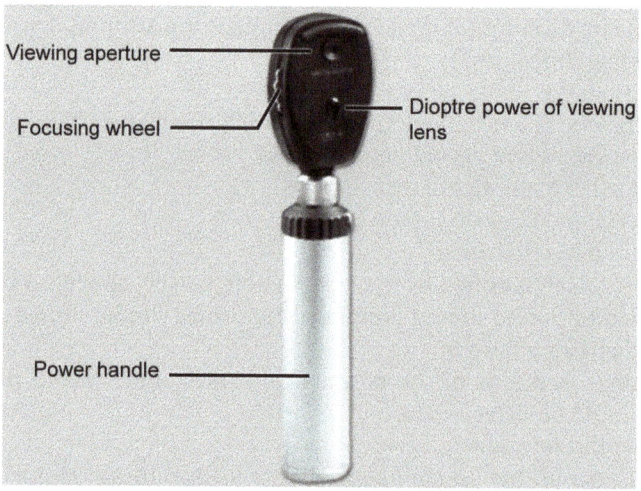

Fig. 3.14: The ophthalmoscope.

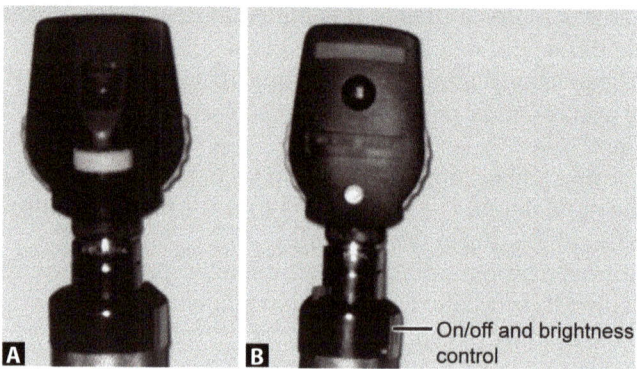

Figs. 3.15A and B: (A) Patient side view of ophthalmoscope; (B) Examiner's side of view.

- In persons with difficulty in fixing the eye and examiner finds it difficult to examine a constantly moving eye, a cross hair mire helps in fixation.
- A green filter helps in red free viewing.

Examination Technique

- Dim the light in the room, so that the patient's pupils dilate a little
- Use mydriatic eye drops to dilate the pupil. Pupils can be dilated using 1 drop of tropicamide 1%, phenylephrine 2.5%, or both (repeated in 5 to 10 minutes if necessary); for longer action, a larger dilated pupil, or both, cyclopentolate 1% can be substituted for tropicamide
- Have patient seated in a comfortable position
- Let the person look at something straight ahead and level over examiner's shoulder
- Hold ophthalmoscope in same hand as eye you are looking at, and looking through (e.g. left hand for examining patients left eye, using your left eye)
- Hold the head steady with thumb above eyebrow, or hold shoulder
- Turn on the ophthalmoscope
- Set the diopter power on the scope to 0
  - Turning the dial to positive (or green) numbers increases the refractive index. Short focal length lens is used for examining cornea, iris, or opacities in vitreous or lens. For example, Start at +20 and use the slit light
  - Turning the dial to negative (or red) numbers decreases the refractive index. This is used for examining retina. start at -10 as you move in and dim the scope light about halfway
- At a distance of 30 cm with ophthalmoscope light on eye, look for red reflex. It appears as an orange glow in the pupillary area
- Follow the red reflex into the eye at an angle of 15° laterally to the person's line of vision. Optic disc can be visible by this way
- If disc is not visible, focus on a vessel and follow blood vessels up to disc
- Examine vessels in all 4 quadrants of eye (upper and lower nasal and temporal quadrants)
- Identify macula—slightly darker pigmented area, 2 optic disc widths lateral away from the optic disc
- In the end, you can ask the patient to look at the light to bring the macula in your focus, however looking at it too long can be irritating to person.

Rule of thumb: You will focus on the retina with same number as your refractive error, then correct for your patient's refractive error. If the examiner is emmetropic, mean not using any correction, examine with 0 power on the ophthalmoscope. If examiner is ammetrope, having correction; example -2, use -2 power on the ophthalmoscope. Similarly if patient has correction, use the same power on the ophthalmoscope.

What to observe:
- The size, shape and borders of the optic disc
- The disc to cup ratio
- The number, relative size of the arteries and veins, width of vessels, and tortuosity

- The texture of the retina
- The color of the retina
- Trace the vascular structure to the equator of the retina.
- Find the macula and note its color and size
- Other findings—hemorrhages, soft and hard exudates, edema

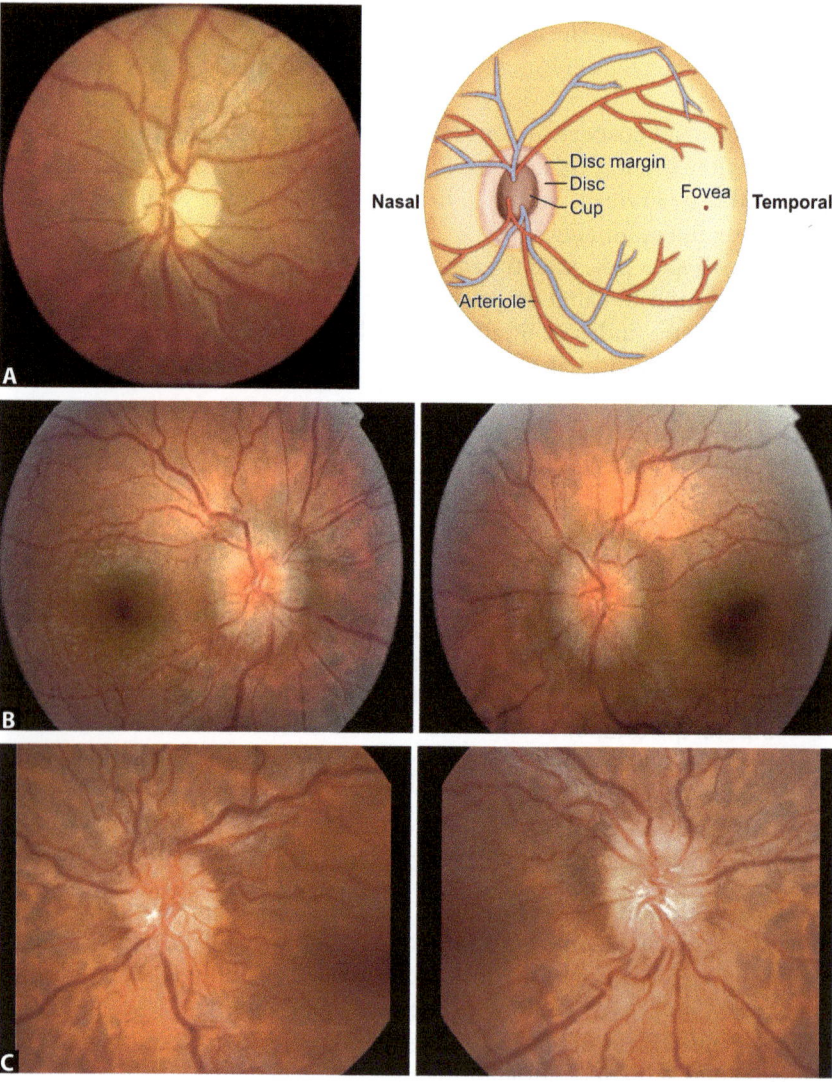

Figs. 3.16A to C: (A) Normal retina with disc, vessels, macula and fovea focused; (B) Swollen disc; (C) Pseudopapilledema.

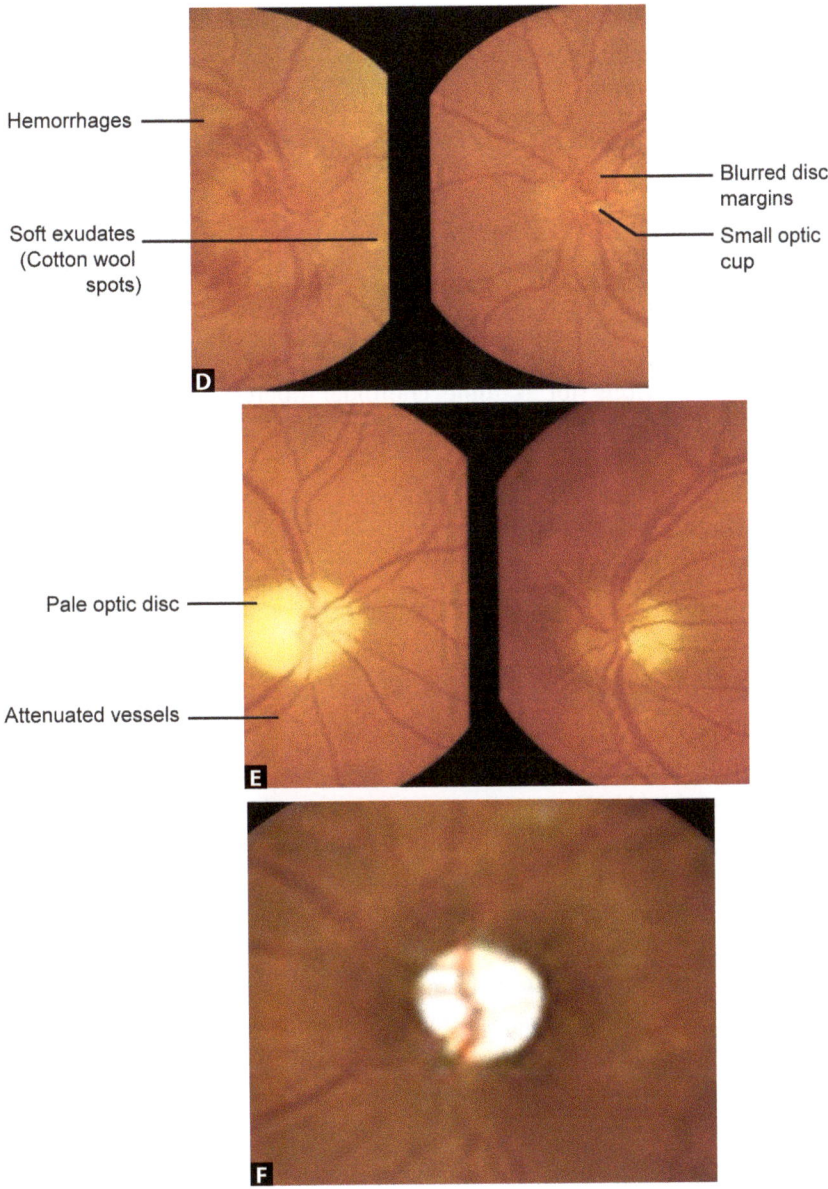

Figs. 3.16D to F: Stages of papilledema.

CLINICAL INTERPRETATION

Abnormalities of ophthalmoscopic findings may be classified for neurological interest as:
- Abnormalities of the disc:

- Swollen disc:
  - Unilateral
  - Bilateral
- Pale disc
- Anomalous disc
- Normal appearing disc with optic neuropathies
• Abnormalities of the retina:
  - Pigmentation
  - Macular dystrophy
  - Cherry red spot
  - Hemorrhages
  - Exudates
  - Other lesions (for example, choroidal tubercle, cysticercal lesions, etc.)
• Abnormalities of blood vessels:
  - Arterial diseases
  - Venous diseases
• Other disorders

Some of these conditions of neurologic interest are discussed.

Unilateral Swollen Disc

- The differential diagnoses include:
  - Inflammatory (optic neuritis, neuroretinitis, sarcoidosis)
  - Vascular (AION, retinal vein occlusion)
  - Compressive lesions (meningiomas, gliomas, paranasal sinus disease, Grave's ophthalmopathy)
  - Optic nerve infiltration (lung or breast carcinoma, lymphoreticular malignancy)
  - *Genetic diseases:* Leber's hereditary optic neuropathy (LHON)
- The characteristic and salient findings in each of these conditions are listed below:
  - *Optic neuritis:* Pain at onset, impaired color vision, contrast sensitivity, relative afferent pupillary defect (RAPD)
  - *Neuroretinitis* (usually infectious like syphilis, etc.): Macular star
  - *Sarcoidosis:* Whitish nodules on disc surface
  - *AION:* Sudden painless visual loss > 55 years of age, sectoral chalky white disc pallor, disc hemorrhages, centrocecal field defect respecting horizontal meridian
  - *LHON:* Peripupillary telangiectasia in the symptomatic and the asymptomatic eyes
- The most common differential diagnoses are presented in Table 3.1.

Table 3.1: Common differential diagnosis of unilateral swollen disc.

	AION	Papillitis	Compressive lesion
Disc color	Chalky white	Congested	Congested
Disc hemorrhages	Common	Rare	Common
Edema location	Sectoral	Diffuse	Diffuse
Visual field defect	Centrocecal respecting the horizontal meridian	Central	Central
Retinal exudates	–	+	–
Optociliary shunts	–	–	Optociliary shunts
Color vision	Impaired disproportionate to acuity	Proportionate loss	Proportionate loss
RAPD	--	+	+
Onset	Sudden	Acute	Insidious
Pain at onset	--	+	+/–

(AION: anterior ischemic optic neuropathy; RAPD: relative afferent pupil defect)

Bilateral Swollen Disc

- The differential diagnoses are:
  - Papilledema
  - Pseudopapilledema
  - Malignant hypertension
  - Diabetic papillopathy
  - Hyperviscosity syndrome
  - Anemia
  - Blood loss
  - Hypotension
  - Bilateral AION
- The differential diagnoses between true papilledema and pseudopapilledema are presented in Table 3.2.

Table 3.2: Differential diagnoses between true papilledema and pseudopapilledema.

	Papilledema	Pseudopapilledema
Disc color	Hyperemic	Normal pink/yellowish
Disc margins	Indistinct, progressing from superior and inferior poles to the rest of the disc	Irregularly blurred
Vessel pattern	Normal distribution	Anomalous pattern, arise from the center of the disc, tortuous, multiple vessels
Spontaneous venous pulsations	Absent	Present
Hemorrhages	Splinter	Subretinal
Hard exudates	+	–
Soft exudates	+	–
Physiological cup	Present	Usually absent

Pale Disc

- Any optic neuropathy can result in optic atrophy, but some features may help in differentiating them
- In primary optic atrophy, the margins are regular and sharp, the retina does not show exudates, hemorrhages and other abnormalities
- In secondary optic atrophy, the margins are blurred and the retina may show exudates and hemorrhages
- A deep cup is typical of glaucoma and also seen in AION
- Temporal pallor and excavation are typical of autosomal dominant optic atrophy.

Normal Appearing Disc with Optic Neuropathy

- *Unilateral disease:* The differentials include:
    - Retrobulbar neuritis
    - Posterior ischemic optic neuropathy
    - Early compressive lesions
- *Bilateral diseases:* The differentials include early stages of the following:
    - Nutritional (B_{12}, folate deficiency)
    - Toxic (tobacco, alcohol, heavy metals)
    - Drugs (INH, ethambutol, etc.)
    - Inherited optic neuropathies.

Pigmentary Retinopathy

- Caused by degeneration of rods and later, cones
- Causes progressive constriction of visual fields
- The classic appearance is described as "bone spicule" like
- The important differential diagnosis are as follows (*Mnemonic:* BRICKS)
    - **B**atten's disease
    - **R**efsum's disease
    - **I**nherited vitamin E deficiency
    - **C**ockayne syndrome
    - **K**earns-Sayre syndrome
    - **S**CA 7.

Caveats

- The pattern of optic disc elevation rarely gives an absolute indication as to the underlying cause.
- The pattern of visual loss, associated symptoms such as pain on eye movements or transient visual obscuration, and other physical signs such as intraocular inflammation or retinal abnormalities must be taken into account.

- The classic features of papilledema like blurred disc margins and spontaneous venous pulsation are not reliable
- The optic disc margins are often indistinct in small or tilted optic discs
- Spontaneous venous pulsation is not always present when the intracranial pressure is normal and has been shown to be present when the intracranial pressure is markedly elevated
- Optic disc pallor is usually a sign of optic nerve disease, but it also occurs secondary to retinal disease.

Answers to the Pretest

1. The ophthalmoscopy showed pigmentary degeneration of macula.
2. This combination of cerebellar ataxia with macular degeneration is typical of SCA-7.
3. Her genetic studies revealed a trinucleotide expansion of the gene encoding ataxin-7 on chromosome 3p14.1.

BIBLIOGRAPHY

1. Balcer LJ. Clinical practice. Optic neuritis. N Engl J Med. 2006;354:1273-80.
2. Balcer LJ. Anatomic review and topographic diagnosis. Ophthalmol Clin North Am. 2001;14:1-21.
3. Balcer L, Prasad S. Abnormalities of the optic nerve and retina. In: Bradley WG, et al. Neurology in Clinical Practice, 5th edition; 2008.
4. Clark D, Kebede W, Eggenberger E. Optic neuritis. In: Lee AG, Brazis PW (Eds). Neurologic clinics. Neuro-Ophthalmology. 2010;28(3):573-81.
5. Galetta SL, Balcer LJ, Liu GT. Neuro-ophthalmologic anatomy and examination techniques. In: Schapira AHV, Samuels MA (Eds). Blue books of Neurology: Neuro-ophthalmology. Butterworth- Heinemann Publications.
6. Kerr NM, Chew SS, Eady EK, et al. Diagnostic accuracy of confrontation visual field tests. Neurology. 2010; 74:1184-90.
7. Whiting AS, Johnson LN. Papilledema: clinical clues and differential diagnosis. Am Fam Physician. 1992;45:1125-34.

OCULAR MOTOR NERVES (III, IV AND VI)

GRK Sarma

PICTORIAL PRETEST

This 57-year-old diabetic patient presented with acute onset squinting of the eyes with double vision on waking up from sleep. There is no headache or vomiting. There is no weakness or sensory loss or ataxia.

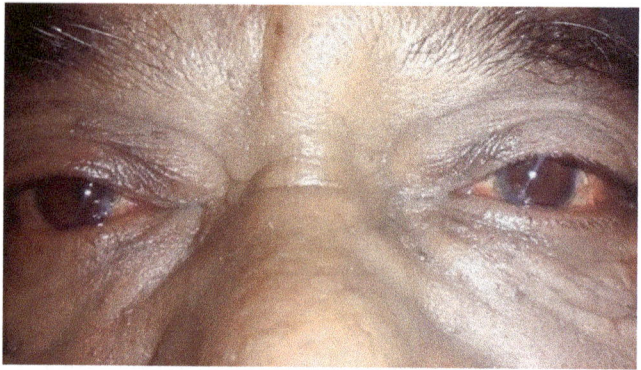

Questions

1. Describe the ocular deviation in this patient.
2. Which anatomical location(s) of lesion(s) can produce this deviation?
3. Which clinical techniques can confirm the lesion localization?

OCULAR MOTOR NERVES

- In this chapter, the anatomy of individual cranial nerves III, IV and VI is presented first.
- Their functions are discussed together as "ocular motor system".
- The examination of the eyelids and pupils is discussed separately.

III Cranial Nerve (Oculomotor Nerve)

- The nucleus is located close to the midline in the upper midbrain (at the level of superior colliculus), just anterior to the aqueduct of Sylvius.
- Each nucleus contains various subgroups of neurons, each innervating different extraocular muscle.
  - *Lateral subnucleus:* Inferior oblique, medial rectus, inferior rectus
  - *Medial subnucleus:* Contralateral superior rectus
  - *Central nucleus (single midline nucleus):* Bilateral levator palpebrae superioris
  - *Edinger-Westphal (EW) nucleus (spread throughout the oculomotor nucleus complex):* Bilateral pupillary sphincter (rostral part of the nucleus) and ciliary muscles (anteromedial part of the nucleus)

- Fibers from the contralateral medial subnucleus, ipsilateral lateral subnucleus, central nucleus and EW nucleus join to form the III cranial nerve
- These fibers travel anteriorly through the red nucleus and substantia nigra and exit the midbrain in the interpeduncular fossa
- The III nerve passes between the posterior cerebral artery and the superior cerebellar artery, parallel to the posterior communicating artery
- It courses close to the medial temporal lobe and enters the cavernous sinus lying close to the lateral wall
- In the anterior part of the cavernous sinus, III nerve separates into a superior and an inferior division
- These divisions enter the orbit through the superior orbital fissure, pierce the annulus of Zinn
- The superior division supplies the superior rectus and the levator palpebrae superioris
- The inferior division supplies the inferior rectus, medial rectus, inferior oblique and the pupil.
- A short root is given off to the ciliary ganglion to supply the pupillary sphincter and the ciliary muscle.

IV Cranial Nerve (Trochlear Nerve)

- The nucleus is located in the lower midbrain at the level of inferior colliculus
- It is situated just caudal to the lateral subnucleus of the III nerve
- The fibers traverse posteriorly and decussate around the aqueduct of Sylvius and exit on the posterior aspect of the midbrain
- The nerve courses forward, encircling the midbrain, passing anteriorly between the superior cerebellar artery and the posterior cerebral artery
- It enters the cavernous sinus, just below the III nerve and exits the sinus to enter the superior orbital fissure to reach the superior oblique
- It does not pass through the circle of Zinn
- It terminates on the contralateral superior oblique muscle.

VI Cranial Nerve (Abducens Nerve)

- Its nucleus is located in the mid or lower pons, in the floor of the IVth ventricle
- It is encircled by the looping fibers of the facial nerve
- It exits anteriorly at the pontomedullary junction and ascends the clivus in the prepontine cistern
- It crosses the petrous apex and enters the cavernous sinus, lying freely within the sinus inferomedial to the III nerve and lateral to the internal carotid artery
- It enters the orbit through the superior orbital fissure, piercing the annulus of Zinn.

PHYSIOLOGIC BASIS OF OCULAR MOTOR SYSTEM

- This chapter deals with the peripheral ocular motor mechanisms. The central mechanisms are discussed in the next chapter.
- A clear knowledge of this system is required while evaluating the following clinical problems:
    - A patient complains of double vision, but there is no prominent or clear abnormality in the ocular alignment
    - A patient presents with obvious ocular misalignment, but the muscle(s) involved is not certain on routine examination. For example, a diplopia in a vertical direction needs to be evaluated systematically, while a lateral rectus palsy is usually obvious.
- The ocular motor system works to place the images of objects of interest on the fovea in various head postures and movements, while perfectly aligning both the visual axes.
- To achieve this, each eye has 6 extraocular muscles yoked in 3 pairs (Tables 3.3 and 3.4, Figs. 3.17 to 3.19).
- Their primary, secondary and tertiary actions are all important in evaluation of diplopia (see the three step test for diplopia). The individual primary movements are also called "ductions". The conjugate movements are called "versions".
- All the three actions of each muscle can be predicted by the anatomical relation of the longitudinal axis of the muscle with the axis of rotation of the globe (Fig. 3.17).
- The recti work as pure elevators or depressors when the eye is abducted to nearly 30°.
- The obliques do the same when the eye are adducted by nearly 45° (to be precise, 51°, but clinically, this precision is not possible).

Table 3.3: Actions of extraocular muscles.

Muscle	Primary	Secondary	Tertiary
• Medial rectus	• Adduction	-	-
• Lateral rectus	• Abduction	-	-
• Superior rectus	• Elevation	• Intorsion	• Adduction
• Inferior rectus	• Depression	• Extorsion	• Adduction
• Superior oblique	• Intorsion	• Depression	• Abduction
• Inferior oblique	• Extorsion	• Elevation	• Abduction

- One muscle of one eye and one muscle of another eye move together to produce a conjugate movement, like the oxen fixed in a yoke (Table 3.4). This knowledge is essential to understand diplopia rules.

Table 3.4: Yoked muscle pairs.

Ipsilateral	Contralateral
• Medial rectus (MR) • Superior rectus (SR) • Inferior rectus (IR)	• Lateral rectus (LR) • Inferior oblique (IO) • Superior oblique (SO)

- These yoked muscle pairs can also be worked out by their anatomic relations, and are representatively shown in the Figure 3.19.

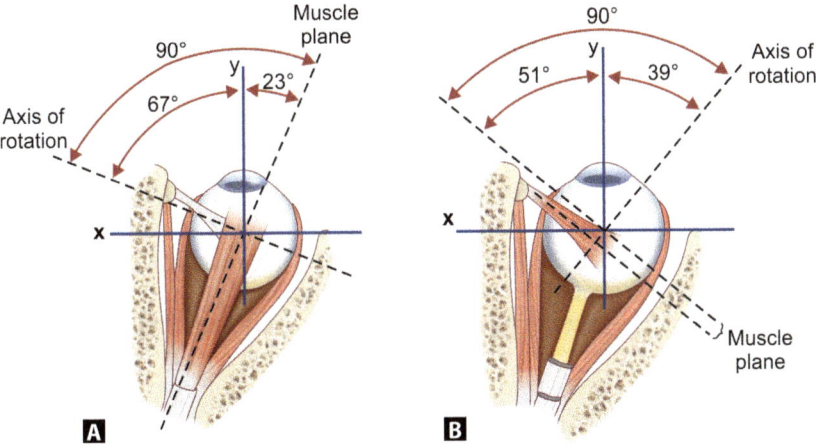

Figs. 3.17A and B: Relationship between the long axes of the rectus and oblique muscles and the rotational axis of the globe. (A) Rectus muscles; (B) Oblique muscles.

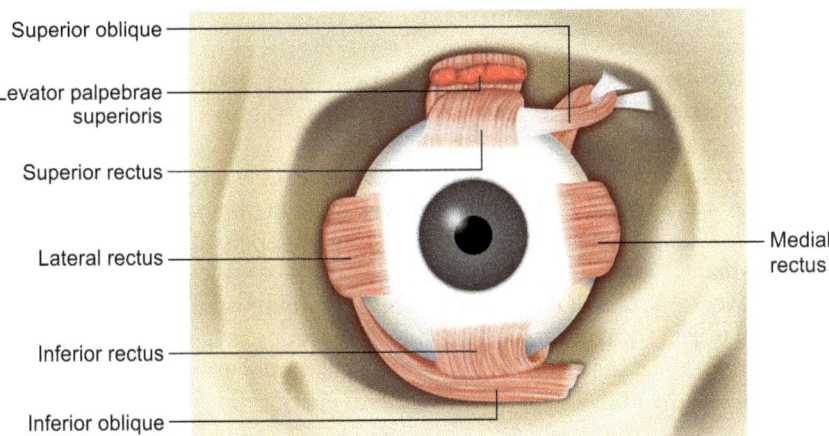

Fig. 3.18: Extraocular muscles of the right eye, to show their insertional positions and directions.

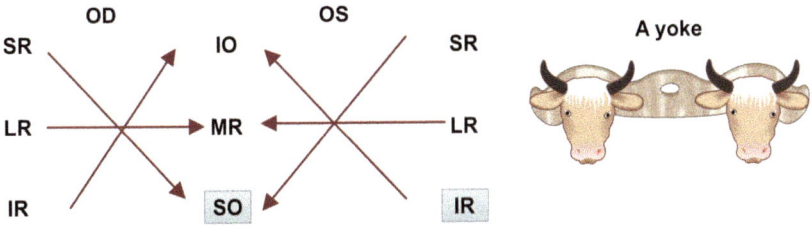

Fig. 3.19: Yoked pairs of muscles (one from the right and one from the left eye) work together to produce a conjugate movement of both eyeballs. SR-IO, IR-SO and MR-LR are like oxen in a yoke. For example, the right superior oblique and the left inferior recti are yoked to move the eyes "down and to the left".

- *Hering's law of dual innervation:* States that the yoked muscles receive equal and simultaneous innervations. (This law comes into action during the cover-uncover test described below) (Fig. 3.19).

CERTAIN TERMS AND RULES

- *Heterophoria:* It is the **latent** tendency for ocular misalignment in the general population.
- *Heterotropia:* When the latent tendency for ocular misalignment becomes **manifest**, it is called heterotropia (for example, fatigue, sedative use, etc.)
- *Esotropia:* It is a heterotropia wherein the eyes are **convergent**
- *Exotropia:* A heterotopia wherein the eyes are **divergent**
- *Hypertropia:* A heterotropia in which the non-fixating eye is higher.
- *Hypotropia:* A heterotropia, in which, the non-fixating is lower.
- *Comitant strabismus:* In this, the degree of **misalignment is constant** in all positions. This is of ocular origin.
- Noncomitant (or paralytic) strabismus; in this the degree of **misalignment varies** with different positions. This is neurological in origin
- *False image:* In patients with paralytic strabismus, the image perceived by the non-fixating eye is the false image. It is displaced in the direction of the paralyzed muscle. For example, if the right lateral rectus is weak, the false image is deviated to the right of the true image (i.e. in a direction opposite to the eye deviation, which is to the left)
- *Uncrossed diplopia:* As in the above instance, in esotropias, the image is shifted outward from the true image resulting in uncrossed diplopia
- *Crossed diplopia:* In exotropia, the opposite happens resulting in crossed diplopia
- *Primary deviation:* It is the angle of misalignment when the patient fixates on an object with his intact eye, while the paretic eye is covered (Fig. 3.20).
- *Secondary deviation:* It is the angle of misalignment when the same patient fixates on the object with the paretic eye (Fig. 3.20).

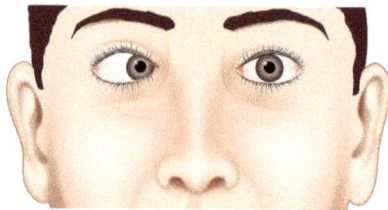
Primary deviation
(left eye fixing)

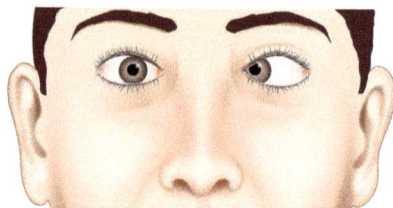
Secondary deviation (right eye fixing; overshoot of sound left eye)

Fig. 3.20: As a rule, the eye that deviates more (secondary deviation) is the normal eye. This is explained by the Hering's law.

- As a rule, the secondary deviation is greater than the primary deviation. This happens because, as stated in the Hering's law, to bring the paretic eye to fixate on an object, the patient overdrives the contralateral yoked muscle. This does not happen with the primary deviation because there is no such overdrive.

Rules for Diplopia Evaluation

To understand and apply these rules, it is useful to visualize three events in ocular motor palsy (Figs. 3.21A to C). Misalignment (A) results in perception of true and false images (B), which triggers compensatory mechanisms (C). All the three events can be assessed to derive the paretic muscle. Tests of 'B' are subjective (need patient cooperation), while 'A, C' are objective.

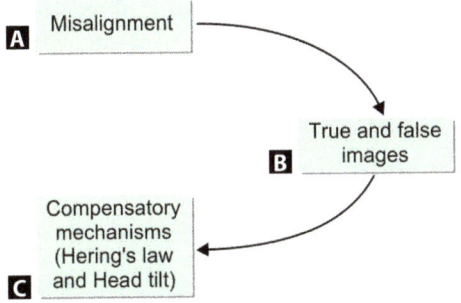

Figs. 3.21A to C: Sequence of events after ocular motor palsy.

Rules

A. *Based on the type of misalignment:*
- If the misalignment varies with the direction of the gaze, it is noncomitant (neurological). If it remains constant, it is comitant (ocular)
- In noncomitant strabismus, the degree of misalignment is maximum in the direction of action of the weak muscle.

B. *Based on true and false images:*
- The false image is displaced in the direction of the paretic muscle
- The false image is the most peripheral image (and is also the fainter image)
- The degree of separation of the two images increases in the direction of the paretic muscle.

C. *Based on compensatory mechanisms:*
- The head is tilted in the direction of the paretic muscle.
- In the cover-uncover test, the secondary deviation is greater than the primary deviation (Hering's law).

Examination Methods to Evaluate Diplopia/Ocular Motor Palsy

The overall scheme of examination is presented below, followed by discussion of each method.

The scheme may be modified and differently prioritized in individual patient.

Examination Scheme

Preparatory tests:	
• Visual acuity • Ptosis • Pupils • Proptosis • Fatigability	
Tests of eye movements	**Tests of ocular misalignment**
• Visual fixation • Duction • Version (saccades, pursuits) • Vergence • OKN (These movements other than ductions are described in the chapter on 'Supranuclear Gaze')	• Head tilt • Gross ocular misalignment • Hirschberg's test • Cover uncover test • Diplopia chart

Examination Methodology

A. *Visual acuity:*
   - If acuity is impaired, patient will not be able to fixate, making it difficult to perform other tests
   - Therefore, checking acuity is the first step before examining eye movements in detail
   - This has been already described in the previous chapter.

B. *Ptosis, proptosis, pupils:*
   - Look for asymmetry in the palpebral fissures
   - Look for the asymmetry in the distance to which the upper eyelid covers the upper cornea
   - Evaluation of ptosis is described in the section on eyelids and pupils
   - Ptosis suggests III nerve palsy
   - Miosis in an apparent VI nerve palsy suggests convergence spasm
   - Proptosis is a clue to orbital infiltration or edema
   - Fatigability is a clue to myasthenia.

C. *Head tilt:*
   - Look for a head tilt or turn
   - The direction of the head tilt is the direction in which the paretic muscle normally acts
   - For example, if the head is turned to the right side, then either the right lateral rectus or the left medial rectus is weak
   - If the head is tilted downwards and to the left, it suggests right superior oblique weakness.
   - Correct the head tilt (forced primary position) for subsequent tests

D. *Ductions and ocular misalignment:*
- Check for ductions in the 9 cardinal positions [these include the primary gaze plus the 8 directions]

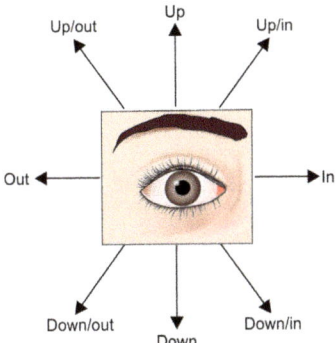

- Look for misalignment in any of these directions
- Observe if the misalignment varies in these various positions (noncomitant) or remains constant (comitant)
- Normally, the eye moves by about 45° to either side of the primary position
- In other words, the amount of movement is 10 mm for adduction, abduction and elevation; and 7 mm for depression
- For practical purposes, the patient must be able to bury the limbus in full lateral and medial gaze
- In some people, a small rim of the sclera may be visible ('sclera show'), but this must be symmetric on both the sides
- In noncomitant strabismus, the degree of misalignment is maximum in the direction of action of the weak muscle
- Horizontal misalignment is usually easier to interpret.

To analyze **vertical misalignment**, the three-step method is used:
- *Step 1:* For example, in a patient with right hypertropia, either the right eye depressors or the left eye elevators are weak. These are marked out:

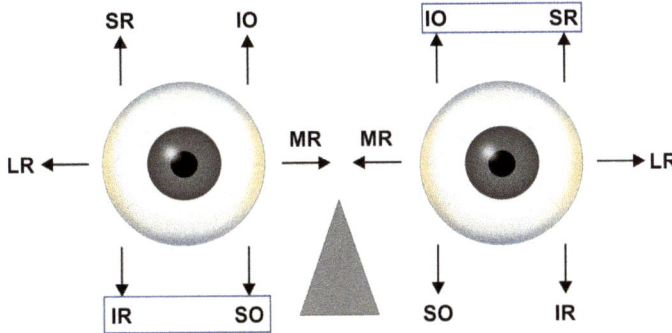

- *Step 2:* if the misalignment (or diplopia) increases on left gaze, muscles acting in this direction are marked out. Note that the left SR and the right SO are marked in both the steps and are the only contenders left at this step.

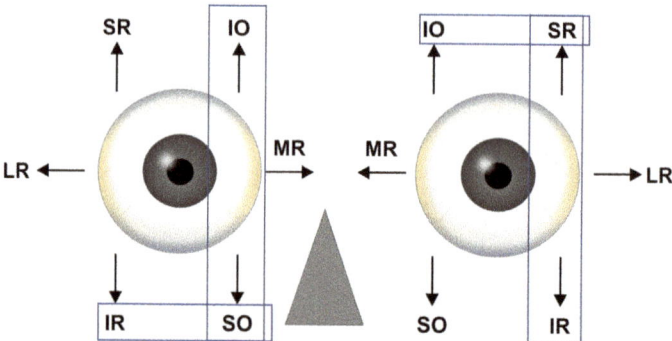

- *Step 3:* The head is tilted to either side. If the misalignment is greater, say, on right head tilt, the muscles involved in opposite movement of the eye (rotation to left and down) are marked out. It can be seen that only the right SO is common to all the three steps, hence this is the paretic muscle.

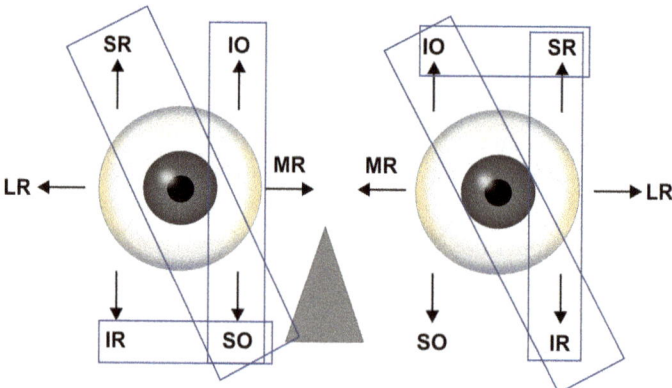

E. *Hirschberg test:*
   - Performed at near vision (distant reflections are too dim)
   - Patient is asked to look at a point of light (pen torch)
   - The reflected light from the cornea of both eyes is observed (corneal light reflex)
   - The amount of deviation of the light reflex from the center of the pupil indicates the degree of ocular deviation
   - Each mm of displacement of light from the center is equivalent to 18° of deviation
   - This test is useful in young children and uncooperative patients.

F. *Cover-uncover test*:
- Ask the patient to fix at an object (both near and distant, i.e. 30 cm and 6 m)
- While he fixates on the object, cover the right eye, and observe the left eye
- If the left eye moves to the target, it suggests that the left eye was not fixating. Note the angle of deviation of the left eye
- As the patient fixates with his left eye, uncover the right eye and cover the left eye. Note the angle of deviation
- Whichever angle of deviation is greater is the secondary deviation, while the lesser angle indicates the primary deviation (Hering's law).
- The eye with the primary deviation is the non-fixating (paretic) eye.

G. *Diplopia chart:*
- This is reliable in the acute stage. Later on in the course of illness, compensation may occur
- One can use spectacles with one glass red and the other green colored. This helps in identifying if the false image is from the right or the left eye

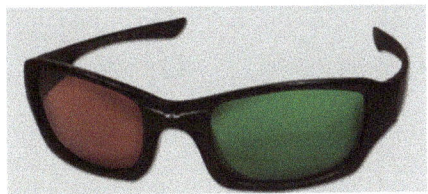

- If colored glasses are not used, the false image is the more peripheral and more blurred image
- Conventionally, the right eye has red glass
- Patient looks at a point light source (for example, torch light) placed in 9 cardinal positions
- The light source must be placed at least 1 meter away from the patient to avoid convergence
- Patient indicates the relative position of the two images in each cardinal position as this information is charted out. This may be done by the patient holding up his two fingers to show the relative position of the two images
- Based on the diplopia rule, the chart is interpreted to derive at the paretic muscle.
- The diplopia rules described above are used to identify the paretic muscle (Figs. 3.22A to F).
    - The false image is displaced in the direction of the paretic muscle.
    - The false image is the most peripheral image (and is also the fainter image).
    - The degree of separation of the two images increases in the direction of the paretic muscle.

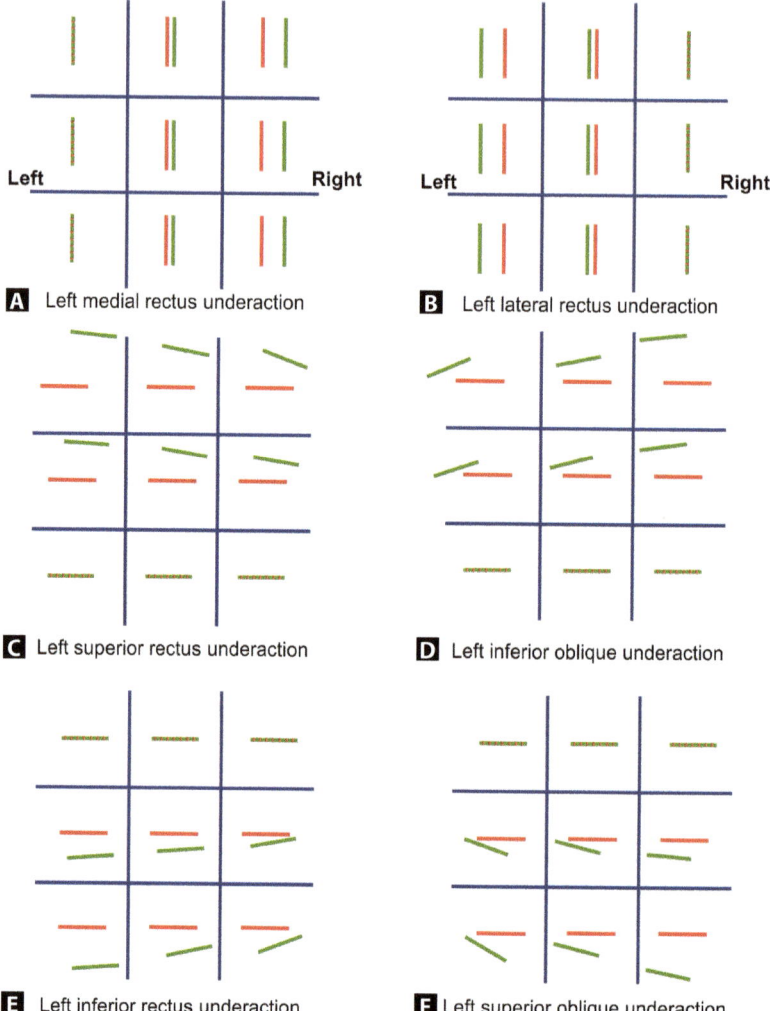

Figs. 3.22A to F: Red is in front of right eye and green in front of left, the horizontal images are used to show the vertical and torsional separation and tilt.

Diplopia Chart

In panel A, for example, the green image is the false image on looking to the right, because, it is the farthest image. As the left eye is covered with green glass, we know that this false image is originating from the left eye. As the misalignment is maximum on right gaze, the muscle that produces this movement, the left medial rectus is the weak muscle.

Similarly, in the last panel, the green image is the false image as it is most peripheral image. The false image is from the left eye (green color). The deviation of the images is maximum in the "down and right direction". The muscle that moves the left eye in this direction is the left superior oblique. Therefore, this is the weak muscle.

Interpretation of Mono-ocular Diplopia

- Some patients report mono-ocular diplopia. These patients need a systematic evaluation (Flowchart 3.1)
- Pinhole test is the 1st step in evaluation of mono-ocular diplopia. Its method has been described in the chapter on Optic Nerve.

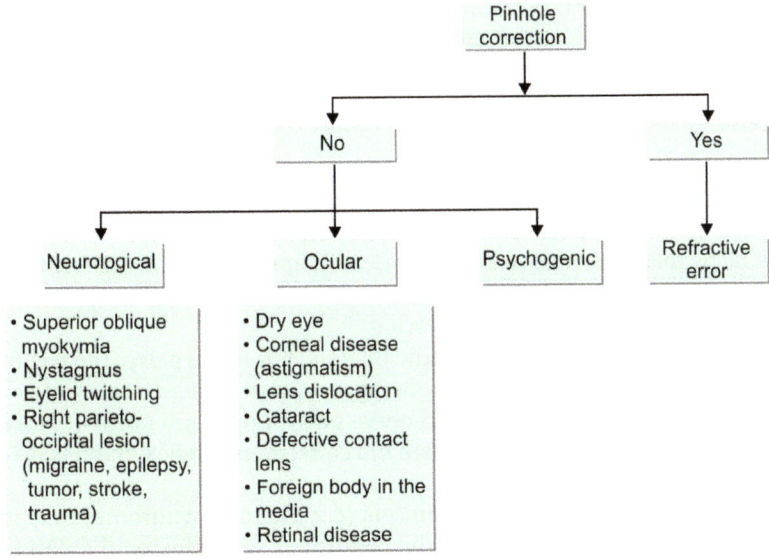

Flowchart 3.1: Approach to mono-ocular diplopia

Interpretation of Ocular Motor Palsies

- Thyroid ophthalmopathy and myasthenia must be considered in all cases of unexplained palsies
- Forced duction test performed under local anesthesia by an ophthalmologist is sometimes necessary to clinch the diagnosis of restrictive conditions like the Duane's or Brown's syndrome. In this test, the globe is mechanically forced to move in a particular direction. Failure to achieve this indicates mechanical restriction rather than a true muscle palsy
- Ophthalmoparesis associated with eye closure weakness (facial nerve innervated) is suggestive of muscle or neuromuscular junction disorder
- In a patient with III nerve palsy, it is difficult to identify additional IV nerve palsy. This is because, the superior oblique produces its depressor action when the eye is adducted, but the latter is impaired due to III nerve palsy. In this situation, one has to look for intorsion of the abducted eye, which is produced by the superior oblique. Intorsion is easily noted by observing the horizontally directed conjunctival vessels for tilting.
- Aberrant reinnervation is a feature of mechanical compressive lesions rather than ischemic lesions
- Bilateral ptosis can occur due to lesion of the unpaired central caudal nucleus of III nerve
- Incomplete lesions of the III nerve suggest a nuclear lesion or the orbital lesion. These can be differentiated by the long tract signs

- Isolated III nerve palsy is likely in lesions of the subarachnoid course of the III nerve
- Involvement of multiple ocular motor palsies suggest the cavernous sinus as the site of the lesion
- IV nerve palsy may present with head tilt and difficulty in climbing down the steps
- VI nerve nuclear lesions produce ipsilateral horizontal gaze palsy because the nucleus contains neurons that project to the MLF
- VI nerve palsy, facial pain and impaired V1 sensation is called Gradenigo's syndrome and is seen in petrous apicitis.

Caveats

- The rules of diplopia evaluation may break down when more than one muscle is affected
- They also break down in the chronic stages following ophthalmoparesis
- Skew deviation can mimic superior oblique palsy. The differentiation is possible by noting the torsional direction. In SO palsy, the eye is extorted, but in skew deviation, it is intorted
- Convergence spasm may mimic bilateral 6th nerve palsy. The pupils give away the correct answer. In convergence spasm, there is miosis (as a part of convergence reflex). In 6th nerve palsy, pupils are normal. Moreover, covering one eye may eliminate the convergence reflex, but has no effect in 6th nerve palsy.
- Mechanical restriction of a muscle (e.g. Duane's syndrome) may mimic ocular motor palsy. This can be confirmed by the forced duction test by the ophthalmologist after instilling local anesthetic drops.

ANSWERS TO THE PRETEST

1. Both the eyes are medially deviated as evidenced by the location of the corneal light reflex and by the increased scleral show on the lateral aspect of both the eyeballs.
2. This can result from (a) paresis of both lateral recti or (b) overaction of both medial recti (convergence spasm) or (c) divergence paralysis.
3. The three conditions can be differentiated by examination of the eye movements, pupil and by one-eye occlusion. In divergence palsy, the individual eye movements are of full range and the pupil is normal. In convergence spasm, the pupils are miotic (as a part of the convergence reflex), but in bilateral abducens palsy, pupils are normal. Moreover, if one eye is occluded, the convergence reflex may (or may not) be abolished and the eye deviation may be normalized. In abducens palsy, eye occlusion has no effect. In this patient, the pupils were miotic, suggesting possible convergence spasm.

   His MRI brain was normal. CSF opening pressure and analysis were normal. He was started on antiplatelets and statins and improved rapidly over next few days. The clinical diagnosis is a possible lacunar infarct in the inferior thalamic region causing convergence spasm.

EXAMINATION OF PUPILS AND LIDS

Pictorial Pretest 1

This 48-year-old man presented with acute left hemiplegia preceded by right frontal and periorbital headache.

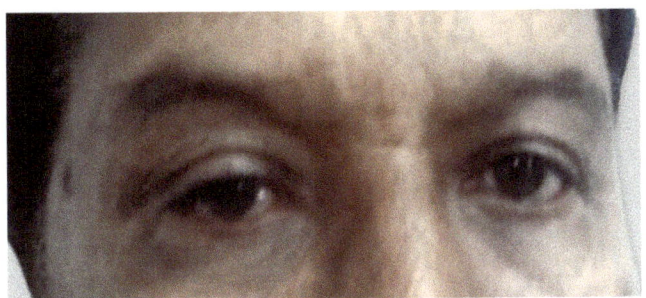

Questions

1. What is the eye finding?
2. What is the lesion location based on this clinical information?

Pictorial Pretest 2

A 55-year-old man presented with widening of his right eye for the last 6 months. There is no eye pain or visual disturbance. He has no past medical illness. His pupils and ocular movements were normal. There were no other neurological deficits. His thyroid function tests were normal and thyroid antibodies were negative. An MRI of the orbit with contrast was normal.

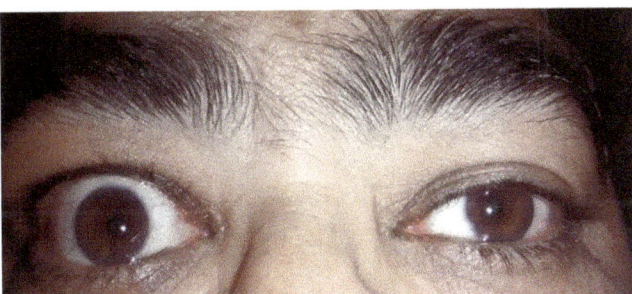

Questions

1. Where is the lesion that has resulted in the ocular appearance?
2. What is the possible etiology?
3. What investigation(s) might help in establishing the diagnosis?

Pictorial Pretest 3

This patient presented with fluctuating ptosis on left side.

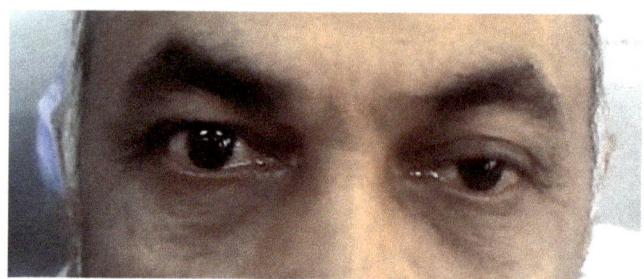

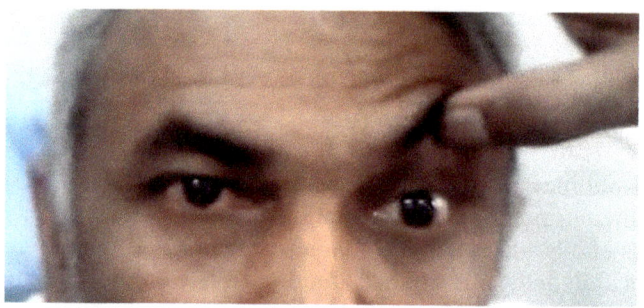

Question

1. What is the sign being elicited?

(Answers are discussed at the end of the chapter)

THE PUPILS

Anatomy and Physiology (Figs. 3.23 and 3.24)

- The function of the pupil is to control the amount of light entering the eye by dilating or constricting.

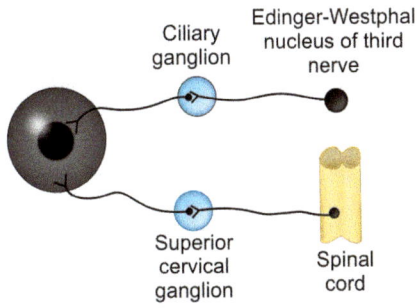

Fig. 3.23: General scheme of autonomic innervations of the pupil.

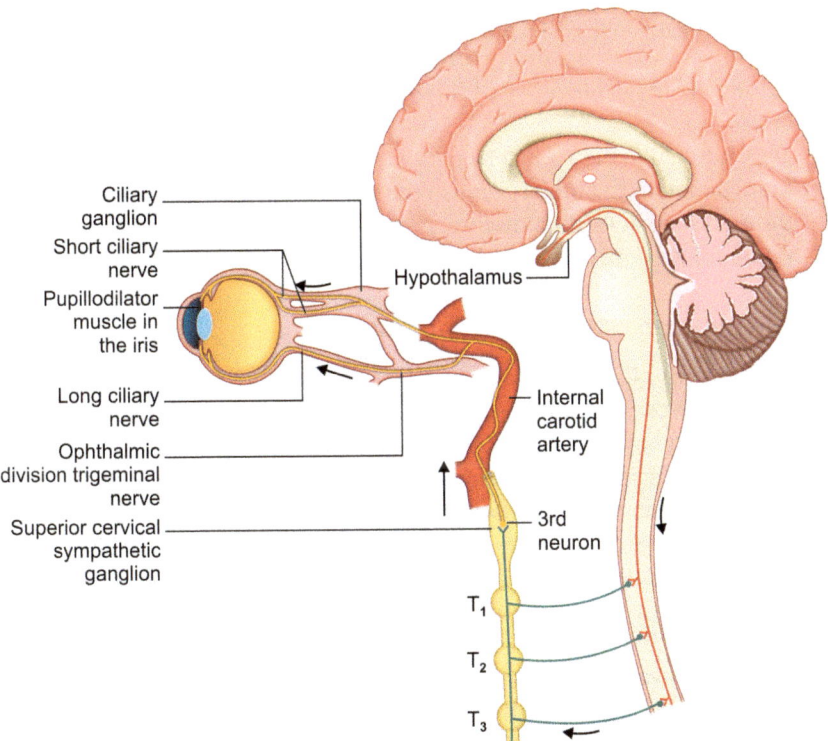

Fig. 3.24: Sympathetic innervation of the pupils.

- Pupillodilator muscle is supplied by the sympathetic fibers (α-1 adrenergic receptors), while the pupilloconstrictor muscle is supplied by the cholinergic fibers (muscarinic M3 receptors) from the Edinger-Westphal nucleus.

Sympathetic Innervation

- The **sympathetic innervation** to the eye begins in the **1st order neurons** in the posterolateral **hypothalamus**
- Their fibers descend through the brainstem, pass through the trochlear nucleus, and upper cervical cord to reach the **2nd order neurons** in the **intermediolateral column** in the C8-T2 cord (ciliospinal center of Budge)
- Their fibers exit through the anterior roots, and pass through the gray rami communicantes, arch over the apex of the lung and beneath the subclavian artery to reach the cervical sympathetic chain
- They further ascend in the sympathetic chain uninterrupted in the stellate ganglion at the apex of the lung, then through the inferior and middle cervical ganglia, to synapse with **3rd order neurons** in **superior cervical ganglion** at the level of carotid bifurcation and the angle of the jaw
- **Postganglionic fibers** of the 3rd neurons lie in the pericarotid plexus on the wall of the common carotid artery
- Fibers destined to facial structures (including sweating) follow the external carotid artery, while those destined to the eye follow the internal carotid artery
- They hitch hike the abducens nerve for a while and reach the nasociliary branch of the Vth cranial nerve in the cavernous sinus and enter the orbit through superior orbital fissure and continue as long ciliary nerve to the pupillodilator muscle.

Parasympathetic Innervation (Fig. 3.25)

- The **preganglionic parasympathetic fibers** arise in the **unpaired Edinger–Westphal nucleus**, which extends throughout the length of the oculomotor complex
- They travel through the III cranial nerve and reach the **ciliary ganglion** in the orbit, from which, **postganglionic fibers** supply the pupillosphincter muscle and the ciliary muscle that is involved in accommodation
- Within the oculomotor nerve, the parasympathetic fibers lie superficially throughout the course. Therefore, they are involved early in compressive lesions and spared in ischemic lesions
- The pupillary light reflex is mediated by the retina, optic nerve, chiasm and the optic tract. The receptive field of this reflex is widespread in the entire retina, with slightly greater representation of the macula
- Therefore, pupillary reflex may be preserved even though the patient may be severely visually impaired in macular lesions.

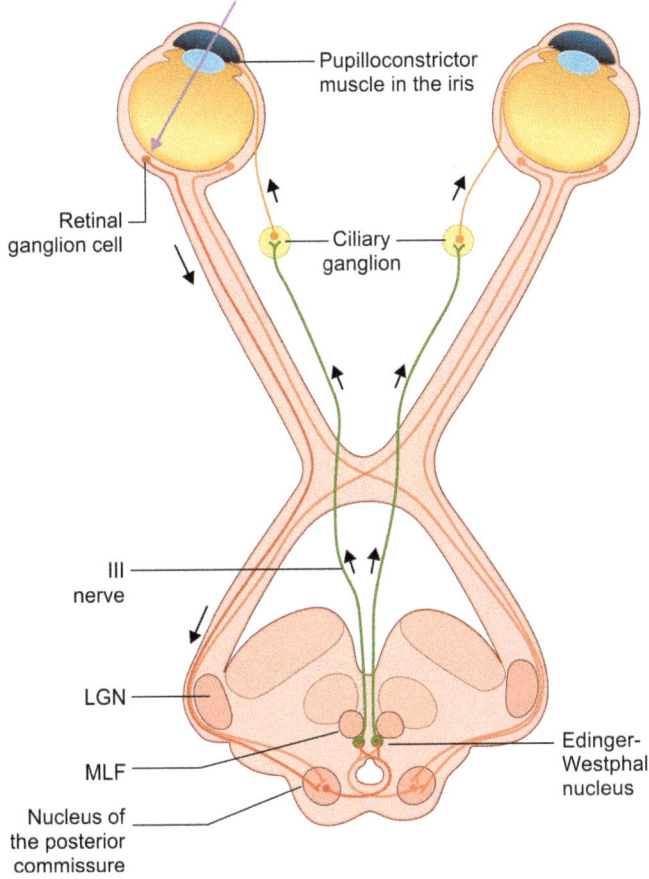

Fig. 3.25: Parasympathetic innervation of the eye.
(LGN: lateral geniculate nucleus; MLF: medial longitudinal fasciculus)

- Pupil afferents leave the optic tract before reaching the lateral geniculate body and synapse in the pretectum.
- Fibers from pretectal region project to the EW nucleus, which mediates cholinergically mediated pupillary constriction. Because of extensive decussation in the posterior commissure, the light reflex is bilateral.
- Swinging flashlight test is a test to compare the integrity of afferent and efferent pathways between the two eyes. If there is miosis on direct light stimulus, but mydriasis on consensual light stimulus, it indicates an afferent pupillary defect in the latter eye. However, false positive RAPD may be seen if light stimulus is projected away from the macula in one eye (e.g. in manifest strabismus), if there is significant anisocoria (less light enters one eye).
- The pathways of accommodation are less well delineated than pupillary reflex.

- Fibers from visual cortex descend through corticotectal tract to near response cells in the pretectum. As these pathways are separate from light reflex pathways, there can be light-near dissociation in certain conditions.
- Healthy subjects with myopia, presbyopia and those with poor motivation may show little or no pupillary constriction on attempted near gaze. Therefore, these individuals may exhibit apparent light near dissociation.

Examination

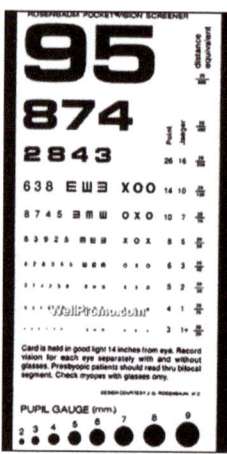 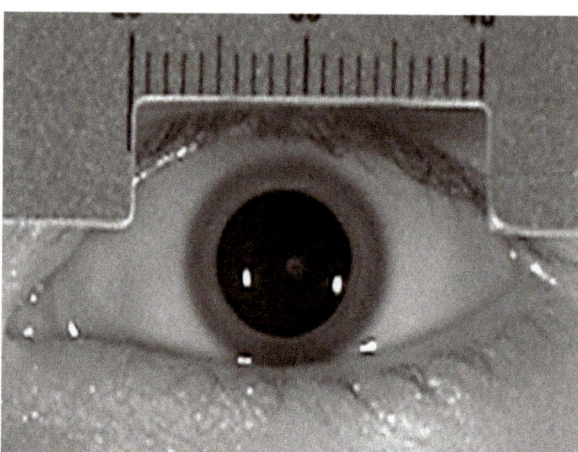

Pupil gauge   Millimeter ruler

Fig. 3.26: Measurement of pupil size.

Examination Method

- *Size:* Measured by pupil gauge or millimeter **ruler** (Fig. 3.26). Measure the pupil at **ambient light**
- *Symmetry:* Compare the size of both pupils by measurement
- *Shape:* Note any irregularity in the shape of the pupil
- *Color:* Note if the color of the iris is abnormal (e.g. heterochromia iridis)
- *Position:* Note the position of the pupil with respect to the iris
- Reflexes:
  1. *Light reflex:*
     - *Direct:* Test in each eye individually
       - Shine the light obliquely into the eye (to avoid convergence reflex)
       - Patient has to fix at a distance to avoid accommodation reflex
       - Normal pupil reflex is brisk constriction followed by slight relaxation.
     - *Consensual:* Test each eye individually
       Observe the pupillary response in one eye after shining light in the other eye.

- *Swinging flashlight test:* Flash the light alternately in to each eye, noting the pupillary response of each eye
- *Redilatation lag:* If a patient has symmetrically miotic pupils, look for prompt dilatation of the pupils after darkening the room. The pupil which takes a longer time to dilate is the abnormal pupil.
2. *Accommodation*:
    - Patient is asked to gaze at a distance and then shift the gaze to a near object (examiner's finger or patient's own tip of nose)
    - Observe for the adequacy of convergence effort by noting the degree of miosis
3. *Light near dissociation:* Note if the response to the light and accommodation reflex is equal or not.
4. Ciliospinal reflex consists of ipsilateral mydriasis on painful stimulation of one side of the neck. As the response is minimal and difficult to see even in normal persons, its utility is limited.

- Response to topical agents:
    - Mainly used in evaluation of Horner's syndrome
    - Use 4–10% cocaine, 2.5–10% phenylephrine, 1–4% pilocarpine
    - Examine the pupil at 30–45 minutes after instillation of the agent
    - Use one drug at a time, and give at least 48 hours between the instillation of different drugs
    - Ensure that the subject does not squeeze out the instilled drops to avoid misinterpretation of test results.

Interpretation

Size:
- *Size:* 2–6 mm is normal
- <2 mm: Miosis
- >6 mm: Mydriasis
- *Miosis may be caused by*:
    - *Ocular causes:* Hyperopia, trauma, iridocyclitis, anterior segment ischemia, synechia
    - *Autonomic disorders:* **Horner's syndrome**, diabetes, neurosyphilis, senile miosis
    - *Central causes:* Pontine hemorrhage
    - *Drugs:* L-dopa, alcohol
- *Mydriasis may be caused by:*
    - *Ocular causes:* Myopia trauma, iris rupture
    - Visual pathway lesions
    - *Autonomic disorders:* Anxiety, fear, pain, Adie's pupil, **III nerve palsy**
    - *Central causes:* Midbrain lesion, cerebral anoxia, terminal coma
    - Drugs

Shape/color:
- *Normal pupil:* Round with smooth regular outline

- *Oval pupil:* Suggests midbrain lesion
- *Grossly abnormal shape:* Usually seen in ocular disease (iritis, previous surgery, synechia, coloboma, trauma)
- Heterochromia iridis occurs in long standing Horner's syndrome from early childhood (intact sympathetic supply is required for normal melanization).

Position:
- *Normal:* pupil is in the center of the iris
- *Corectopia (eccentric pupil):* Midbrain lesion or ocular disease

Equality:
- Asymmetry up to 0.7 mm is normal (95% limits). Rarely, asymmetry of 1.5 mm may be seen in healthy persons. Asymmetry beyond this is unequivocally abnormal
- Unequal pupils, both reacting well to light and dark, with constant asymmetry: Physiological anisocoria
- *Pathological anisocoria:* The poorly reacting pupil in response to light or dark is the abnormal one. In other words, if the asymmetry increases in the bright light, the larger pupil is abnormal (as in 3rd nerve palsy). If the asymmetry is more in the dark, the smaller pupil is abnormal (as in Horner's syndrome). See Flowchart 3.2 for approach to anisocoria.
- *Reaction to light:* See below
- *Reaction to near reflex:* See below
- *Reaction to drugs:* See below
    - When the pupil reacts to low concentrations of topical agents (1% phenylephrine, 0.1% pilocarpine), it is considered as supersensitivity. This indicates muscle denervation
    - *Caveat:* This also occurs in dry eyes when drug penetration into the eye is increased
    - Absence of pupillary response to topical agents is abnormal, but also occurs when the drug is squeezed out by an uncooperative subject
    - About 4-10% cocaine blocks the reuptake of norepinephrine at sympathetic neuroeffector junctions in the dilator muscle and causes mydriasis in normal persons. Failure of mydriasis indicates sympathetic palsy (Horner's syndrome), but does not localize the lesion
    - About 1% hydroxyamphetamine releases norepinephrine from sympathetic nerve endings and causes mydriasis in normal persons and in those with preganglionic Horner's syndrome. Failure to do so in a patient with Horner's syndrome localizes the lesion to the postganglionic level
    - *Caveats:* At least 48 hours must elapse between instillation of different topical agents to allow for wash out of the previous agent.

Clinical Scenarios

- The usual pupillary syndromes that occur with lesions at various levels are summarized in Figure 3.27

Cranial Nerves

Flowchart 3.2: The approach to a patient with anisocoria.

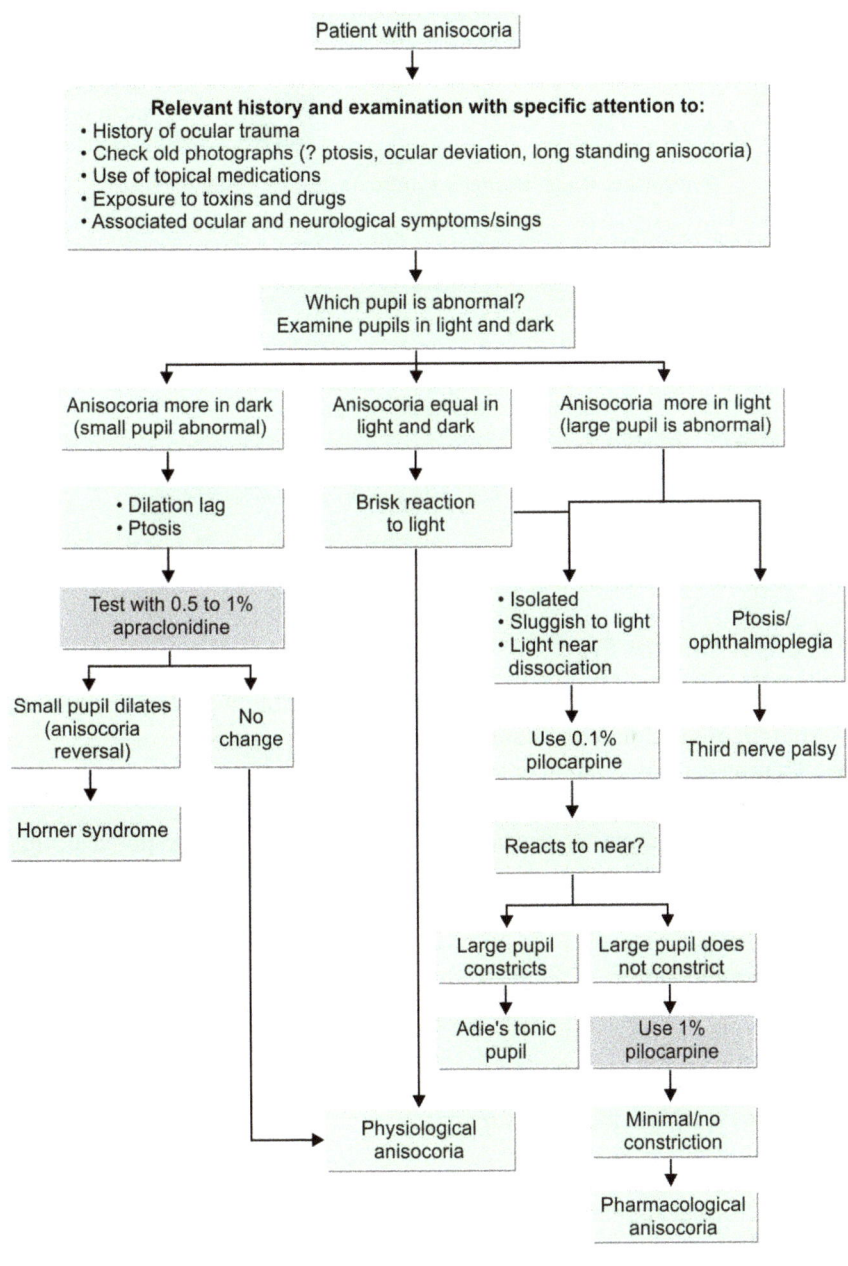

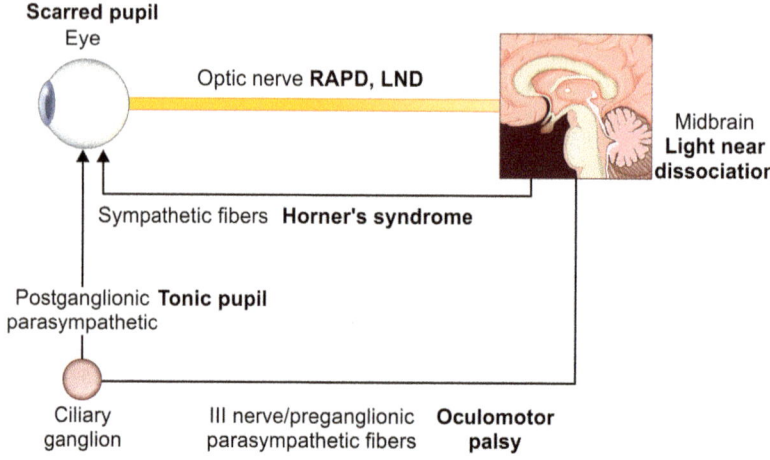

Fig. 3.27: Pupillary abnormalities with lesions at various sites.
(RAPD: relative afferent pupil defect; LND: light near dissociation)

- It may be remembered that a given syndrome may be caused by lesions at more than one level.

Lesions Within the Eye

- If the pupil abnormality does not fit in any plausible neurologic condition, obtain ophthalmologist's opinion to exclude local cause
- Trauma can cause small or large misshapen pupil
- Active inflammatory disease causes miosis
- Chronic inflammatory disease can cause irregular, poorly responsive pupil to light/near response
- *Iris ischemia* (DM, angle closure glaucoma, etc.): Stiff unresponsive pupil with irregular margins
- *Hyperopia:* Miosis
- *Myopia:* Mydriasis.

Visual Pathway Lesions [Relative Afferent Pupillary Defect (RAPD) and Light Near Dissociation (LND)]

- *RAPD is characterized by:*
  - Normal appearing symmetric pupils
  - Impaired direct pupillary response to light, preserved consensual light reflex
  - Preserved near response
  - Normal response to all topical agents
- RAPD results from impaired direct pupillary reflex on the side of the visual pathway lesion and preserved consensual reflex from the intact eye

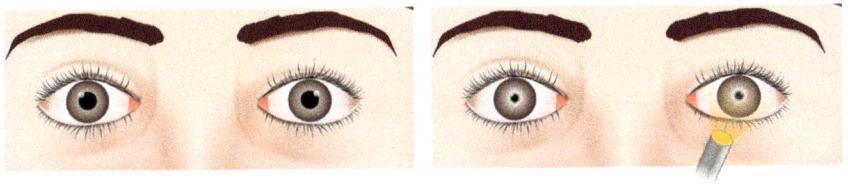

No light   Normal response to light

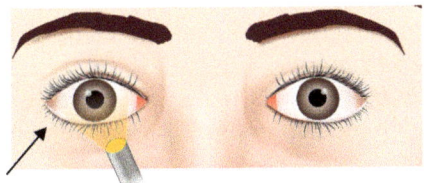

Positive RAPD of right eye

Fig. 3.28: Elicitation of RAPD.

- In lesions of retina or optic nerve, RAPD is seen, but in unilateral or asymmetric visual impairment due to media opacities like cataract/corneal scar, RAPD is not seen (these lesions merely scatter the light degrading acuity. As the pupillary light reflex is dependent on the total amount of retinal receptors being activated rather than on the macular stimulation, light reflex appears normal)
- In bilateral visual pathway lesions, RAPD indicates asymmetric lesion, while its absence suggests symmetric lesions
- *Chiasmal lesions:* No effect on pupillary light reflex if symmetrical
- *Optic tract lesions:* No significant RAPD
- *Retrogeniculate lesions:* No significant RAPD
- The degree of attenuation of pupillary light response correlates with the extent of visual field loss and not acuity
- For example in advanced glaucoma, the response is sluggish because of extensive field loss, but acuity is still preserved (pupillo-visual dissociation)
- Conversely, in macular disease, there is severe visual loss, but pupillary response is brisk (may be mistaken as malingering)
- In LHON also, there is preserved pupillary response in the presence of visual loss due to sparing
- Subtle RAPD is often present before loss of visual acuity or fields in optic nerve disease
- RAPD can also be detected in patients with previous optic neuritis who have improved in fields and acuity. This ability to detect subclinical visual pathway lesions makes the swinging flash light test the "**poor man's VEP**"
- Therefore, swinging flash must be a part of the routine examination of pupillary reflexes.

Brainstem Lesions

Lesions in midbrain

- *Classic syndrome of light near dissociation:*
    - Large pupils
    - Impaired light reflex with preserved accommodation reflex
    - Preserved vision
- *Other signs:*
    - Collier's sign (lid retraction on attempted upgaze)
    - Vertical saccadic palsy
    - Skew deviation
    - Convergence retraction nystagmus (involvement of adjacent rostral interstitial nucleus of Cajal).

  The combination of the above signs together constitute Parinaud's syndrome (dorsal midbrain syndrome) which is seen in pineal tumors and hydrocephalus.
- The syndrome of light near dissociation results from the fact that the pupillary fibers are located dorsal to the aqueduct of Sylvius (in the posterior commissure) while the fibers for accommodation are located ventral to it.
- It may be noted that light-near dissociation can occur at lesions at 4 levels (Table 3.5):
    - Visual pathway
    - Dorsal midbrain
    - Argyll Robertson pupil
    - Postganglionic parasympathetic pathway (Tonic pupil)

The differentiating features of these syndromes are tabulated below.
- Visual pathway lesions are differentiated by the presence of visual loss and RAPD. The resting pupil size is normal because of the intact consensual light reflex. In brainstem lesions, the resting pupil size is bilaterally large (bilateral decussating pupillary fibers are involved) and the vision is normal, and RAPD is not seen
- In postganglionic parasympathetic lesions, the pupil size is small, and irregular because of aberrant innervation of ciliary muscle by the pupillary

Table 3.5: Differential diagnosis of light-near dissociation.

	Optic nerve lesion	Brainstem lesion	Argyll Robertson pupil	Tonic pupil
Pupil size	Normal	Large	Small (inhibitory pathways to EWN)	Small
Pupil shape	Normal	Normal	Irregular	Irregular
Vision	Abnormal	Normal	Normal	Normal
RAPD	Present	Absent	Absent	Absent
Other brainstem signs	Absent	Present	Present	Absent

fibers. In brainstem lesion, in contrast, the light near dissociation is associated with large pupils
- *Argyll Robertson pupil* is a combination of brainstem and postganglionic parasympathetic lesions in syphilis. Therefore, its appearance is similar, but there are additional brainstem signs and the pupillary changes are bilateral. Similar pupils can be seen in chronic alcoholism, diabetes, MS, sarcoidosis, myotonic dystrophy, degenerative dementias
- *Inverse ARP:* also seen in midbrain disease (depends on which pathways are affected and which are spared).

Sympathetic Lesions/Horner's Syndrome

- Comprises of miosis, ptosis, inverse ptosis, anhydrosis
- *Also:* Congestion of the conjunctival vessels, low IOP
- Some clinical signs and syndromes may help in localization of lesion in Horner's syndrome
- Pharmacological testing of Horner's syndrome (Fig. 3.29 and Table 3.6) helps to localize the lesion to pre- or postganglionic level
- Sometimes, it is clinically impossible to do so and extensive imaging of head, neck and chest may be the only way to localize the lesion
- Various possible levels of lesion and the typical syndromes are depicted in the Figure 3.30.

Some salient clinical features to be remembered are listed below:
- Anhydrosis of entire ipsilateral face occurs in preganglionic lesions. Anhydrosis of only supraorbital skin occurs in postganglionic lesions.
- *Harlequin syndrome:* T1 or T2 root lesions impair sweating of the ipsilateral face and neck
- *Pancoast syndrome:* Lesions of lung apex cause ipsilateral hand wasting and Horner's syndrome

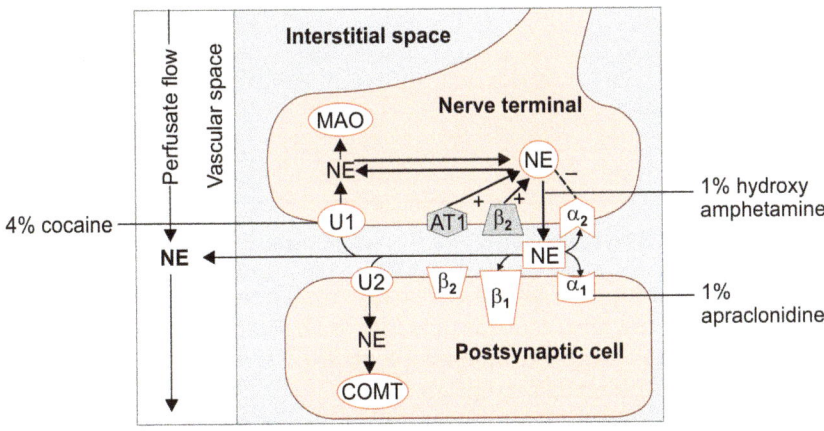

Fig. 3.29: Horner's pharmacology.

Table 3.6: Horner's pharmacology.

	Is NA released?	Are there presynaptic stores of NA?	Is there denervation supersensitivity
Preganglionic (1st, 2nd order neuron)	No	Yes	No
Postganglionic (3rd order neuron)	No	No	Yes
Drug used for test	4% cocaine	1% hydroxy amphetamine	1% apraclonidine

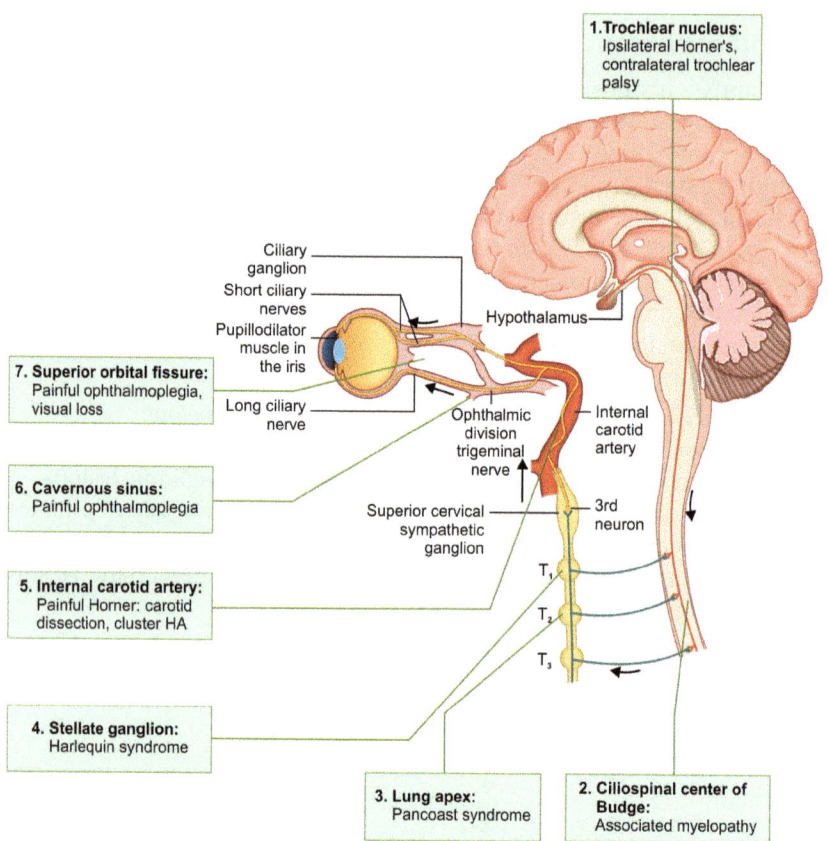

Fig. 3.30: Localization of Horner's syndrome to various levels.

- Contralateral superior oblique palsy in central horner's (midbrain lesion of ipsilateral trochlear nucleus through which sympathetic fibers pass)
- Similar brainstem syndromes with obvious long tract signs help in localizing the lesion to appropriate level
- Heterochromia iridis: Early onset Horner's syndrome
- Isolated painful Horner's: Carotid dissection, cluster headache
- Painful Horner's, visual loss, ophthalmoplegia: Infiltrative lesions of cavernous sinus

- Bilateral Horner's: Especially in elderly, is easily mistaken for senile miosis. It is best detected by redilatation lag. Seen in DM, amyloidosis, pure autonomic failure (PAF), hereditary sensory and autonomic neuropathy (HSAN).
    - About 4% cocaine inhibits reuptake of Norepinephrine by sympathetic nerve terminals. Normal persons show mydriasis, while Horner's syndrome at any level impairs this mydriasis (as no NE is released)
    - About 1% hydroxyamphetamine releases NE from nerve terminals. Normal people and preganglionic Horner's patients show mydriasis. In postganglionic Horner's syndrome, this is impaired.
    - About 1% apraclonidine does not produce a response in normal persons and in preganglionic Horner's syndrome. In postganglionic Horner's syndrome, due to denervation supersensitivity, apraclonidine produces brisk response.

Lesions in the Parasympathetic System

- The origin and the course of parasympathetic fibers to the eye have already been described
- Within the oculomotor nerve, the parasympathetic fibers lie superficially throughout the course. Therefore, they are involved early in compressive lesions and spared in ischemic lesions
- However, it is too simplistic to state that "pupil spared = noncompressive lesion, pupil involved = compressive lesion", because there are exceptions to these rules.

Rule	Exception
In compressive III nerve palsy, pupil is involved	It may not be involved in the **early stages** (first few days to weeks)
In noncompressive lesions, pupil is spared	In ischemic **complete** III nerve palsy, pupil may be involved

- Therefore, we need to add some qualifiers to these "rules":
    1. In partial III nerve palsy, if pupil is involved, compression is highly likely
    2. In complete III nerve palsy, if pupil is spared, compression is highly unlikely
- The main differences between pre- and postganglionic parasympathetic palsy are discussed in Table 3.7.
- The peculiarities in postganglionic lesion are explained by the following facts:
    - In these lesions, there is aberrant reinnervation that sprouts from the ciliary ganglion level
    - These aberrant fibers innervate the pupillary sphincter muscle in an irregular fashion, leading to irregular pupil
    - Since these aberrant fibers are originally meant for accommodation, they cause pupillary constriction in response to accommodation, but not to the light (light near dissociation)

- As part of the sphincter is not successfully reinnervated, there is sector palsy
- The pupil also becomes small because of the aberrant reinnervation.
- The reverse phenomenon (reinnervation of ciliary muscle by sympathetic fibers) does not occur in Horner's syndrome because of the long distance that separates the sympathetic ganglion and the eye.

Table 3.7: Difference between preganglionic and postganglionic parasympathetic palsy.

	Preganglionic	Postganglionic
Size	Dilated	Initially large, later small
Shape	Round	Irregular
Selective paresis of a meridian	No	Sector palsy, vermiform movements with moving light
Light reflex to direct	Absent	Absent
Light reflex to consensual	Absent	Absent
Accommodation	No miosis	Exaggerated miosis (aberrant reinnervation)
Tonic pupil (shifting gaze from near to far)	No	Yes

- Tonic pupil results from postganglionic parasympathetic lesions. Its causes are:
    - *Unilateral:* Local (trauma, neoplasms, inflammatory conditions).
    - *Bilateral:* Generalized autonomic neuropathies (amyloidosis, Sjögren's syndrome, PAF, paraneoplastic state)
    - When no cause is evident and there is associated tendon areflexia in a young female, it is called Holmes-Adie syndrome.

EYELIDS
Physiological Basis
- Five muscles act on the eyelids:
  1. The upper eyelid is held in position by the levator palpebrae superioris, a voluntary muscle innervated by the superior division of the III cranial nerve.
  2. The upper and lower eyelids are also supplied by the tarsal muscle, a smooth muscle, innervated by the sympathetic fibers.
  3. The globe is held forward in the orbit by the Muller's muscle, also innervated by sympathetic fibers
  4. Frontalis muscle is partially inserted in to the orbital margins and can indirectly help in eye opening
  5. Orbicularis oculi.
- Examination of the eyelids thus can assess the three components: III, VII and sympathetic fibers.

Methodology and Observations
General Observations

- **Head thrust**: It is compensatory to ptosis. Correct any upward head thrust to make ptosis more obvious
- **Forehead wrinkling**: It is also compensatory to ptosis. Fix the frontalis to bring out ptosis
- **Enophthalmos**: Check if the globe appears drawn in it is a feature of Horner's syndrome
- Compare with patient's old photographs for long standing ptosis that often goes unrecognized in early stages.
- Examine the family members for ptosis if possible.

Eyelid Examination
- Look for asymmetry in the width of palpebral fissures
- Use a millimeter ruler for accurate measurement of palpebral fissure width
- Inspect if pupil is partly or completely covered by the upper eyelid (the defining feature of ptosis)
- Check if patient can overcome the ptosis with effort
- Check if the ptosis is fatigable on prolonged staring for at least 1 minute
- Check for see-saw ptosis in this, if one eyelid is passively lifted, ptosis on the other side increases and vice versa. This happens in myasthenia wherein, the frontalis overaction partly compensates for the ptosis. When one eyelid is passively lifted, the frontalis overaction is released causing increased ptosis in the other eye
- Ask the patient to close his eye tightly and try to passively open his eyes. This assesses the orbicularis oculi strength

- Ask the patient to close his eyes tightly and then to open them, while looking for myotonia
- Ask the patient to open the mouth and look for synkinetic movements of the lids.

Interpretation

Normal Appearance

- Normal palpebral fissure width is 9–12 mm from upper to lower lid margin
- The normal upper lid crosses the iris 1–2 mm below the limbus (junction of iris with the sclera)
- The normal lower lid touches or slightly crosses the limbus
- Sclera is not normally visible above the limbus. If it is visible, it indicates lid retraction/lid lag
- One-third of normal population show some asymmetry in palpebral fissure width
- Palpebral fissure width may be decreased (ptosis) or increased (lid retraction) in disease states.

Ptosis

- One-third of normal population show some asymmetry in palpebral fissure width
- Bilateral partial ptosis may be of benign familial nature
- If the patient can overcome the drooping completely with voluntary effort, it is pseudoptosis. This suggests paralysis of upper tarsal muscle as in Horner's syndrome
- Elevation of lower eyelid and enophthalmos indicate Horner's syndrome
- Absence of wrinkling may suggest hysterical ptosis
- Fatigable ptosis suggests myasthenia (mild fatigue can be seen in non-myasthenic ptosis also)
- Ptosis at rest and lid retraction on jaw opening are seen in the congenital Gunn phenomenon
- Nonfatigable ptosis that cannot be overcome with voluntary effort indicates weakness of levator palpebri superioris
- Presence of weakness of eye opening (ptosis) as well as eye closure suggests a myopathy
- Ptosis and myotonia are seen in myotonic dystrophy.
- Various lesions from peripheral structures to central structures can cause ptosis.
  - *Ocular causes mimicking ptosis:* Trauma from contact lens, blepharitis, lid edema, lid tumors
  - Levator dehiscence disinsertion (LDD) occurs in old age and causes pseudoptosis. However, the levator function is normal when formally tested

- *Muscle diseases:* Usually cause weakness of both eye opening and closure:
  - Congenital ptosis
  - Mitochondrial
  - Ocular myopathy
  - *Myotonic dystrophy:* Patient may find it difficult to open his tightly close eyes due to eyelid myotonia
- *Myasthenia:* Prominent fatigability is suggestive
- 3rd nerve palsy: Total unilateral ptosis occurs in 3rd nerve palsy, but not in Horner's syndrome
- *Sympathetic palsy (Horner's):* If the patient can overcome the drooping completely with voluntary effort, it suggests paralysis of upper tarsal muscle as in Horner's syndrome
- *Aberrant reinnervation (Gunn phenomenon):* Characterized by ptosis at rest and lid retraction on jaw opening
- *Midbrain lesion:* Causes bilateral ptosis due to involvement of unpaired central caudal nucleus
- *Cerebral ptosis:* 30-40% of hemispheric strokes can manifest unilateral or bilateral ptosis
- *Hysterical ptosis:* Absence of wrinkling, over action of orbicularis oculi may suggest hysterical ptosis.

Lid Retraction

- Thyroid eye disease (causes both retraction on primary gaze and lid lag on downward gaze)
- Posterior commissure lesions (cause only retraction but not lag)
- Sympathomimetic drugs
- Aberrant reinnervation of 3rd nerve can cause lid retraction on attempted adduction (opposite of Duane syndrome)
- Mechanical causes (trauma, surgery)
- Müller muscle inflammatory (irritative) lesion.

ANSWERS TO THE PRETEST 1

1. This patient has right Horner's syndrome. Two important differential diagnoses of painful Horner's syndrome are (a) acute attack of cluster headache (b) carotid dissection.
2. In this patient with right Horner's syndrome and left hemiplegia, a right carotid dissection or thrombosis is most likely. His MRA confirmed the diagnosis (Figure 3.31).

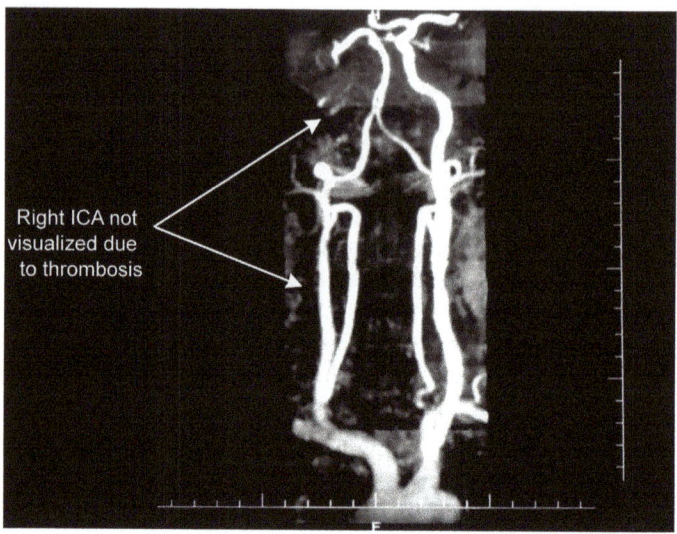

Fig. 3.31: MR angiogram shows right carotid thrombosis.

ANSWERS TO THE PRETEST 2

1. This patient has right lid retraction, suggestive of Muller muscle over action.
2. The usual cause is thyroid disease (thyroid ophthalmopathy). However, normal thyroid functions and negative thyroid antibodies suggest that alternate diagnosis has to be searched for.
3. Inflammatory irritative lesions of the Mueller's muscle can result in lid retraction. An MRI brain with contrast was performed and showed meningeal enhancement in the middle cranial fossa and pituitary region, typical of sarcoidosis (Fig. 3.32). His ACE levels were marginally elevated. CSF study was normal. Patient refused Müller muscle biopsy but responded well to empirical steroid therapy. There is a single published case report of biopsy proven Müller muscle sarcoid granulomatous inflammation, presenting with isolated lid retraction.

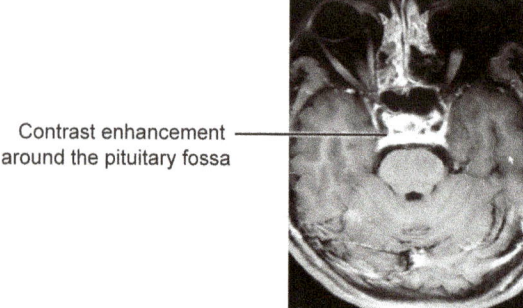

Fig. 3.32: Enhancing sarcoid lesion.

ANSWER TO THE PRETEST 3

1. The sign elicited is see saw ptosis, which is described in myasthenia. On passively opening the ptotic eye, frontalis overaction on right side is no longer required and the eyelid on that side started to droop.

BIBLIOGRAPHY

1. Averbuch-Heller L. Neurology of the eyelids. Curr Opin Ophthalmol. 1997;8:27-34.
2. Behbehani R, Nipper KS, et al. Systemic sarcoidosis manifested as unilateral eyelid retraction. Arch Ophthalmol. 2006;124(4):599-600.
3. Biousse V, Newman NJ. Third nerve palsies. Semin Neurol. 2000;55-74.
4. Brazis PW. Isolated palsies of cranial nerves III, IV & VI. Seminars Neurol. 2009;29:14-28.
5. Jacobson DM. Pupil involvement in patients with diabetes associated oculomotor nerve palsy. Arch Ophthalmol. 1998;116:723-7.
6. Kaeser PF, Kawasaki A. Disorders of pupillary structure and function. Neurol Clin. 2010;28:657-77.
7. Kwon JH, Kwon SU, Ahn HS et al. Isolated superior rectus palsy due to contralateral midbrain infarction. Arch Neurol. 2003;60:1633-5.
8. Leigh RJ, Zee DS. The neurology of eye movements. New York: Oxford University press; 2006.
9. Mughal M, Longmuir R. Current pharmacologic testing of Horner's syndrome. Curr Neurol Neurosci Rep. 2009;9(5);384-9.
10. Nadeau SE, Trobe JD. Pupil sparing in oculomotor palsy: a brief review. Ann Neuro. 1983;13:143-8.
11. Reede DL, Garcon E, Smoker WRK, et al. Horner's syndrome: clinical and radiological evaluation. Neuroimaging Clin N Am. 2008;18(2):369-85.
12. Prasad S, Volpe N. Paralytic strabismus. Neurol Clin. 2010;28:803-33.
13. Thompson HS, Kardon RH. The Argyll Robertson pupil. J Neuroophthalmol. 2006;26(2):134-8.

EXAMINATION OF GAZE DISORDERS

GRK Sarma

PRETEST

The Figures represent the saccadic eye movements in various conditions.

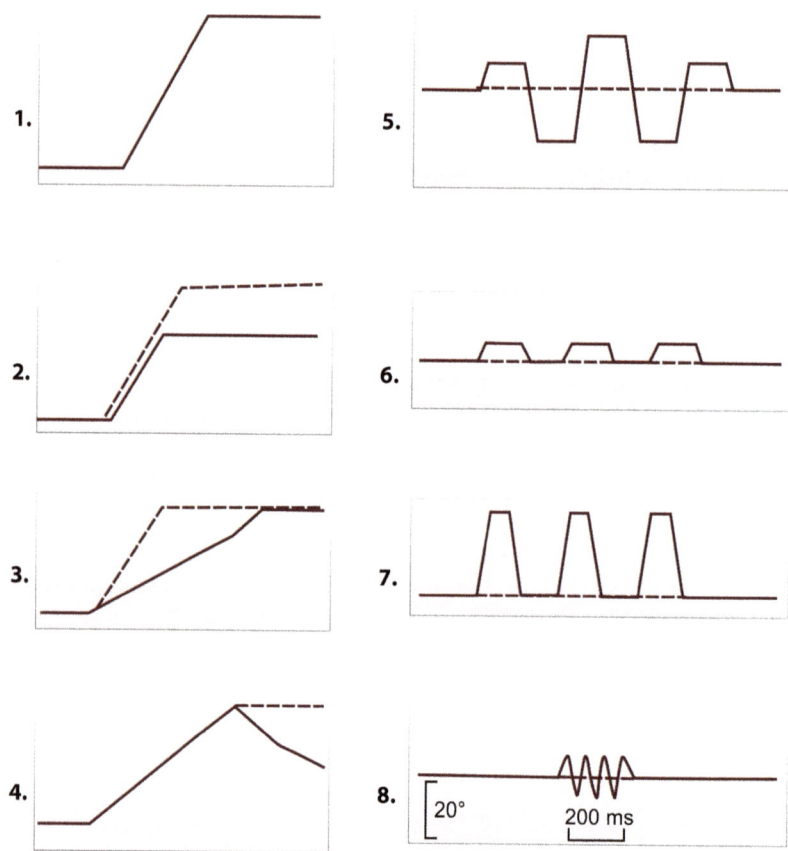

Question

1. Comment on each one of them and identify the physiologic and then anatomic substrates that lead to the defective saccades.

SACCADES

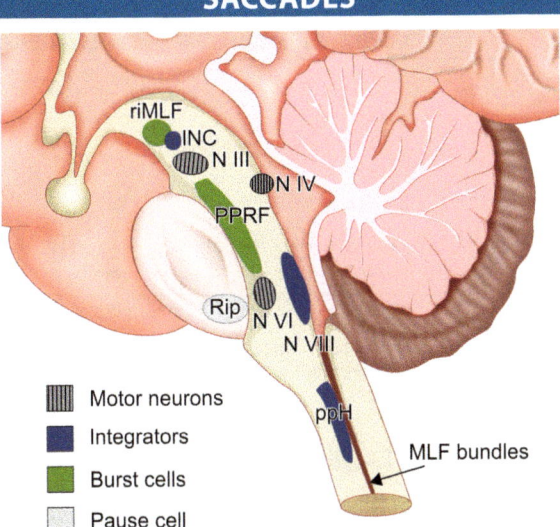

Fig. 3.33: Sagittal view of brainstem saccadic centers.

(riMLF : rostral interstitial nucleus of medial longitudinal fasciculus; INC: interstitial nucleus of Cajal; NIII: Nucleus of III cranial nerve; PPRF: parapontine reticular formation; NVI: nucleus of VI cranial nerve; N VII: nucleus of VII cranial nerve; ppH: prepositus hypoglossi; MLF: medial longitudinal fasciculus)

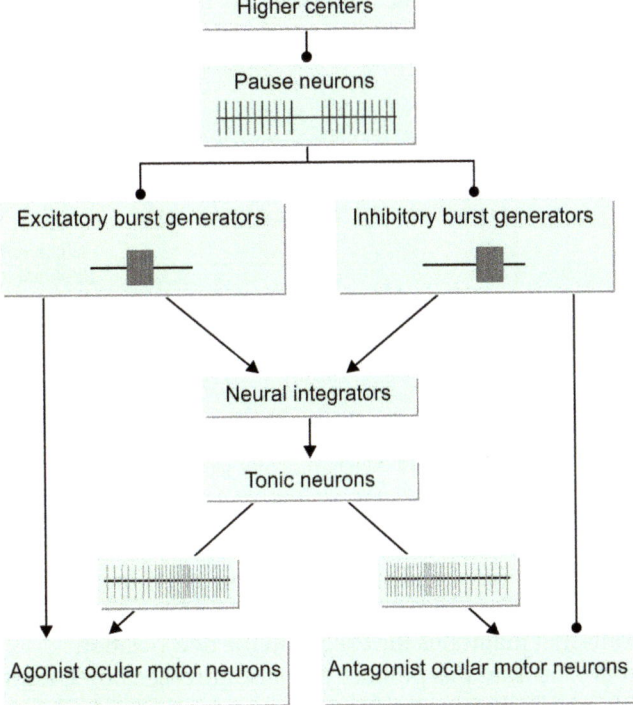

Fig. 3.34: General organization of saccadic control.

Table 3.8: Various centers in horizontal and vertical saccades.

	Horizontal saccades	Vertical saccades
EBN	PPRF	riMLF, caudal PPRF
IBN	Nucleus para-gigantocellularis (caudal to VI nucleus)	riMLF
Integrator	ppH/MVN	INC
Pulse calibrator	Fastigial nucleus, dorsal vermis	Fastigial nucleus, dorsal vermis
Step calibrator	Flocculus	Flocculus

(ppH: prepositus hypoglossi; MVN: medial vestibular nucleusl; NC: interstitial nucleus of Cajal; PPRF: paramedian pontine reticular formation; riMLF: rostral interstitial nucleus of medial longitudinal fasciculus; EBN: excitatory burst neurons; IBN: inhibitory burst neurons)

PHYSIOLOGIC BASIS (TABLE 3.8)

- Saccades are rapid (up to 900° per second) re-fixation movements of the eyes that refocus a peripheral visual image on the center of the retina where it can best be seen
- They are classified into different categories based on the generating mechanisms. These have different anatomical substrates and thus help in neurological localization
- To understand the saccadic abnormalities in a patient, it is essential to understand the mechanics and the anatomical substrates of saccades

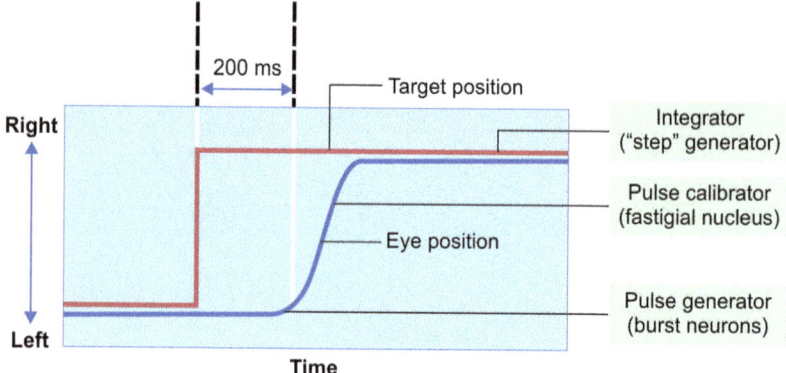

Fig. 3.35: Mechanics of a saccade.

- A saccade comprises of a **pulse** and a **step** (Fig. 3.35). Abnormalities can occur in various components of this sequence of events
- "Pulse" is a brief (few tens of milliseconds), rapid burst of neurons that shifts the eyeball to a new position, while a "step" is a tonic, sustained burst of neurons that maintains the eyeball in the new position
- The group of neurons that produce the pulse are called **burst neurons**. There are anatomically distinct excitatory (to the agonists) and inhibitory (to the antagonists) burst neurons for horizontal and vertical eye movements

- The group of neurons that produce the "step" are called "**integrators**" because the conversion of the pulse to step signal requires mathematical integration. Again, there are distinct integrators for horizontal and vertical movements
- The cerebellum (fastigial nucleus and vermis) plays key role in precise calculation of pulse size and duration. Failure to do so results in hypo- or hypermetric saccades. Flocculus is important in "step" phase maintenance. Its failure leads to gaze evoked nystagmus
- The pause neurons inhibit all the burst neurons (EBN and IBN) at rest to maintain a neutral eye position. Brief inactivity of the pause neurons releases the burst neurons to initiate the saccade
- Figure 3.34 provides an over view of how the saccadic system is organized at the level of brainstem lower centers. Saccadic control by higher centers is described below.

Higher Level Anatomical Substrates

The following regions play important role in the control of saccades:
- Frontal cortex
- Parietal occipital cortex
- Basal ganglia, thalamus
- Superior colliculus
- Cerebellum.

Cortical Control (Fig. 3.36)

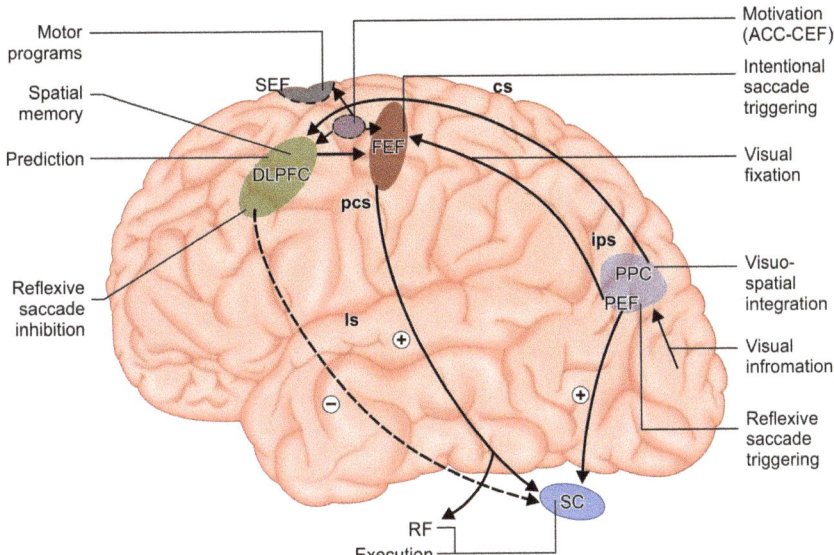

Fig. 3.36: Various cortical areas and their role in saccadic generation.
(DLPFC: dorsolateral prefrontal cortex; FEF: frontal eye field; PEF: parietal eye field; PPC: posterior parietal cortex; SC: superior colliculus; SEF: supplementary eye field)

Various cortical regions and their role in saccadic eye movements are summarized below:
- Frontal eye field (area 6, 4) in middle frontal gyrus: Intentional saccades to visible targets, predictive saccades to the opposite side
- Parietal eye field (areas 39, 40) in the supramarginal gyrus: Visually guided reflexive saccades.
- Supplementary eye field (in supplementary motor area): Memory guided saccades with vestibular input (as in head or body motion)
- Dorsolateral prefrontal cortex (area 46): Inhibition of saccades (as in anti-saccade paradigms).

Superior Colliculus, Basal Ganglia and Cortical Interactions

- The superior colliculus (SC) is a **key center** on which various cerebral, cerebellar and visual inputs converge to control the saccades. It achieves visuo-motor integration by these converging inputs
- The **caudal SC** facilitates saccade production by exciting the burst neurons, while the **rostral SC** suppresses it
- It is excited by the cortical inputs through a direct pathway and an indirect pathway (Fig. 3.37)
- The indirect pathway includes cortico-striatal (excitatory), striatonigral (inhibitory) and nigro-collicular (inhibitory) connections
- In addition, the **rostral SC** has foveal representation, is active during visual fixation, and therefore suppresses saccade generation by inhibiting caudal SC and stimulating the omnipause cells.

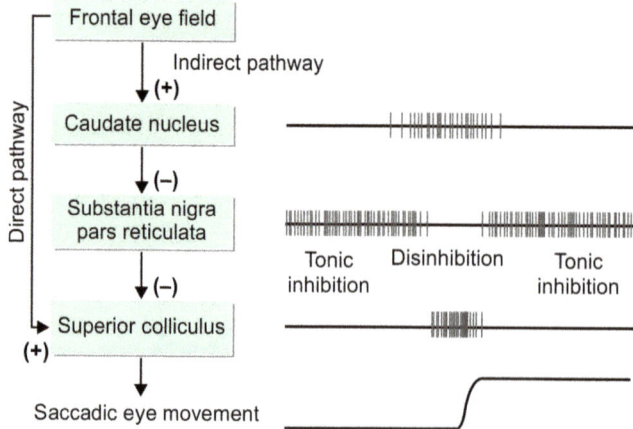

Fig. 3.37: Superior colliculus, basal ganglia and cortical interactions in saccadic generation.

Cerebellum (Fig. 3.38)

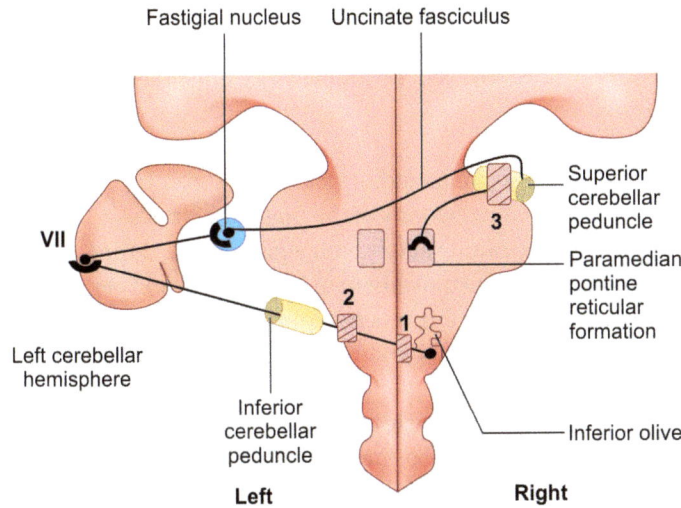

Fig. 3.38: Schematic diagram of cerebellar influence on saccades.

The cerebellum influences the saccades by its connections with the SC and various brainstem centers. It coordinates both the pulse and the step phase of the saccade.
- The dorsal vermis normally inhibits the underlying fastigial nucleus
- Output from one fastigial nucleus crosses to the opposite side, passes through brachium conjunctivum to reach the contralateral PPRF to produce a saccade
- Fastigial nucleus thus is responsible for **contralateral** saccadic **pulse** amplitude regulation
- Dorsal vermis, brachium conjunctivum play the opposite role, i.e. **ipsilateral** saccadic **pulse** amplitude regulation
- *Flocculus:* Saccadic **step** maintenance by its connections with the nucleus prepositus hypoglossi and medial vestibular nuclei
- Nodulus regulates the vestibulo-ocular reflex. Its lesion results in periodic alternating nystagmus.

METHODOLOGY

- Examine saccades in horizontal and vertical directions.
- Examine in a hierarchical fashion:
    - Quick phase of optokinetic nystagmus (OKN) (or swivel chair)—tests the premotor burst neurons in the brainstem
    - Reflexive saccades in response to sudden visual stimulus in the visual field

- To command (for example, look down) (loss of voluntary saccades with preserved reflexive saccades and quick phase of OKN is typical of ocular motor apraxia).
- To visual cues (for example, look at my finger and nose quickly and alternatively).
- Predictive saccades:
  - Hold two fingers up on either side
  - Instruct the patient to look at the finger that moves
  - Move the fingers alternately with a predictable timing
  - Randomly miss the movement of a finger. Normal persons produce a saccade even if the finger is not moved at the expected time. Failure to do so is common in Parkinson's disease.
- Antisaccades:
  - Hold two fingers up on either side
  - Ask the patient to look at the finger that does not move
  - Randomly move either finger
  - Failure to perform in this test suggests prefrontal lesion.

INTERPRETATION

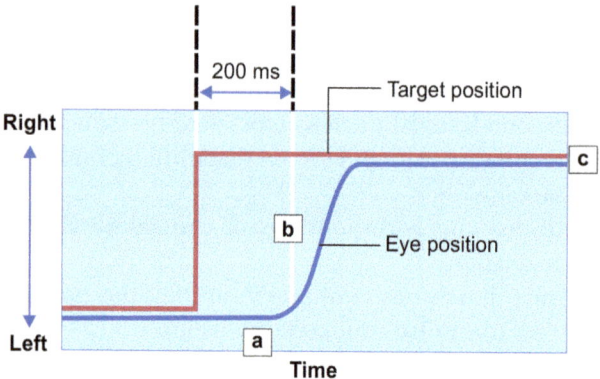

Fig. 3.39: Schematic diagram of mechanics of saccadic generation.

- The abnormality may involve:
  - Saccade initiation (pulse generator dysfunction)
  - Saccade velocity/amplitude/trajectory (pulse calibrator dysfunction)
  - Gaze holding (step generator dysfunction)
  - Unwanted saccades
- Defects of first three categories are summarized in the Table 3.9:

Table 3.9: Various abnormalities of saccades and their anatomical physiological correlates.

Observed defect	Physiologic substrate	Lesion location
Slow saccades with restricted range of movement	Motor neurons (Final motor pathway lesion)	Oculomotor nerve palsies
Horizontal slow saccades with preserved range of movement	Pre-motor neurons	Burst neurons in PPRF
Vertical slow saccades with preserved range of movement	Pre-motor neurons	Burst neurons in riMLF
Slow saccades in all directions	Dis-inhibition of inhibitory burst neurons	Omnipause cells in reticular nuclei
Opsoclonus	Dis-inhibition of excitatory burst neurons	Omnipause cells
Dysmetric saccades	Pulse calibrator dysfunction	Fastigial nucleus and connections
Horizontal gaze evoked nystagmus	Leaky neural integrator	NPH, MVN
Vertical gaze evoked nystagmus	Leaky neural integrator	INC
Gaze evoked nystagmus in all directions	Step calibrator dysfunction	Flocculus and connections
Periodic alternating nystagmus	Delayed vestibular responses	Nodule and connections
Impaired voluntary saccades	Frontal eye field defect	Frontal eye filed
Impaired visual reflexive saccades	Parietal eye field defect	Posterior parietal cortex
Impaired all voluntary and reflexive saccades	Lesion involving all converging pathways	Superior colliculus
Impaired short latency saccades (express saccades)	Superior colliculus	Superior colliculus
Impaired saccades only on command, preserved reflex and voluntary saccades	Ocular apraxia	Posterior parietal lesion, basal ganglia

(riMLF: rostral interstitial nucleus of medial longitudinal fasciculus; PPRF: parapontine reticular formation; NPH: nucleus prepositus hypoglossi; MVN: medial vestibular nucleus; INC: interstitial nucleus of Cajal)

- **Saccadic intrusions: these are of two types—**
  - I. **With inter-saccadic interval**
    - *Square wave jerks:*
      - The image perceived by the retina quickly disappears if it remains constant on the same area, due to receptor adaptation. To avoid this, the square wave jerks are produced, shifting the vision away from the target and bringing it back to the target after few milliseconds (one can verify this by constantly staring at a point on a wall for few seconds, by when, it starts to fade away and even disappear)
      - The square wave jerks are small amplitude (1-5°) saccades with inter-saccadic interval of 200 ms, that return the eye balls to the base line position.

- These are seen in normal individuals up to 20-30 per minute
- They are decreased during attentional tasks and by voluntary will
- They have widespread neural substrates including frontal regions, cerebellum, and their connections with superior colliculus
- In frontal and collicular lesions, the square wave jerk frequency is increased (more than 40-50/min), with the amplitude remaining small
- With cerebellar lesions, the amplitude is increased upto 30°
- *Macrosquare wave jerks:* These are larger in amplitude (up to 30°) and have smaller intersaccadic interval of 50-150 ms. These are seen in cerebellar lesions with a mechanism similar to that of square wave jerks
- *Macrosaccadic oscillations:* Unlike macrosquare wave jerks, these saccades over shoot the base line eye position and oscillate about the target with an interval of 200 ms. These are described with fastigial nucleus lesions.

II. **Without inter-saccadic interval**
- *Ocular flutter:* It is a burst of small amplitude (1-5°) to and fro saccades without intersaccadic interval. This can be seen in normal individuals and in same conditions that produce opsoclonus
- *Opsoclonus:* It is a burst of large amplitude, multidirectional saccadic movement without intersaccadic interval. This indicates a lesion in the omnipause neurons which normally suppress all the burst neurons. This is seen in various conditions in Box 3.1.

Box 3.1: Causes of opsoclonus.

- Viral encephalitis
- Meningitis
- Paraneoplastic(lung/breast cancer, neuroblastoma)
- Intracranial tumors
- Trauma
- Hypoxia
- Thalamic hemorrhage
- Multiple sclerosis
- Drugs: phenytoin, benzodiazepines, lithium
- Toxins: organophosphates, toluene, thallium
- Systemic disease: AIDS, hepatitis
- Psychogenic

Cranial Nerves   147

ANSWER TO THE PRETEST

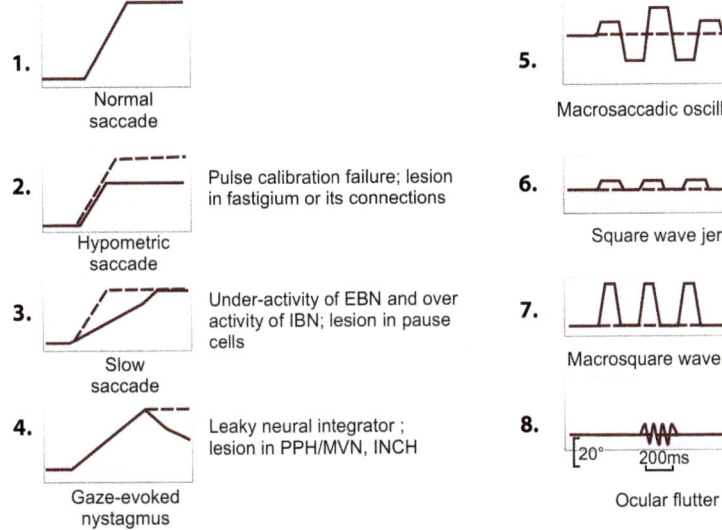

1. Normal saccade
2. Hypometric saccade — Pulse calibration failure; lesion in fastigium or its connections
3. Slow saccade — Under-activity of EBN and over activity of IBN; lesion in pause cells
4. Gaze-evoked nystagmus — Leaky neural integrator; lesion in PPH/MVN, INCH
5. Macrosaccadic oscillations
6. Square wave jerks
7. Macrosquare wave jerks
8. Ocular flutter

THE PURSUIT SYSTEM

GRK Sarma

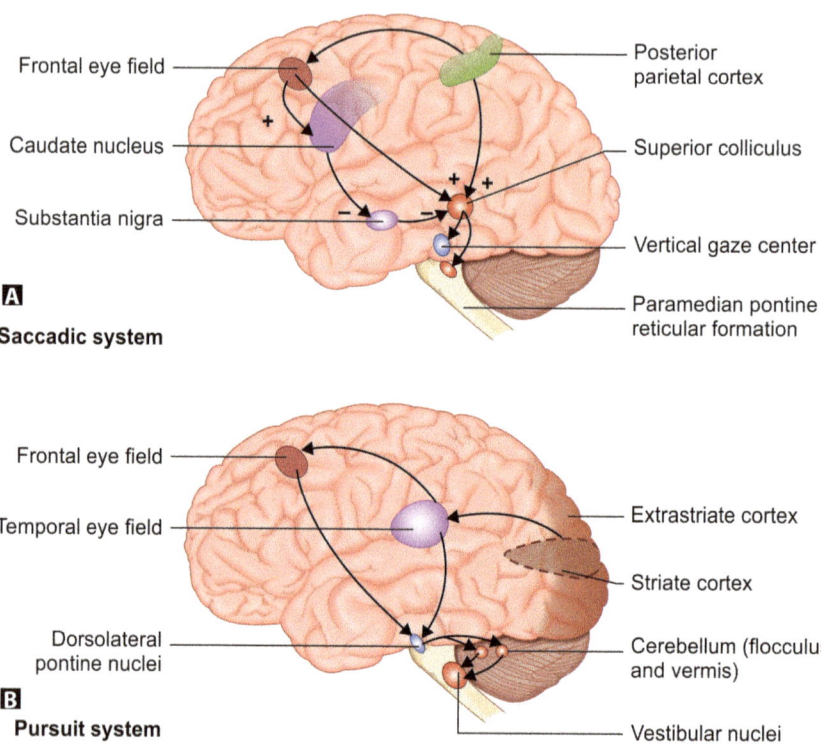

A Saccadic system

B Pursuit system

Figs. 3.40A and B: Different pathways involved in control of saccades and horizontal pursuits. Note that the PPRF is involved in saccades, but not in pursuits. (A) The voluntary saccades circuit; (B) The smooth pursuit circuit.

Cranial Nerves 149

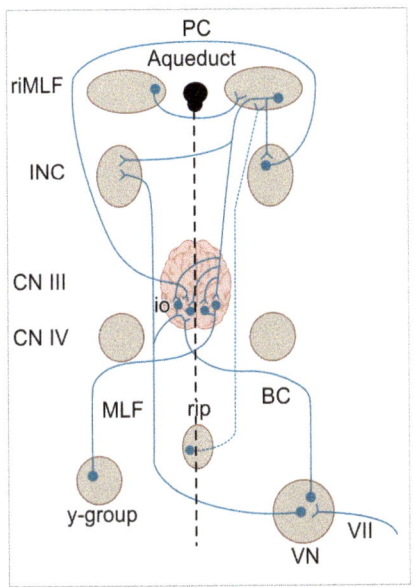

Fig. 3.41: Pathways for upward eye movements.

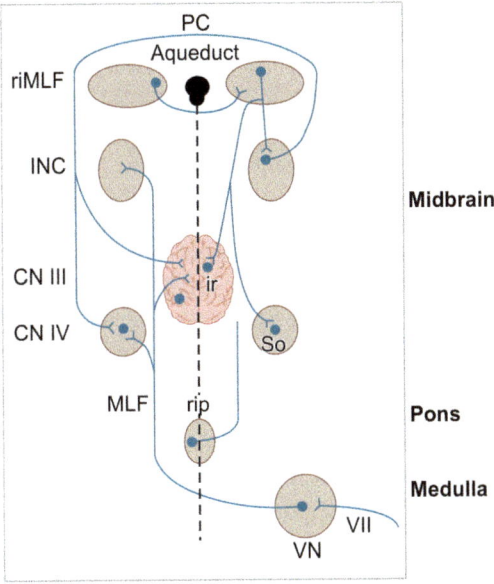

Fig. 3.42: Pathways for downward eye movements.

SMOOTH PURSUIT SYSTEM

Physiologic Basis

- These are **slow** (<40°/second), **involuntary**, conjugate eye movements, that are produced to retain the image of a moving target of interest on the fovea. Vergence movements also achieve the same objective, but by dysconjugate movements
- Unlike saccades, pursuit movements cannot be produced voluntarily
- The pursuit system consists of visual afferents, central processing regions and efferents
- Retinal afferents carry information on the direction and speed of the target through the lateral geniculate body to the striate cortex, which sends this information to the temporal visual cortex and lateral occipital cortex and angular gyrus
- These cortical regions project information to the homologous regions of the contralateral hemisphere through the splenium of corpus callosum, tapetum and forceps major. From here, the information is relayed to the posterior parietal cortex (PPC) (in the ventral bank of intraparietal sulcus) that subserves visual attention
- The PPC projects to the frontal eye field (FEF), which projects through the internal capsule, and the cerebral peduncle to the ipsilateral dorsal pontine nuclei. Fibers from DLPN **decussate** and pass through the middle cerebellar peduncle to the flocculus, and dorsal vermis of cerebellum
- Efferents from the cerebellar nuclei, project to the ipsilateral medial vestibular nucleus, whose projections **once again decussate** in the pons close to the 4th ventricle to reach the abducens nucleus
- This **double decussation** results in the control of pursuit movements to one side by the ipsilateral hemisphere
- The pathways for upward and downward pursuits are different from horizontal pursuits distal to the vestibular nuclei
- Efferents from the vestibular nuclei travel through the MLF and brachium conjunctivum to reach the nucleus of Cajal. The efferents from the iNC for upward pursuit decussate in the posterior commissure (PC) to reach the oculomotor nuclei. The iNC efferents for downward pursuit do not traverse the PC and descend directly to the oculomotor nuclei
- The fastigial nucleus and dorsal vermis contribute to the onset of the pursuit and the flocculus/paraflocculus sustain the pursuit
- When a patient is tracking a target by rotating his head as well as moving his eyes (as in a revolving chair), the pursuit system and vestibular ocular reflex work in opposite directions. The latter has to be suppressed adequately to produce a smooth pursuit movements. Failure of VOR suppression results in broken pursuits and corrective saccades.

Examination Methodology

- Hold a pencil tip or other small object 1 meter away from the patient

- Ask him to track the moving object in horizontal and vertical directions
  - Catch up saccades (in the direction of moving object) indicate low pursuit gain
  - Back up saccades (opposite to the direction of the moving object) indicate excess gain
- Rotate an optokinetic drum (or use a tape) and assess the pursuits in the 4 directions:
  - Pursuit asymmetry indicates an ipsilateral posterior hemispheric lesion (it may be confusing because this appears as contralateral reduced saccadic amplitude)
  - Pursuit reversal suggests congenital nystagmus (pursuit movement occurs opposite to the direction of drum rotation)
- Test VOR cancellation using swivel chair. Ask patient to stretch out his clasped hands with thumbs pointing upwards. He needs to fix his gaze on the tips of the thumbs as the swivel chair is rotated first in one direction and later in the other. Normal persons continue to maintain their fixation on thumb.
An inadequate VOR cancellation (pursuit followed by corrective saccades) in one direction indicate ipsilateral pursuit gain deficit.

Interpretation

- Lesion in the striate cortex or middle temporal gyrus causes impaired horizontal pursuit in both directions in the contralateral visual field (due to scotoma)
- Lesion in the medial superior temporal gyrus causes ipsilateral pursuit defect when the stimulus is in either hemifield
- Lesion in the NRTP causes upward pursuit defect
- Bilateral flocculus lesions: No effect on the pursuits
- Unilateral lesions in ventral paraflocculus (VPF): Ipsilateral horizontal and vertical pursuit defect and VOR cancellation
- Bilateral lesions of the flocculus and VPF: Severe defect in horizontal and vertical pursuits and VOR cancellation
- Lesions in the vermis: Ipsilateral horizontal pursuit defect
- Lesions in the fastigial nucleus: Contralateral pursuit deficit
- Unilateral horizontal pursuit defect: Implies one of the following:
  - Ipsilateral lesion in the parietal/frontal region/thalamus/internal capsule/midbrain
  - Either ipsilateral or contralateral pontine lesion. Here, the direction of saccadic defect provides the lesion location (this defect is always ipsilateral to the pontine lesion)
  - **Contralateral cerebellar lesion.**
- *Bilateral impaired pursuit defect:* Implies
  - State of decreased attention (for example, sedative use)
  - Diffuse diseases like PSP, Gerstmann-Sträussler-Scheinker syndrome and HIV infection

- Bilateral occipital lesions (abolish the pursuits)
- Bilateral cerebellar damage
- *Impaired upward pursuit:*
  - Medial longitudinal fasciculus (MLF) lesion
  - Interstitial nucleus of Cajal (INC) lesion
  - Superior collicular lesion
- *Impaired downward pursuit:*
  - MLF lesion
  - INC lesion
- Impaired horizontal pursuits with impaired VOR; indicates pontomedullary lesion.

Table 3.10: Localization of cerebellar eye movement abnormalities.

Structure	Function	Disorder
Flocculus and paraflocculus	Retinal image stabilization [smooth tracking with head still of free suppression of inappropriate vestibular nystagmus, holding positions of gaze, adaptive control of the vestibulo-ocular reflex (VOR) and pulsc-step match]	Impaired smooth pursuit, VOR cancellation and fixation suppression of caloric nystagmus; gaze evoked, rebound, centripetal and downbeat nystagmus; postsaccadic drift; inappropriate amplitude or direction of the VOR
Nodulus and ventral uvula	Control of low-frequency response of the VOR	Periodic alternating nystagmus, impaired tilt suppression of postrotatory nystagmus, positional nystagmus, impaired habituation of the VOR, increased duration of vestibular responses
Dorsal vermis and posterior fastigial nucleus	Saccade accuracy, smooth-pursuit eye alignment	Saccadic dysmetria, impaired pursuit, esodeviations

(VOR: Vestibulo-ocular reflex)
Source: Zee DS, Walker MF. Cerebellar control of eye movements. In: Challepa LM, Wemer JS (Eds). The visual neurosciences. Cambridge, MA: MIT press, 2003, pp. 1485-98.

VERGENCE SYSTEM

PHYSIOLOGIC BASIS

- Vergence system consists of convergence and divergence movements
- Visual cortical areas 19 and 22 of the occipital lobe may induce the vergence
- Vergence premotor neurons are located in the midbrain, dorsal and lateral to the oculomotor nucleus and also in the medial pontine reticular formation
- The midbrain nuclei are involved in fast convergence movements and the pontine nuclei are involved in slow (<2°/second) convergence movements
- The convergence and divergence neurons project to the medial and lateral recti respectively, through pathways outside MLF
- Cerebellar flocculus coordinates the vergence movements.

METHODOLOGY

- Ask patient to focus on a near point and suddenly remove the object from the visual field. In patients with convergence spasm, the convergence remains even after the object has been removed
- Move the object back and forth towards and away from the patient. Watch for convergence spasm
- To differentiate convergence spasm from abducens palsy (unilateral or bilateral), look at the pupil size. In convergence spasm, but not in abducens palsy, there will be miosis. This miosis may resolve if one eye is occluded.

INTERPRETATION

- **Convergence insufficiency**
    - The initial convergence is normal, but fatigues after few minutes of sustained convergence as in reading. This manifests as eye strain and headache
    - Seen in the teenagers and in the elderly
    - Also seen in non dominant parietal lobe lesions.
- **Convergence paralysis**
    - Causes diplopia at near gaze, with normal adduction.
    - Lesion is in the midbrain convergence centers
    - Seen in Parkinson's disease, PSP, dorsal midbrain infarct/hemorrhage/tumors and in paramedian thalamic lesions
    - Unilateral loss of convergence occurs in thalamotectal lesion, by disrupting the descending cortical inputs for convergence that decussate in thalamotectal areas.
- **Convergence spasm**
    - Defined as a triad of:
        - Intermittent/sustained convergence
        - Miosis especially on attempted abduction usually released by a blink
        - Accommodative spasm
    - It is seen in:
        - Brainstem lesions (as part of dorsal midbrain syndrome)
        - Diencephalic lesions
        - Metabolic encephalopathies (Wernicke's encephalopathy)
        - Arnold Chiari malformation
        - Functional disease (produces isolated convergence spasm that is unusual in structural lesions)
- **Divergence paralysis**
    - It is unknown if there is a distinct divergence center. But, divergence insufficiency and divergence paralysis have been reported for a long time

- *Divergence paralysis is characterized by:*
  - Acute onset, uncrossed diplopia
  - Diplopia beyond 70 cm (diplopia increases as the object is moved away and decreases or disappears at close distance)
  - Comitancy
  - No end point nystagmus
  - No change in lateral gaze
  - Normal eye movements
  - No miosis
- *Seen in:*
  - Raised intracranial pressure
  - Meningitis
  - Intracerebral hemorrhage
  - Posterior fossa tumors
  - Head trauma
  - Demyelinating disease.

NYSTAGMUS

PHYSIOLOGIC BASIS (FIG. 3.43)

- Nystagmus is defined as a biphasic ocular oscillation containing slow eye movements (with or without fast movement) that initiate and maintain the oscillation.
- Three mechanisms are normally involved in maintaining the eyes in primary position:
  a. Visual fixation
  b. The vestibulo-ocular reflex, and
  c. The neural integrator.
- If any of these mechanisms are defective, there results an abnormal eye drift away from the primary position, followed by corrective saccade, manifesting as nystagmus.
- **Neural integrator:** When the eye is turned in an eccentric position in the orbit, the fascia and ligaments that suspend the eye exert an elastic force to return toward the primary position. To overcome this force, a tonic contraction of the extraocular muscles is required. A gaze-holding network called the neural integrator generates the signal.
- The neural integrators are:
  - Nucleus prepositus hypoglossi and medial vestibular nucleus for horizontal gaze
  - The interstitial nucleus of Cajal for vertical gaze
  - Vestibulocerebellum, which optimizes gaze holding
  - Ocular motor nuclei.

Different types of nystagmus have different pathophysiological basis and are discussed briefly as follows:

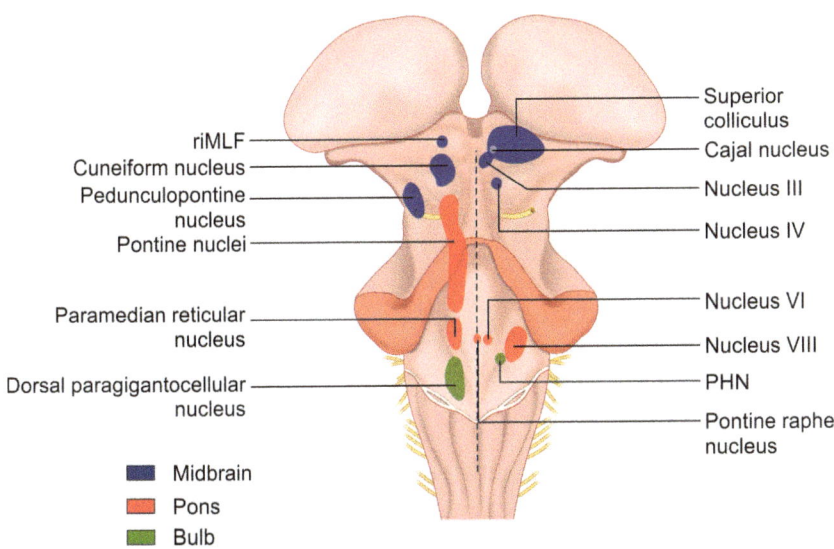

Fig. 3.43: Brainstem nuclei and reticular formation involved in eye movement generation. (riMLF: rostral interstitial nucleus of medial longitudinal fasciculus; PHN: perihypoglossal nucleus)

- **Congenital nystagmus**: There is no accepted model to explain congenital nystagmus. Though 5 different models have been proposed, each has its opponents
- **Pendular** nystagmus may be due to **impaired cerebellar feedback to the neural integrator**. This is somewhat akin to the **pendular knee jerk** in cerebellar lesions, where the oscillations are not appropriately inhibited by the cerebellum. Thus, lesions involving inferior olive, central tegmental tract, medial vestibular nuclei or the paramedian tracts can cause pendular nystagmus. The same lesions can cause palatal myoclonus and these two often co-exist
- **Gaze paretic** nystagmus is due to a **leaky (fatiguing or tiring) neural integrator.** A leaky integrator (Fig. 3.44) is a system that takes a constant input, but gradually leaks a small amount of output over time. When the neural integrator output declines over time, it fails to maintain a constant output to the gaze center involved in an eccentric gaze. As the output exponentially decreases, the eyes drift from the eccentric gaze and a corrective saccade in the direction of gaze is produced
- **Periodic alternating nystagmus** is due to **instability in the velocity storage mechanism** and lesions in the GABAergic Purkinje neurons in the cerebellar nodulus. Velocity storage is a central vestibular mechanism that stores (accumulates) incoming velocity information over time about head and body movement and activates the oculomotor system. Velocity storage has been modeled as an integrator, with inputs from the canals, visual and somatosensory systems and generates a low frequency component of eye velocity that compensates for motions that activate these systems.

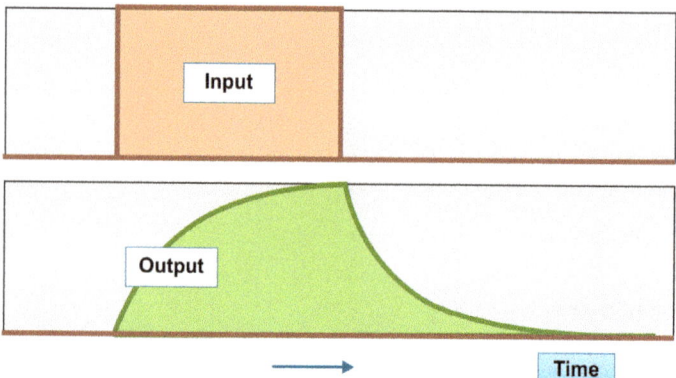

Fig. 3.44: Schematic representation of leaky neural integrator.

- **See-saw nystagmus** (Fig. 3.45) is due to impaired **ocular counter rolling reflex**. This reflex is dependent on the visual pathway inputs to the inferior olive and the interstitial nucleus of Cajal. Therefore, patients with chiasmatic lesions, severe visual loss, and brainstem lesions may develop this nystagmus.

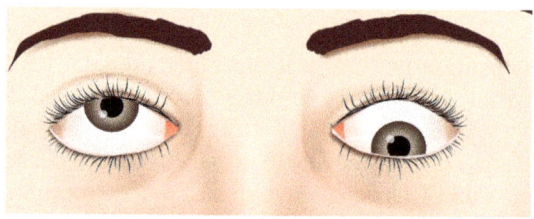

Fig. 3.45: See-saw nystagmus.

- **Upbeat nystagmus:** Normally, the **superior vestibular nucleus**, through the **ventral tegmental tract** provides a tonic excitatory input to the nucleus of superior rectus (III cranial nerve). If this pathway **is hypofunctional** due to a lesion, the eyes drift downwards with a corrective upward saccade, resulting in upbeat nystagmus. A number of brainstem and posterior fossa lesions can cause UBN
- **Down beat nystagmus:** The same pathway, i.e. **superior vestibular nucleus-ventral tegmental tract**, becomes **hyperactive** if there is a lesion in the cerebellar flocculus (the latter normally inhibits this pathway by GABA ergic mechanism). The overactive SVN-VTT pathway causes upward drift of the eyes with corrective downward saccades manifesting as downbeat nystagmus (Fig. 3.46)
- **Latent** nystagmus (that manifests when one eye is covered or is suppressed): Normally each **nucleus of optic tract (NOT)** receives input from the both eyes and both NOT are in balance even if one eye is closed. In patients with latent nystagmus, each NOT receives input only from the contralateral eye. Thus, when one eye is covered, there is an imbalance in the output of the NOT, generating the nystagmus (Fig. 3.47).

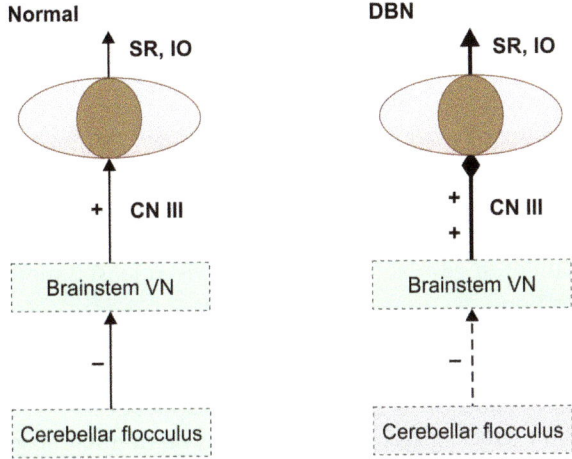

Fig. 3.46: Mechanism of vertical nystagmus.

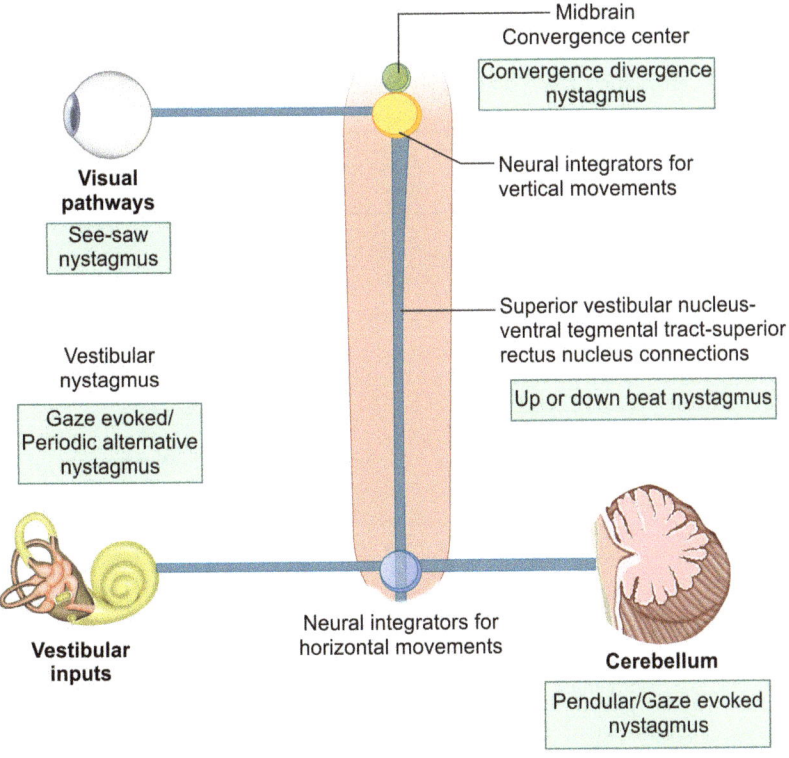

Fig. 3.47: Schematic diagram to show various types of nystagmus and their localization.
(PAN: periodic alternating nystagmus)

METHODOLOGY AND OBSERVATIONS

- Check the visual acuity in both the eyes (visual deprivation nystagmus)
- Look for head tilt or oscillations
- Look for range of extraocular movements and strabismus, including convergence
- Use optokinetic drum or tape and elicit OKN in horizontal and vertical planes
- Ask the patient to gaze at an object which is at least 2 meters away in a central position
- Identify if the involuntary eye movement is initiated by a slow eye movement (true nystagmus) or fast movement (saccadic intrusion)
- Cover each eye and check if the nystagmus appears
- Low amplitude nystagmus will be seen only on ophthalmoscopy
- Also use Frenzel's/Michael's lenses to bring out peripheral vestibular nystagmus
- Repeat the examination in all 9 cardinal directions of gaze
- Classify the nystagmus according to the scheme in the Flowchart 3.3. This shortens the list of differential diagnoses

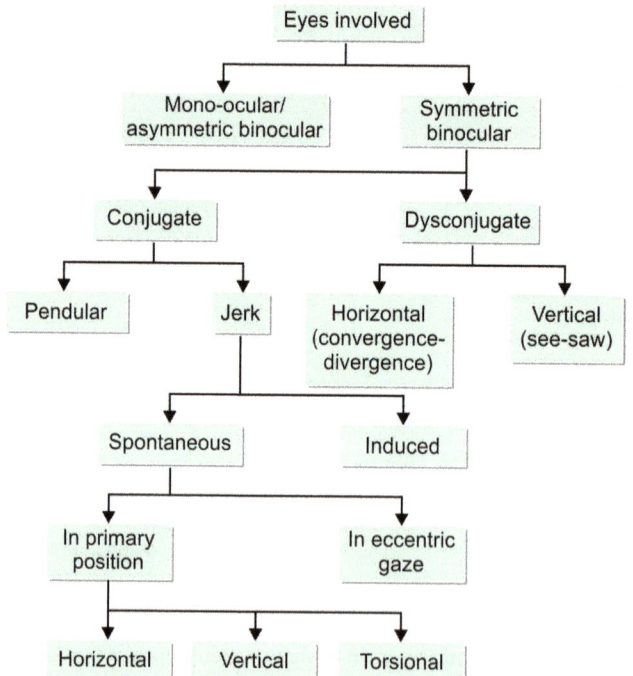

Flowchart 3.3: A clinical classification of nystagmus to narrow the differential diagnoses.

- Note all the characteristics of nystagmus: laterality, symmetry, conjugate/dysconjugate, pendualr/jerk, primary gaze or eccentric gaze, horizontal/vertical/torsional, and provoking or suppressing maneuvers
  Also try to answer the following questions about the patient's nystagmus:
- Does the nystagmus disappear at <30° angle of gaze? (physiologic nystagmus)
- Does the nystagmus increase if one eye is covered? (Latent nystagmus)
- Is there a null zone (a direction of gaze in which the nystagmus is minimal or absent)?
- Does convergence alter the nystagmus? (see below)
- Look for ocular albinism (congenital PAN)
- Is there a paradoxical response to OKN? (fast phase of OKN in the direction of drum rotation)
- Are there involuntary movements in other regions (e.g. palatal myoclonus)
- Observe at least for 2 minutes to identify if the nystagmus changes direction (PAN)
- Does the nystagmus change with prone and supine postures?

Etiologies of each subtype are listed in the subsequent Boxes 3.2 to 3.9.

Box 3.2: Causes of mono-ocular or asymmetric binocular nystagmus.

Ophthalmic/ocular causes
- Visual deprivation
- Restrictive syndromes of extraocular muscles
- Partial weakness of extraocular muscles
- Superior oblique myokymia

Neurological causes
- Spasmus nutans
  - Idiopathic
  - Lesional (optic pathway, III ventricle, thalamic tumors)
- Inter nuclear ophthalmoplegia (INO)/pseudo INO
- Mono-ocular down beating nystagmus (MS/CVA)
- Epileptic nystagmus

Box 3.3: Causes of bilateral symmetric, vertically disconjugate nystagmus (see- saw).

- Congenital
- Optic pathway lesions: **Usually pendular**
  - Septo-optic dysplasia, retinitis pigmentosa
  - Parasellar masses
- Brainstem lesions (interstitial nucleus of Cajal—vestibular nuclei connections: **Usually jerky**
  - Stroke (lateral medullary infarction)
  - Demyelination
  - Arnold-Chiari malformation (type I)
  - Syringobulbia
  - Paraneoplastic (anti-Ta antibodies)
  - Irradiation

Box 3.4: Causes of bilateral symmetric horizontally disconjugate nystagmus.

Convergence nystagmus
A. *Jerky convergence-retraction nystagmus:*
  - Dorsal midbrain lesions:
    ♦ Stroke
    ♦ Arnold-Chiari malformation (ACM)
    ♦ Pretectal lesions
    ♦ Pineal tumors (Parinaud's syndrome)
  - Epileptic seizure
B. Pendular convergence nystagmus
  - Whipple's disease

Divergence nystagmus
- ACM
- Hepatic coma
- Seizures

Box 3.5: Causes of bilateral symmetrical pendular nystagmus.

- Congenital nystagmus
- Optic neuropathy (MS)
- Dentate-rubro-olivary pathway lesions:
  - Multiple sclerosis (MS) lesions
  - Stroke
  - Tumors
- Pelizaeus-Merzbacher disease
- Adrenoleukodystrophy
- Toluene addiction
- Oculopalatal myoclonus

Box 3.6: Bilateral symmetric spontaneous jerk nystagmus.

Horizontal
- Congenital
- Latent
- Vestibular
- Periodic alternating
- Drug induced
- Epileptic

Box 3.7: Causes of periodic alternating nystagmus (uvulonodular lesions causing imbalance between neural integrators).

- Cerebellar degeneration (e.g. SCA 6)
- Ataxia telangiectasia
- Cerebellar infections (syphilis)
- Encephalitis
- CJD
- Cerebellar mass
- Brainstem infarction
- MS
- Visual loss
- Epileptic
- Drug induced (Phenytoin, lithium)
- Hepatic encephalopathy

Cranial Nerves

Box 3.8: Causes of vertical nystagmus, either upbeat or down beat nystagmus (lesions of superior vestibular nucleus- ventral tegmental tract- superior rectus nucleus pathway).

- Craniovertebral junction anomalies
- Cerebellar degeneration
- Multiple system atrophy (MSA)
- Posterior fossa tumors
- Brainstem stroke
- Encephalitis
- HTLV-1 infection
- MS
- Syringomyelia/bulbia
- Wernicke's encephalopathy
- B_{12} deficiency
- Drugs: Toluene, lithium, phenytoin

Box 3.9: Causes of gaze-evoked nystagmus (leaky/fatiguing/tiring neural integrator).

- End point/physiological nystagmus
- Brainstem/cerebellar disease
- Brun's nystagmus
- Drug induced nystagmus

INTERPRETATION

- *Oscillopsia:* Usually acquired nystagmus
- Convergent–divergent nystagmus: Whipple's disease, chiari malformation, MS, brainstem stroke
- Elliptical pendular nystagmus on oculography: Pelizaeus Merzbacher disease
- Pendular convergence movements along with rhythmic, synchronous jaw contractions are called oculomasticatory myorhythmia-diagnostic of Whipple's disease
- Symmetric gaze paretic nystagmus is usually due to drugs/alcohol. Asymmetric gaze paretic nystagmus is usually due to structural lesions
- Infantile nystagmus is suppressed by convergence, and may increase when one eye is covered. It also exhibits a null zone wherein the nystagmus is minimal or absent (usually in convergent position) and worsens on lateral gaze. Thus, child may learn to intentionally converge his eyes to improve his nystagmus
- *Downbeat nystagmus:* Flocculus lesion (cervicomedullary junction lesion), episodic ataxia type 2 (EA-2), drugs
- *Periodic alternating nystagmus:* Nodulus lesion (cervicomedullary junction lesion)
- *Upbeat nystagmus:* Lesion involving the superior vestibular nucleus and the ventral tegmental tract (bilateral pontomesencephalic or pontomedullary lesion)
- *Pendular nystagmus:* Paramedian pontine lesions, deep cerebellar nuclear lesions-fastigial nucleus, especially MS and CVA

- *See-saw nystagmus:* Visual pathway lesion/mesodiencephalic lesion
- *Brun's nystagmus:* Large cerebellopontine angle lesion
- *Paradoxical response to OKN:* Congenital nystagmus (infantile nystagmus syndrome)
- *Horizontal jerk nystagmus in primary gaze:* Most often it is PAN. This is often missed because the patient is not observed for long enough duration (2–3 minutes)
- *Nystagmus that improves in supine position:* Cerebellar lesion (these patients may prefer to lie supine while reading). This worsens in prone position
- *Nystagmus attenuated by visual fixation:* Likely vestibular
- *Nystagmus accentuated by visual fixation:* Congenital
- *Nystagmus that remains horizontal in all gaze angles:* Congenital
- *Nystagmus that changes direction when alternate eyes are covered:* Congenital
- *Effect of convergence:* May increase or decrease the vertical jerk nystagmus.

CAVEATS

- Myasthenic patients may exhibit gaze paretic nystagmus, as the extraocular muscles in eccentric position start to fatigue
- In some patients, nystagmus is not grossly visible and only a direct ophthalmoscopy can demonstrate the nystagmus
- Some forms of nystagmus vary with time (e.g. PAN). So a several minutes of examination may be warranted
- Nystagmus may be seen only in a particular direction of gaze. Therefore, examination in all directions of gaze for nystagmus is important
- It is important to examine the eye not only in eccentric gaze, but also after returning to primary gaze. Rebound nystagmus is seen only after returning to primary gaze.

BIBLIOGRAPHY

1. Anderson T. How do I examine for a supranuclear gaze palsy? Movement Disorders Clinical Practice. 2015;2(1):106.
2. Bhidayasiri R, Plant GT, Leigh RJ. A hypothetical scheme for brainstem control of vertical gaze. Neurology. 2000; 20:54:1985-93.
3. Jacobson DM. Divergence insufficiency revisited: natural history of idiopathic cases and neurologic associations. Arch Ophthalmol. 2000;118(9):1237-41.
4. Leigh RJ, Zee DS. The neurology of eye movements. New York: Oxford University press; 2006.
5. Newby RE, Lewis M. Convergence spasm: a novel diagnostic tool. J Neurol Neurosurg Psychiatry. 2012;83:A27.
6. Thurtell MJ, Leigh RJ. Nystagmus and saccadic intrusions. Handb Clin Neurol. 2011;102: 333-78.
7. Wong A. Eye movement disorders. Oxford University press; 2007.

Cranial Nerves

TRIGEMINAL NERVE (V N)

GRK Sarma

PICTORIAL PRETEST

A 45-year-old lady with left facial pain was examined. The figures show the appearance of her face with mouth closed and then opened.

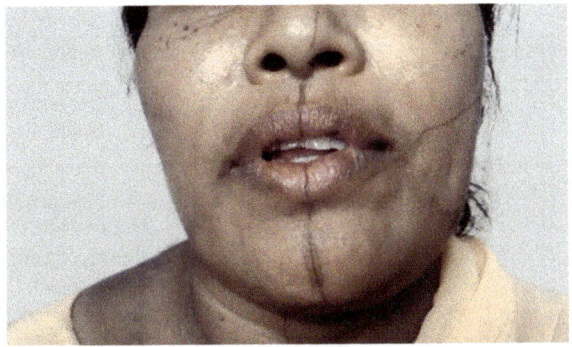

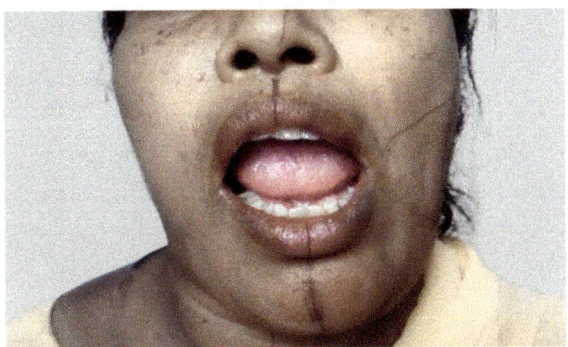

Questions

1. What is the abnormality?
2. What is the anatomical localization?

PHYSIOLOGICAL BASIS

- The V nerve nucleus consists of motor and sensory components
- The motor nucleus lies in mid pons and supplies muscles of mastication
- The sensory nuclei are divided into three components
- The principal sensory nucleus is located in the mid-pons and subserves touch sensation
- The spinal nucleus subserves pain and temperature and lies in pons, medulla and upper cervical cord (up to C2 or 3 or 4 level)

- The mesencephalic nucleus lies in midbrain and subserves proprioception from masticatory muscles.

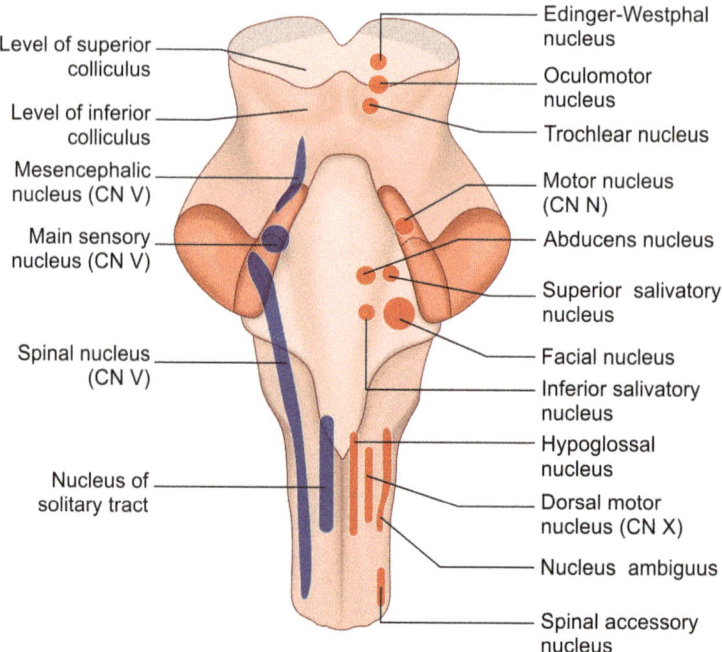

Fig. 3.48: Schematic coronal view of brainstem to depict various cranial nerve nuclei.

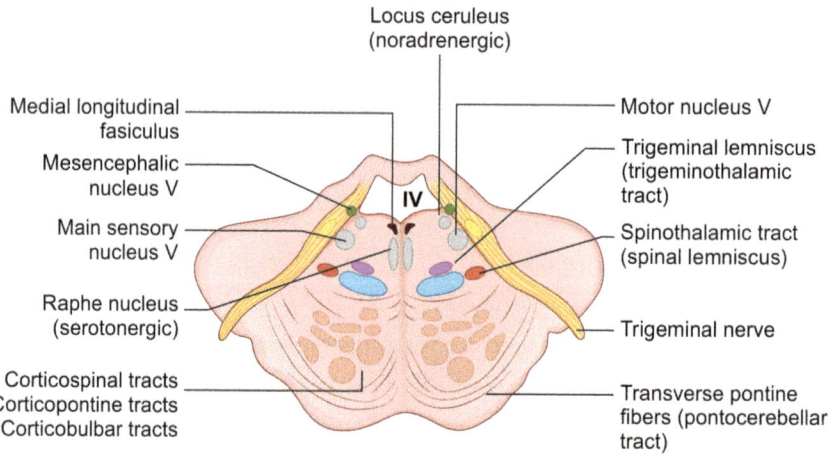

Fig. 3.49: Schematic axial view of pons to depict trigeminal nuclei and their relationship with other structures.

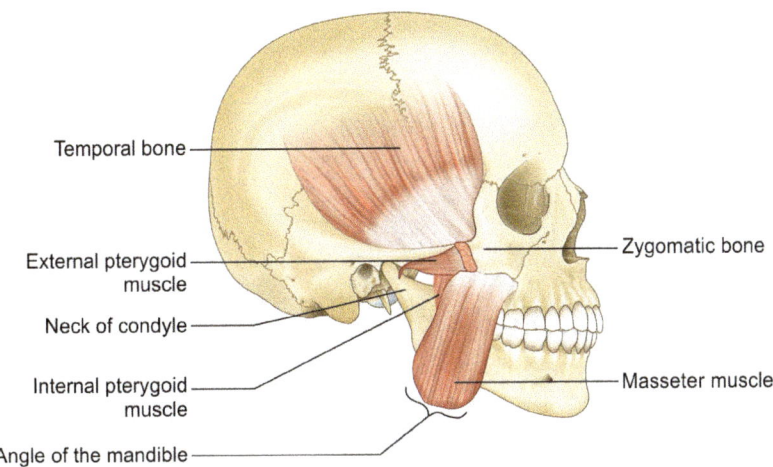

Fig. 3.50: Muscles of mastication

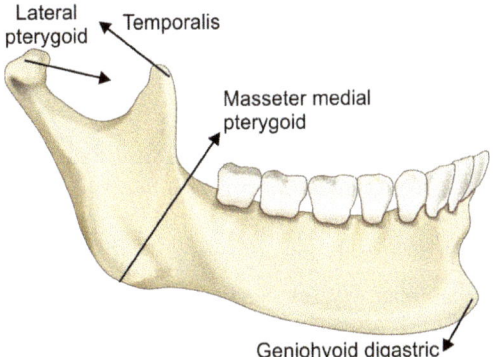

Fig. 3.51: Areas of insertion of muscles of mastication on the mandible and the direction of action of various muscles.

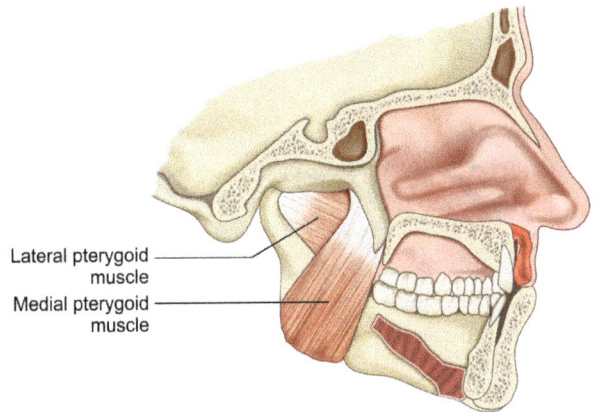

Fig. 3.52: Perpendicular orientation of lateral and medial pterygoids explains their opposite actions.

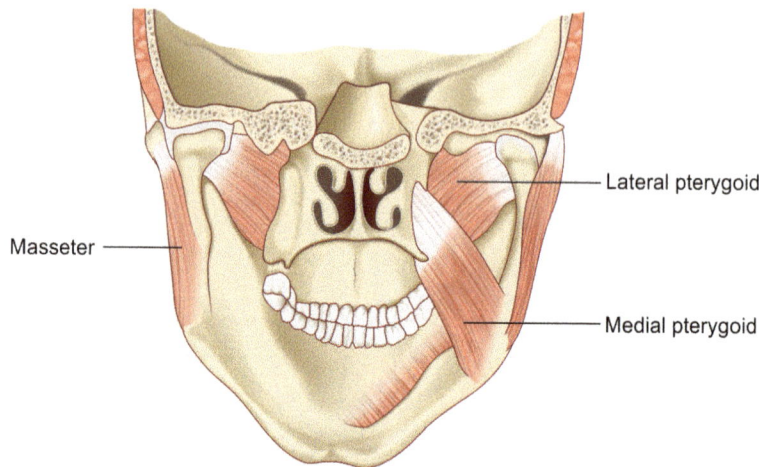

Fig. 3.53: Coronal view to understand the different orientation of pterygoids.

MOTOR NUCLEUS

- The motor nucleus receives projections from bilateral motor cortex, but predominant control is from contralateral cortex (lower third of motor homunculus)
- Motor fibers exit the pons and pass beneath the Gasserian ganglion, exit the skull through foramen ovale to supply masseter, temporalis, the pterygoids, anterior belly of digastrics and mylohyoid muscles
- The main movements of the jaw are opening/closing, protrusion/retraction and side to side movement
- All the muscles except lateral pterygoids close the jaw because their origin is above the level of insertion into the mandible. The lateral pterygoid's origin is below the level of insertion on the mandible and thus, it opens the jaw
- The masseter and medial pterygoids are somewhat parallel to each other, with their origin anterior to their insertion on the mandible. Thus they protrude the jaw, while the temporalis retracts it, because its origin is posterior to its insertion into the coronoid process
- Both the pterygoids originate from the base of the skull and insert into the mandible on its inner aspect. Both pull the mandible to the contralateral side. Their weakness leads to deviation of the jaw to ipsilateral side (towards the weak side).

SENSORY PORTION (FIGS. 3.54 A TO C)

- The trigeminal ganglion lies in the Meckel's cave in the petrous apex just lateral to the internal carotid artery and the posterior part of the cavernous sinus. Lesions involving these structures commonly produce : V cranial nerve involvement
- 3 modalities are carried in the trigeminal nerve: Light touch and pressure, pain and temperature and finally the proprioceptive sensations from the muscles supplied by the trigeminal nerve
- Light touch and pressure sensations are carried to the main sensory nucleus in the pons. Second order neurons cross and ascend in the ventral trigeminothalamic tract to the ventral posterior medial nucleus of thalamus. Uncrossed fibers ascend in the dorsal trigeminothalamic tract
- Pain and temperature sensations are carried to the nucleus of spinal tract of the trigeminal nerve, that extends from mid pons to the 3rd or 4th cervical segment inferiorly. Second order neurons cross to the ventral trigeminothalamic tract and ascend to the VPM of thalamus
- The different routes taken by the touch and pain sensations results in dissociated sensory loss in intrinsic brainstem lesions
- Somatotopic organization of the spinal nucleus is such that V1 is represented most anteriorly and V2 and V3 most posteriorly
- In addition, perioral sensations are represented in the rostral part and peripheral areas of face are represented in the caudal part of the nucleus of spinal tract. This can result in onion skin type sensory loss with intrinsic cord or brainstem lesions
- Proprioceptive fibers pass through the gasserian ganglion without synapsing, to reach the mesencephalic nucleus. These fibers mediate the jaw jerk and also join the trigeminothalamic tract.

TRIGEMINAL NERVE DIVISIONS

1. Ophthalmic division runs forward in the lateral wall of cavernous sinus. It gives a small branch to the tentorium cerebelli just after leaving the gasserian ganglion. It then enters superior orbital fissure and divides into terminal branches, namely, frontal, lacrimal and nasociliary nerve branches. The frontal branch supplies sensation to the upper face (Fig. 3.55). The ciliary nerves supply sensation to the cornea, ciliary body and the globe.

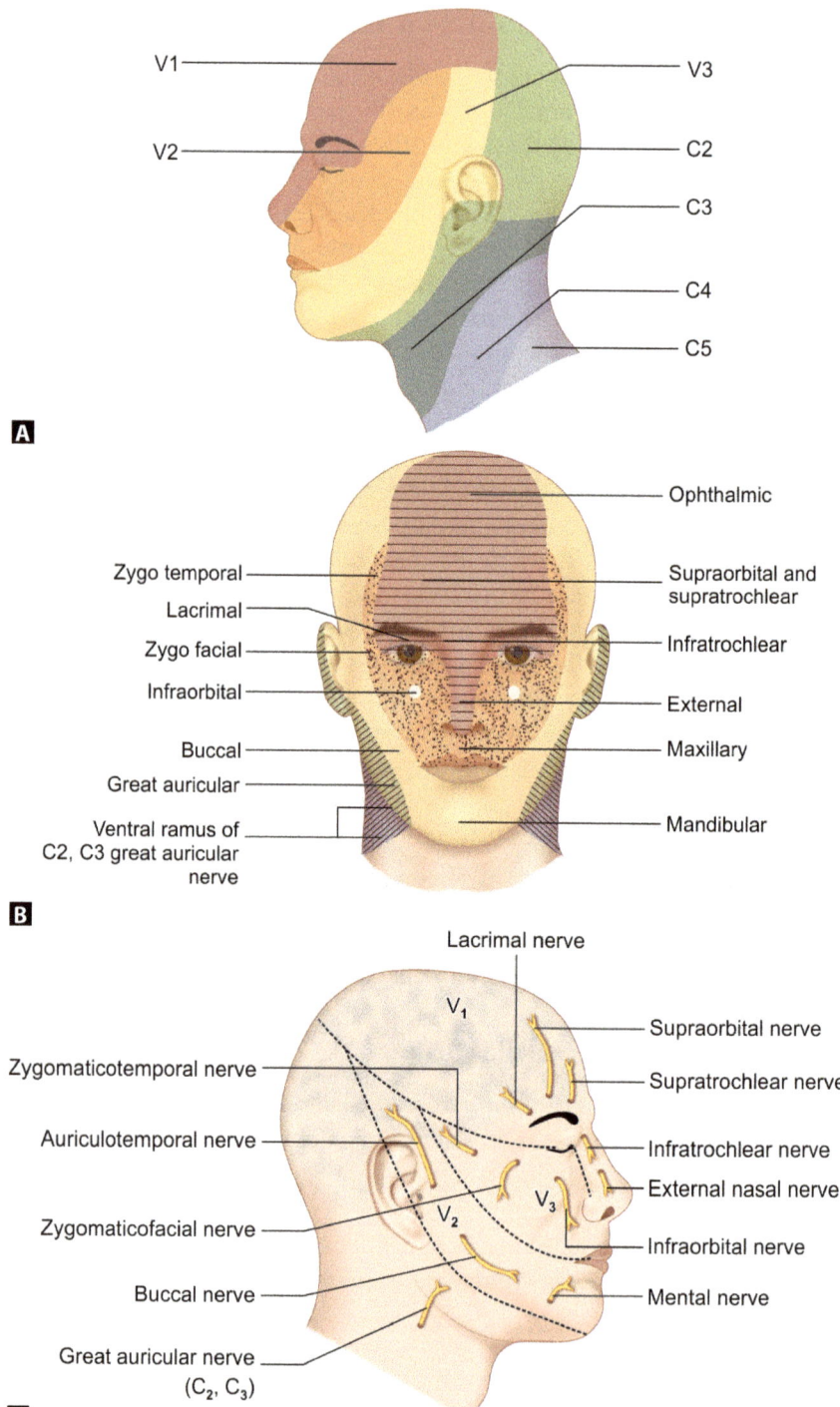

Figs. 3.54A to C: Sensory innervation of face. (A) Segmental innervation; (B) Area of innervation by individual branches of V nerve; (C) Terminal branches of V nerve.

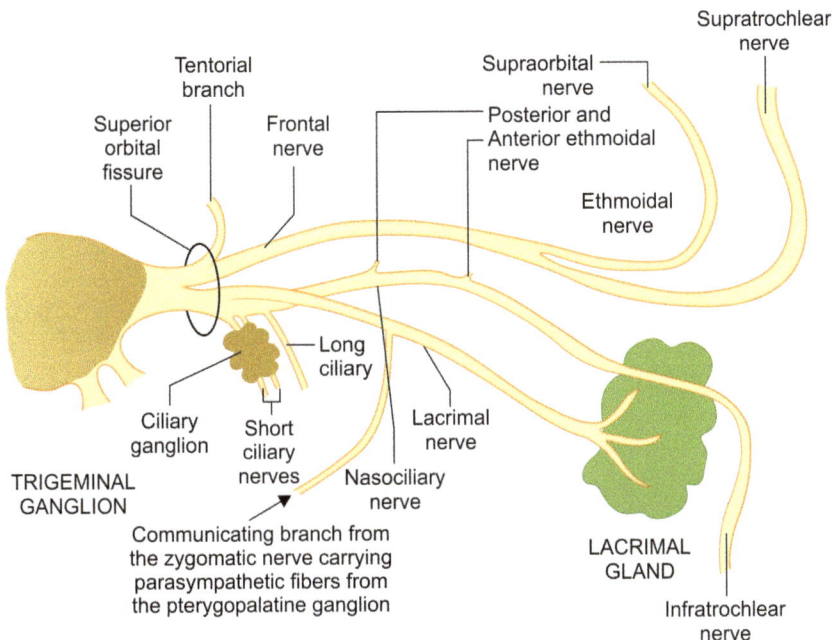

Fig. 3.55: Ophthalmic nerve.

2. Maxillary nerve gives meningeal branch to the middle cranial fossa, passes in the lateral wall of cavernous sinus and exits through foramen rotundum. It crosses the pterygopalatine fossa where pterygopalatine (sensory) branches are given to the palate. It then gives zygomatic and superior alveolar branches and enters the orbit through the inferior orbital fissure and transits the infraorbital canal and exits the infraorbital foramen as the infraorbital nerve. This supplies the sensation to the cheek area (Fig. 3.56) and its lesions cause numb cheek syndrome. Additional loss of sensation from upper gums and teeth indicates a more proximal (maxillary nerve) than the infraorbital nerve lesion. Mapping the sensory loss over the distribution of the branches of maxillary nerves suggests the location of the lesion (main trunk versus terminal branches).
3. Mandibular gives meningeal branch and exits through the foramen ovale. It gives of nervous spinosus, a recurrent meningeal branch to the middle and anterior cranial fossae. It gives motor fibers to the pterygoids and sensory branches namely buccal, lingual, inferior alveolar and auriculotemporal branches. It then enters the mandibular canal and exits through the mental foramen as the mental nerve. Lesions at this site can cause numb chin syndrome. However, a notch at the angle of the jaw is spared because it is supplied by the greater auricular nerve (C2,3) (Fig. 3.57).

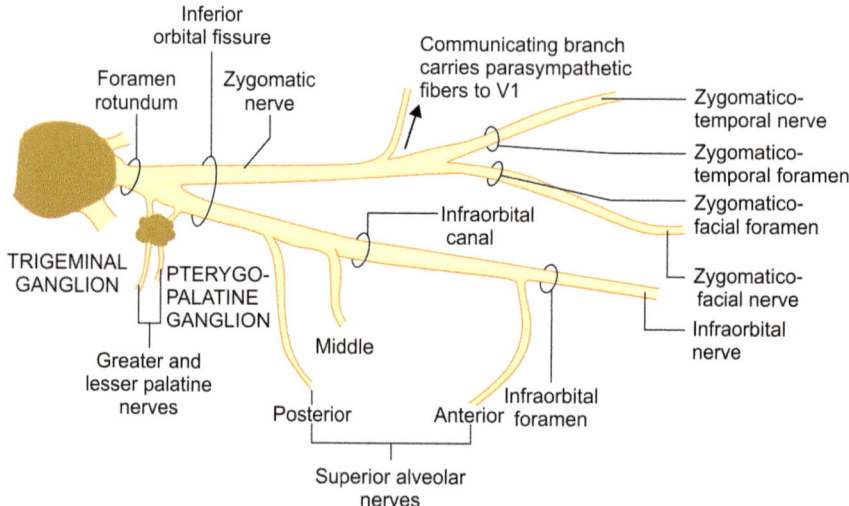

Fig. 3.56: Maxillary nerve.

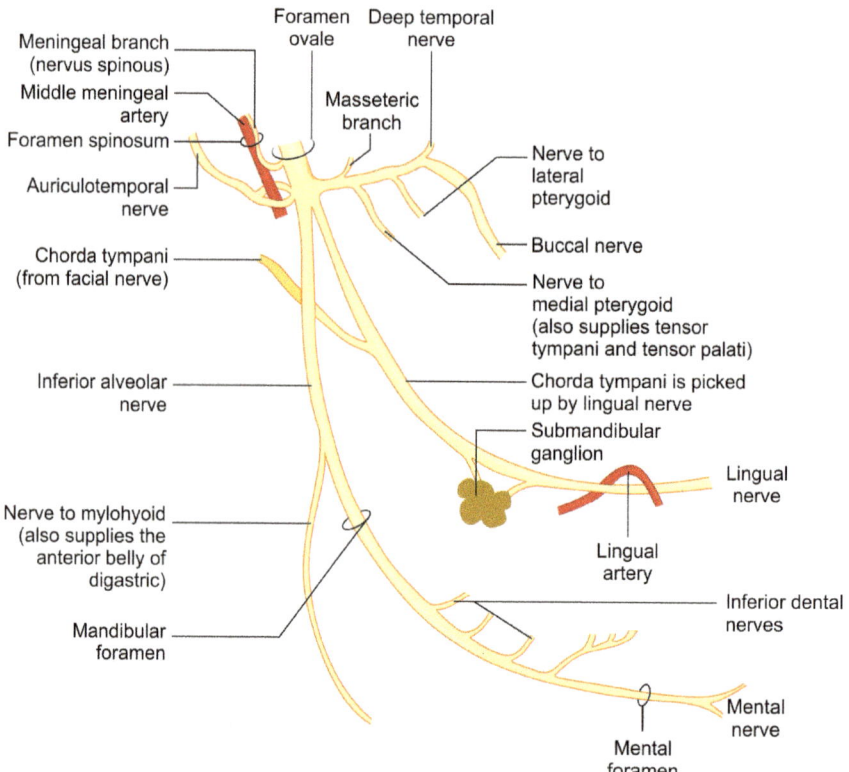

Fig. 3.57: Mandibular nerve.

EXAMINATION METHOD

Examination of trigeminal nerve includes motor, sensory and reflex assessment.

Motor Functions

Inspect

- Wasting, fasciculations of muscles of mastication
- Flattening of jaw line
- Hollowing of the temporal fossa
- Dropped jaw
- Jaw deviation at rest
- *Ask the patient to open the jaw.* The inter-incisural notches (notches between incisor teeth in the midline of upper and lower jaws) and the tip of the nose should be in one line. Deviation of jaw to one side indicates weakness of the ipsilateral pterygoids (contralateral strong pterygoids push the jaw to the weak side)
- Involuntary movements (tremor, dystonia, trismus, dyskinesia).

Palpation

- Feel the masseters and temporalis at rest and on jaw closure. Note any thinning and flabbiness
- Place a finger on the anterior border of masseter and ask the patient to clench his jaw. The masseter muscle pushes the examining finger forward. Asymmetry of this movement indicates weakness of the ipsilateral masseter
- Ask the patient to move the jaw sideways to each side against resistance. Weakness of pterygoids on one side will manifest as inability to move the jaw sideways to the opposite side.

Percussion for Jaw Jerk

- Place the index finger over the patient's chin in the middle with the mouth open and relaxed and tap the finger with the reflex hammer
- Look for the upward jerk of the jaw
- Normally, this movement is absent or minimal
- It is exaggerated in lesions of the corticobulbar fibers above the motor nucleus
- It is depressed in infranuclear lesions in the reflex arc (consisting of the trigeminal sensory fibers, mesencephalic nucleus and trigeminal motor fibers)
- *Afferent:* Ia afferent fibers in mandibular division
- *Nuclei:* Mesencephalic nucleus, motor nucleus of V nerve
- *Efferents:* Motor fibers in mandibular division
- Lesions in the reflex arc diminish the reflex, supranuclear lesions make it brisk.

Blink reflex (Glabellar reflex)
- Percuss over the supraorbital ridge, look for orbicularis oculi contraction
- *Afferents:* Reach sensory and spinal nucleus of V nerve
- *Efferents:* Facial nerve.

Examination of Sensory Function
- Examine touch, pain and temperature
- Examine the face in three patterns:
    1. Vertically, checking all the three divisions, i.e. V 1,2,3 (comparing with contralateral side)
    2. Horizontal plane, comparing peri-oral versus lateral face sensations (for onion peel loss)
    3. In individual branch distribution (example: mental nerve/infra-orbital nerve areas)
- Examine the gums, anterior tongue and inside of cheeks with a swab stick, comparing both the sides (for involvement of terminal branches of maxillary and mandibular nerves).

Examination of Reflexes
1. *Corneal reflex:*
    - Ask patient to look to one side.
    - With a clean wisp of cotton, gently touch the cornea at its junction with sclera at its upper and lower limbus.
    - Look for reflex blink of both eyes on stimulating each eye (direct and consensual reflexes).
    - Contralateral thalamic/parietal lesions can suppress the corneal reflex on one side.
    - Lesions of brainstem trigeminofacial connections can suppress both direct and consensual reflexes.
    - High cervical lesions can also suppress the corneal reflex by involvement of spinal nucleus of trigeminal nerve.
    - *Caveat:* Corneal reflex may be impaired in long-term use of contact lens.
2. *Jaw jerk:* Please see above.

Interpretation of Sensory Dysfunction
- Impaired touch sensation with preserved pain: Main sensory nucleus lesion
- Impaired pain with preserved touch: Lesion of the nucleus of spinal tract of trigeminal nerve
- Impairment of all modalities in all three divisions: Lesion proximal to gasserian ganglion
- Impaired sensation over nose: V1 lesion (specifically anterior ethmoidal branch)

- Impaired sensation over cheek: Infra-orbital nerve lesion
- Impaired sensation over cheek and gum of the posterior (beyond canines) upper jaw: V2 lesion
- Impaired sensation over chin: Mental nerve lesion (numb chin syndrome)
- Impaired sensation over chin and anterior tongue: V3 lesion
- Impaired corneal reflex on stimulation of upper limbus: V1 lesion
- Impaired corneal reflex on stimulation of lower limbus: V2 lesion
- Trigeminal neuropathy with marked xerophthalmia/xerostomia: Consider Sjögren's syndrome (mild impairment in secretory functions may be seen with trigeminal neuropathy of any cause because of impaired secretory reflex afferent arc).
- V1 facial pain with ipsilateral VI nerve palsy: Petrous apex lesion (Gradenigo's syndrome)
- V1 or V2 pain with Horner's syndrome: Cavernous sinus lesion (no anhydrosis)
- V1 dysfunction with ocular motor palsy; superior orbital fissure lesion.

Caveat

- Proximal lesions in the skull base/meninges can also produce numb chin syndrome due to preferential involvement of V3 fibers
- Peri-sylvian parietal lobe lesions can also cause loss of contralateral corneal reflex (suprasegmental influence)
- Facial nerve lesions cause loss of corneal reflex on paralyzed side on stimulation of either side.

Interpretation of Motor Function Examination

- Bilateral jaw weakness with brisk jaw jerk indicates bilateral UMN lesion (pseudobulbar palsy)
- Deviation of protruded jaw to one side indicates weakness of ipsilateral trigeminal innervated muscles (UMN or LMN)
- LMN lesions result in more severe weakness than UMN lesions (bilateral innervations by UMN fibers)
- Unilateral masticatory muscle weakness with sensory loss over V1-V3 indicates trigeminal nerve involvement. Rarely, pontine lesions can present with this deficit, without long tract signs
- Above syndrome with contralateral hemiparesis: Dorsal pontine lesion extending to involve basis pontis
- Above 'syndrome' with contralateral hemianesthesia: Lesion extending to spinothalamic tract
- With ipsilateral tremor: involvement of brachium conjunctivum
- Above with INO: MLF lesion

- Hemimasticatory spasm (similar to hemifacial spasm) may be due to dorsal pontine tumors/demyelination.
- Loss of pain near midline/peri-oral region: Rostral lesions (pontomedullary junction)
- Loss of pain over lateral face: Caudal lesions (caudal medulla or upper cervical)
- Dissociated sensory loss in V1, V2: Ventral aspect of spinal nucleus and tract of V
- Dissociated sensory loss in V2, V3: Dorsal aspect
- Dissociated sensory loss over V1-V3: Complete lesion
- Loss of pain on ipsilateral face, arm, leg: Spinothalamic and ventral trigeminothalamic tract involvement
- Involvement of V with VI, VII, VIII without long tract signs: Lesion in cisternal portion/CPA
- Bilateral trigeminal neuralgia: suspect multiple sclerosis.

ANSWERS TO THE PRETEST

1. There is jaw deviation to the left on opening the mouth. This can be better appreciated if a line is drawn over the midline of upper and lower jaws (using incisors as the landmark). These lines would be aligned when mouth is closed, but the alignment is broken when the jaw is opened as in this patient.
2. Jaw deviation to the left indicates ipsilateral pterygoid weakness. In addition to this motor deficit, there is sensory loss over V2 and 3 areas (demarcated in the Figure). This suggests a left trigeminal neuropathy. Her MRI revealed a large schwannoma of the left trigeminal nerve.

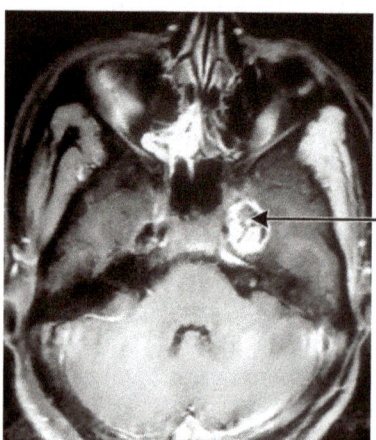

Schwannoma identified on gadolinum enhanced MRI

BIBLIOGRAPHY

1. Brazis PW, Masdeu JC, Biller J. Localization in clinical Neurology, 6th edition. Philadelphia: Wolters Kluwer/Lippincott Williams and Wilkins; 2011.
2. Campbell WW. DeJong's the Neurologic examination, 7th edition. Wolters Kluwer/Lippincott Williams and Wilkins; 2013.
3. Campbell WW Jr. The numb cheek syndrome: a sign of infraorbital neuropathy. Neurology. 1986;36: 421-3.
4. Kim JS, Lee JH, Lee MC. Patterns of sensory dysfunction in lateral medullary infarction. Clinical-MRI correlation. Neurology. 1997;49:1557-63.
5. Lecky BRF, Highes RAC, Murray NMF. Trigeminal sensory neuropathy: a study of 22 cases. Brain. 1987;110:1463-85.
6. Onella MC, Fischbein NJ, So YT. Disorders of the trigeminal system. Semin Neurol 2009;72: 297-9.

THE FACIAL NERVE (VII N)

GRK Sarma

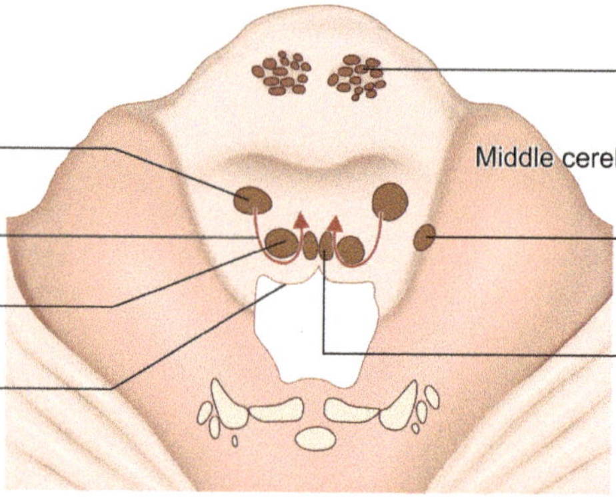

Fig. 3.58: Anatomy of facial nuclei.

PHYSIOLOGIC BASIS

- The facial nerve subserves following functions:
    - Muscles of facial expression
    - Muscles of scalp and ear
    - Platysma, buccinators
    - Stylohyoid, posterior belly of digastrics and stapedius
    - Parasympathetic secretory fibers to submandibular, sublingual and lacrimal glands, mucous membranes of oral and nasal cavities
    - Taste from anterior 2/3 of the tongue
    - Sensations from the ear drum and external ear canal
- It is divided into seven segments along its course:
    1. Brainstem segment (from the facial nucleus to the exit point)
    2. Cisternal segment (from exit point to internal auditory meatus)
    3. Canalicular segment (through the internal auditory canal to the entry into facial canal)
    4. Labyrinthine segment (from facial canal to geniculate ganglion)
    5. Horizontal segment (from geniculate ganglion to the pyramidal eminence on posterior wall of tympanic cavity)
    6. Mastoid segment (from pyramidal eminence to the exit from stylomastoid foramen)
    7. Extratemporal segment (after exiting from stylomastoid foramen)
- The part of the facial nucleus supplying the upper part of the face has bilateral representation, while the remaining part receives predominantly contralateral innervations. Thus in unilateral upper motor neuron lesions, the upper facial muscles are relatively spared.
- Some corticobulbar fibers to the facial nucleus leave pyramidal tract in crus cerebri and descend along medial lemniscus (**aberrant pyramidal**

tract), decussate in medulla and ascend upwards to reach facial nucleus. Thus in lateral medullary syndrome, one may observe ipsilateral facial weakness of upper motor neuron type, though the lesion is below the level of facial nucleus
- The motor fibers arising from the facial nucleus travel posteriorly and loop around the VI nucleus (facial colliculus) and then anterolaterally close to NTS, spinal tract and nucleus of trigeminal nerve to exit the lower pons between olive and inferior cerebellar peduncle
- The exiting facial nerve also consists of **nervus intermedius** which is formed by sensory fibers destined to the NTS and spinal nucleus of V and secretomotor fibers from the superior salivatory and lacrimal nuclei
- The facial nerve enters the internal auditory meatus lying superior to the vestibulocochlear nerve, close to the anterior inferior cerebellar artery. The subarachnoid space extends along the facial nerve up to the geniculate ganglion.

METHODOLOGY

Facial nerve has to be examined by testing its following functions:
- Motor functions
- Sensory functions
- Reflexes
- Secretory functions

Motor Functions

Inspection

- From above downwards: Symmetry of forehead furrows, palpebral fissures, nasolabial folds, angles of mouth
- Observe for facial asymmetry under spontaneous emotions during conversation (e.g. smiling)
- Facial expression
- Blink rate
- Atrophy of facial muscles
- Fasciculations
- Synkinetic movements
- Other involuntary movements.

Muscle Strength Assessment

- Upper face assessment: Ask patient to raise eyebrows, frown, close eyes tightly while you try to open them
- Lower face assessment: Ask patient to smile/grin broadly, puff the cheeks, whistle, evert the lower lip (looking for platysma activation).
- Ear muscles: Ask patient to look outwards in extreme lateral gaze and watch for movement of opposite ear (may be absent in normal persons).

Sensory Function

- Bedside testing of taste sensation to sweet and salt substances is adequate.
- Other tastes include bitter, sour and Umami (certain amino-acids like l-glutamate) and can be tested for more detailed assessment
- Place before the patient, 4 cards with "sweet" "salt", "sour", and "bitter" written on them
- If a patient is illiterate, give alternate instructions on nonverbal communication to indicate a particular taste (e.g. raise your right hand if you feel sweet and left hand for salt)
- Keep 4 packets or containers with sugar, salt, citrus juice to asafetida and applicator sticks ready
- Ask patient to protrude the tongue and instruct him not to retract it. If patient is unable to hold it there, use a gauze piece and hold it from retracting into the mouth (to ensure that we test the taste from anterior 2/3 of the tongue)
- With the applicator stick, apply one substance at a time to the dorsum of anterior tongue and ask patient to indicate the taste
- Avoid the tip of the tongue, which has fewer taste buds than the dorsum
- Test the bitter taste in the end.

Reflexes

- Bell's phenomenon: Ask patient to close his eyes tightly. Try opening the eyes passively to see the uprolled eyeballs (normal response)
- Orbicularis oculi reflex: Tap the forehead over supraorbital ridge or glabella and watch for bilateral blinking. Watch for its normal suppression with repeated tapping
- Orbicularis oris reflex: Tap over the upper lip or side of the nose and watch for elevation of the angle of the mouth, protrusion of lower lip and puckering of the chin (mentalis contraction)
- Frontal release reflexes (palmomental, snout and suck reflexes)
- Corneal reflex.

Secretory Function

- History of xerostomia and xerophthalmia or excess tearing and sialorrhea
- Tearing is assessed by Schirmer's test using commercially available filter papers. The filter paper is inserted in the inferior conjunctival sac and left for 5 minutes. The advancing edge of the moisture indicates the extent of tearing. Normal values are greater than 15 mm. A reading of less than 5 mm indicates severe xerophthalmia
- Salivation is assessed by quantitative salivary flow by oral surgeons. It is impaired only in bilateral lesions, central or systemic causes and not with unilateral lesions.

INTERPRETATION

- The first step in the analysis of facial weakness is to differentiate upper and lower motor neuron types of palsy.

	Lower motor nerve	Upper motor nerve
Degree of weakness	Severe	Mild to moderate
Upper face	As weak as lower face	Less weak or totally spared
Bell's phenomenon	Present	Absent
Corneal reflex	Absent/reduced	Preserved
Orbicularis oculi reflex	Absent/reduced	Preserved
Spontaneous emotions	Impaired	May be preserved

Localization of Upper Motor Nerve Facial Palsy

- In upper motor neuron type of facial palsy, if volitional and emotional movements are affected to a different degree, it is called dissociated facial weakness and indicates that the two pathways are affected to a different extent.
- In emotional/mimetic palsy, voluntary movements are preserved. This indicates a lesion in lesions of supplementary motor area, thalamic/striato-capsular area and rarely the brainstem.
- In contrast, in voluntary facial palsy, the voluntary movements are more severely affected, and spontaneous emotions are relatively preserved. This indicates a lesion in lower part of the pre-central gyrus, or the corticobulbar fibers up to the level of pons above the facial nucleus. The lower half of face is innervated by bilateral supranuclear fibers, but only contralateral volitional fibers. This explains the dissociation.

Localization of Lower Motor Nerve Facial Palsy (Distal to Proximal)

- Weakness of some but not all facial muscles indicates a lesion distal to the stylomastoid foramen (parotid tumor, trauma, Hansen's disease, etc.) that involves individual branches of facial nerve
- Facial palsy with impaired taste in anterior 2/3 of the tongue suggests lesion between stylomastoid foramen and origin of nerve to stapedius from the horizontal or vertical segment of the facial nerve at the medial or posterior border of the tympanic cavity
- Facial palsy, impaired taste and hyperacusis indicates lesion between geniculate ganglion and the origin of nerve to stapedius
- Facial palsy, impaired taste, hyperacusis and impaired lacrimation suggests lesion at or between geniculate ganglion and internal auditory meatus

- Facial palsy, tinnitus, deafness, ataxia and facial sensory disturbance suggests lesion in the cerebellopontine angle. (Thus, facial palsy can be associated with either deafness in proximal lesions or hyperacusis in more distal lesions)
- Facial palsy with ipsilateral VI nerve palsy or horizontal gaze palsy, contralateral hemiparesis suggests lesion in the intrapontine region
- Neuralgic, paroxysmal pain involving the deep aspect of the ear, with or without radiation to face suggests irritative lesion in the geniculate ganglion (geniculate neuralgia/tic douloureux of chorda tympani).

CAVEATS

Myasthenia gravis can produce markedly asymmetric weakness of facial muscles and mimic Bell's palsy. Variability of weakness during examination and presence of fatiguable ptosis give a clue to the diagnosis.

BIBLIOGRAPHY

1. Brazis PW, Masdeu JC, Biller J. Localization in clinical neurology, 6th edition. Philadelphia: Wolters Kluwer/Lippincott Williams and Wilkins; 2011.
2. Campbell WW. DeJong's the neurologic examination, 7th edition. Wolters Kluwer/Lippincott Williams and Wilkins; 2013
3. Gilchrist JM. Seventh cranial neuropathy. Semin Neurol. 2009;29:5-13.
4. Keane JR. Bilateral seventh nerve palsy: analysis of 43 cases and review of literature. Neurology. 1994;44:1198-202.
5. May M, Klein SR. Differential diagnosis of facial nerve palsy. Otolaryngol Clin North Am. 1991;24: 613-45.
6. Tzafetta K, Terzis JK. Essays on the facial nerve part I. Microanatomy. Past Reconstr Surg. 2010:125:879-89.
7. Urban PP, Wicht S, et al. The course of corticofacial projections in the human brainstem. Brain. 2011;124 (pt 9):1866-76. .

VESTIBULOCOCHLEAR NERVE (VIII N)

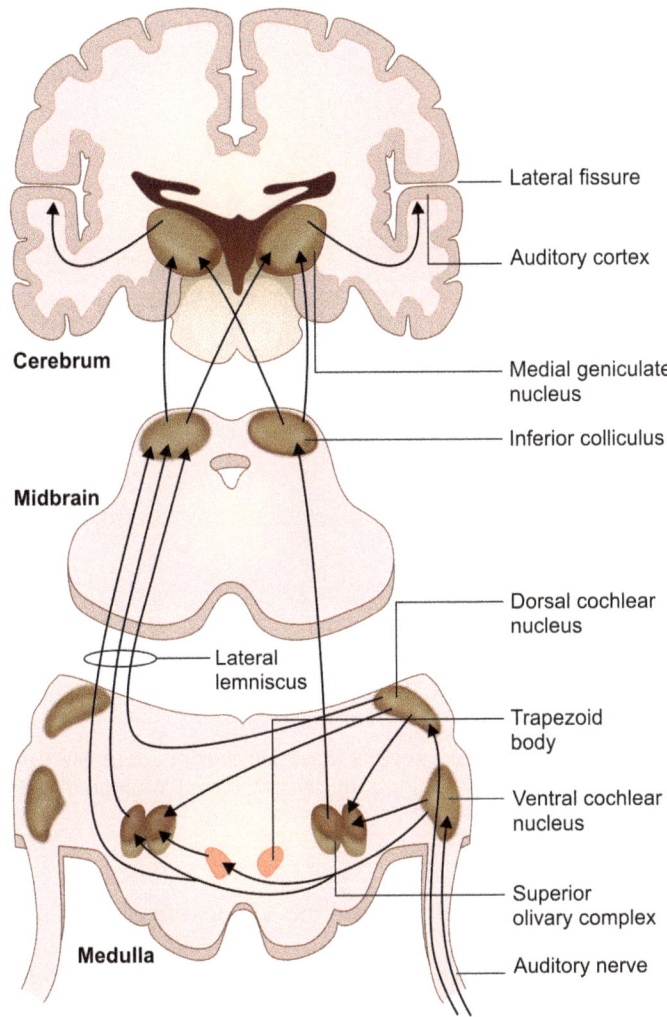

Fig. 3.59: The auditory pathway.

PHYSIOLOGICAL BASICS (FIGS. 3.59 AND 3.60)

The VIII cranial nerve consists of 2 components—cochlear and vestibular nerves for auditory function and equilibrium respectively.

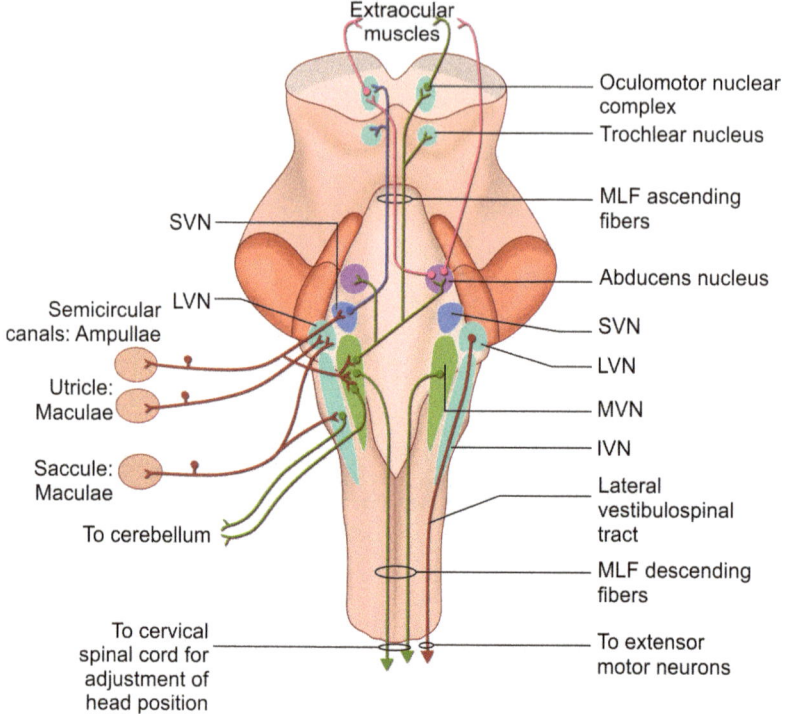

Fig. 3.60: Longitudinal view of brainstem to depict the vestibular nuclei and connections.
(SVN: superior vestibular nucleus; LVN: lateral vestibular nucleus; MVN: medial vestibular nucleus; IVN: inferior vestibular nucleus; MLF: medial longitudinal fasciculus)

Auditory Pathways

- **Receptors** are **the hair cells** of the organ of Corti. The apex of the cochlea responds to low frequency sounds and the base to high frequency sounds
- **First order neurons** are located in the **spiral ganglion** located close to the base of the bony spiral lamina. Their axons form the auditory nerve that enters the pontomedullary junction.
- **Second order neurons** are located in the dorsal and ventral **cochlear nuclei** at pontomedullary junction. These nuclei give rise to certain projections that form the contralateral **lateral lemniscus**:
  - Dorsal acoustic striae
  - Intermediate acoustic striae
  - Ventral acoustic striae. This is a part of the trapezoid body that ends in the superior olivary complex. The latter gives rise to fibers that join the lateral lemniscus
- **Third order neurons** are located in the **inferior colliculus** situated in the midbrain tectum, which receives both ascending (lateral lemniscus) and descending pathways.

- **Fourth order neurons** are located in the **medial geniculate body** of thalamus. It gives rise to auditory radiations that pass through the posterior putamen and adjacent white matter to reach the auditory cortex (Heschl's gyrus in superior temporal gyrus).

Vestibular Pathways

- **Receptors** are the **hair cells** in the membranous labyrinth of the cristae of semicircular canals and maculae of utricle and saccule. The semicircular canals respond to angular acceleration while the utricle and saccule respond to linear acceleration.
- **First order neurons** are located in the **vestibular ganglion of Scarpa** located in the internal acoustic meatus. Axons of these neurons enter the pontomedullary junction along with the auditory fibers.
- **Second order neurons** are located in the medial, lateral, inferior and superior vestibular nuclei in the lower pons and upper medulla. The semicircular canals project mainly to the superior and medial vestibular nucleus, while utricle and saccule project to medial and inferior vestibular nuclei.
- The outputs from the vestibular nuclei project to:
  - The medial longitudinal fasciculus to control the eye movements during head motion
  - Medial vestibulospinal tract to control muscle tone
  - Lateral vestibulospinal tract to control axial muscle tone
  - Reticular formation to control muscle tone
  - Posterior ventral nucleus of thalamus and thence to the vestibular cortex of the temporal lobe.
- In the central pathways, the vestibular fibers for horizontal, vertical and torsional movements diverge. For this reason, central vertigo is accompanied by pure horizontal, vertical or torsional nystagmus, while peripheral vertigo is accompanied by mixed nystagmus.

COCHLEAR NERVE

Methodology and Interpretation

- Examine the general appearance of the patient, response to environmental sounds, head turning while listening, lip reading, speaking in loud voice
- Examine the external ear by otoscope for integrity of tympanic membrane and the external auditory canal
- Perform the CALFRAST and tuning fork tests—Schwabach, Rinne, Weber.

Calibrated Finger Rub Auditory Screening Test (CALFRAST)

- Rub your fingers to test yourself in three positions—arm extended fully, elbow flexed, and then as close to the ear as possible without touching the

ear. If patient can hear at the farthest position, there is no need to test at closer distances.
- Compare your hearing with patient's at approximately same distance
- If patient can hear the softest rub that the examiner can hear with arm extended, his hearing is most likely normal
- If the patient cannot hear the strongest rub that the examiner can hear with arm extended, his hearing is most likely impaired
- Examination at closer distances gives an approximate estimate of the degree of hearing loss.

Schwabach's Test

- Use the tuning fork (256 or 512 Hz) at the patient's ear with the other ear closed by pressing the tragus. Once patient reports inability to hear the sound, check if you can still hear the sound. This indicates impaired hearing in the patient's tested ear
- Repeat the test on the other side.

Rinne Test

- This test compares patient's bone conduction with his air conduction in each ear
- Activate the tuning fork and pace it on the mastoid
- When the patient no longer hears the sound, place it next to his ear.
- If the patient still hears the sound, this implies that his air conduction is better than bone conduction. This has to be reported as "Rinne test positive" or "Rinne test is normal".
- If the patient hears longer over the mastoid than near the ear, it implies that his bone conduction is better than air conduction. This is reported as "Rinne negative" or "abnormal Rinne test".
- Normally, a person can hear twice longer near the ear than over the mastoid
- Positive Rinne is seen in normal persons and in sensorineural hearing loss
- Negative Rinne is seen in conductive hearing loss.

Weber Test

- Place the activated tuning fork over the midline (vertex/forehead/external occipital protuberance)
- Patient has to report if he can hear the sound (not the vibratory sensation) and in which area he can hear the sound
- If the patient reports the origin of sound in the center (midline) area, it implies equal hearing in both ears
- If he can hear it in one ear, it is reported as "Weber's test lateralized" to that side
- If Weber's test is lateralized to one side, it indicates better hearing in that ear. This indicates either conductive hearing loss in that ear or sensorineural hearing loss in the contralateral ear.

Caveats

- If a patient has bilateral conductive or sensorineural hearing loss, Weber's may not be lateralized
- In severe sensorineural hearing loss, bone conduction may be totally absent, while air conduction is minimally preserved
- Thus, Rinne, Weber's test, CALFRAST and Schwabach tests must be used in combination before reaching a conclusion (Table 3.11).

Table 3.11: Interpretation of tuning fork tests.

	Auditory acuity	Rinne test	Weber test
Normal	Preserved	Positive (normal)	Not lateralized
Unilateral CHL	Decreased on one side	Negative (abnormal) on ipsilateral side	Lateralized to the side with decreased hearing
Bilateral CHL	Decreased bilaterally	Bilaterally negative	Lateralized to the more severely affected side or may not lateralize if symmetric
Unilateral SNHL	Decreased ipsilaterally	Positive (normal) both sides	Lateralized to the side with normal hearing
Bilateral SNHL	Decreased bilaterally	Positive (normal bilaterally)	Lateralized to the less affected ear or may not lateralize if hearing loss is symmetric

(CHC: conductive hearing loss; SNHL: sensorineural hearing loss)

VESTIBULAR NERVE

Methodology

The main components to be examined are:
- Vestibulospinal reflexes (past pointing, Romberg, Unterberger-Fukuda stepping test)
- Vestibulo-ocular reflexes (oculocephalic reflex, head impulse test, caloric responses)
- Nystagmus
- Dix hallpike maneuver and static positioning
- Gait.

Vestibulospinal Reflexes

Past Pointing

Methodology
- Patient sits or stands directly in front of the examiner at arms distance

- Examiner and patient stretch their arms forward so that their index fingers just touch each other
- The patient fully raises or lowers his arm and brings it back to original position to touch examiner's finger
- This is repeated several times on one side and then the other side. Both arms can also be tested simultaneously
- Test is done with eyes open and then with eyes closed.

Observation
- Watch for drifting of arm outward from the target (examiner's finger tip)
- Subtle drift is accentuated with eye closure
- The more number of times the test is repeated, the greater is the drift.

Interpretation
- If the ipsilateral arm drifts **outwards** (away from the midline) from the target, it suggests ipsilateral lesion (the normal, more active vestibular system pushes the limb to the abnormal hypoactive side)
- This drift occurs to the hypoactive side when tested with upper limb of either side
- In bilateral symmetrical vestibular disease (as in chronic bilateral vestibulopathy of the elderly), no arm drift will be seen
- Arm drift also resolves with time in vestibular disease due to compensation
- In cerebellar lesions, arm drift can be elicited, but only with the upper limb of the side of the lesion.

Romberg's Test

Methodology
- Patient is asked to stand first with eyes open and then with eyes closed
- If the patient tends to fall to one side, the test is repeated with head turned to ipsilateral side and then to the contralateral side, while noting the direction of falling tendency.

Observations and Interpretation
- If there is marked swaying or fall with eye closed compared to eye open state, it is considered a positive Romberg's test
- This indicates ataxia due to sensory deprivation (impaired joint position sensation or vestibular dysfunction). It is also seen in severe ataxia of any cause including cerebellar lesion
- In vestibular lesion, the direction of falling tendency changes with the direction of head turning before closing the eyes. If there is a left vestibular lesion, the falling tendency will be to the left side with head held straight. It is backward when the head is turned to left, and forward when the head is turned to the right (this occurs because the intact right vestibular system pushes the body **towards** the diseased left vestibular system.

Caveats

Romberg's test may be negative in milder cases. In such circumstances, tandem Romberg (standing with one foot infront of the other with eyes closed) may bring out the deficit.

Unterberger-Fukuda Stepping Test

Methodology
- Patient stands with eye closed
- He has to march at one place with eyes closed for 1 minute.

Observation and interpretation
- Normal person will continue to face more or less in the same direction after marching for 1 minute
- Patient with acute vestibulopathy will slowly rotate to the side of lesion.

Caveats

In chronic vestibulopathy, this test may be normal because of compensation.

Vestibulo-ocular Reflexes

Oculocephalic Reflex

- Used in the evaluation of comatose patients
- Turning of head to one direction normally causes the eyes to move in opposite direction
- This normal response requires the integrity of pathways connecting the vestibular nuclei in the medulla to the nuclei of ocular motor nerves in the pons and midbrain.

Head Thrust (Head impulse) Test

- This test is done in an awake patient
- Ask the patient to look at an object straight ahead
- Suddenly move his head to one direction and then to the other. Notice if the eyes continue to fix on the target during these rapid movements
- If there is impaired vestibule ocular reflex on one side, the eyes move away from the target in the direction of head thrust, followed by visually corrected saccade to refix on the target, in opposite direction to the head thrust.

Caloric Tests

- This can be done in either awake or comatose patients
- In comatose patients, the head is flexed by 30° in supine position. In awake patient, the same position can be used, or the head may be extended towards the ceiling in sitting position

- In comatose patients, 20-50 mL ice cold water is used, while in awake patients, 2-10 mL ice cold water is used
- Ice cold water acts like a temporary lesion of the ipsilateral vestibular system
- This causes a tonic deviation of the eyes to ipsilateral side by the intact contralateral vestibular system
- In an awake patient, this tonic deviation is accompanied by nystagmus with fast component towards the normal side
- A difference of >20% in the duration of nystagmus suggests a lesion on the side with decreased response.

NYSTAGMUS IN VESTIBULAR LESION

Spontaneous Nystagmus

- In acute vestibular disease like labyrinthitis, the spontaneous nystagmus is to the opposite side, as the involved vestibular system is hypoactive. However, in benign aroxysmal positional vertigo (BPPV), the direction is ipsilateral because the lesion is irritative and not destructive
- As three different semicircular canals are involved, the nystagmus is fine and its direction is usually not purely horizontal or vertical, but has a rotary component. In contrast, central nystagmus is usually coarse and is purely horizontal or vertical
- Third degree nystagmus (one which occurs with fast component in the direction of gaze) is usually seen only with vestibular lesions
- Nystagmus that is suppressed by visual fixation is typical of peripheral nystagmus. This suppression can be prevented by using Frenzel's glasses, using which, the typical rotary nystagmus is well visualized
- Failure of visual fixation to suppress the nystagmus suggests central cause for the nystagmus.

Provocative Maneuver (Dix-Hallpike) for BPPV

- The patient is seated on the cot. The head is turned to one side by 45° and the patient is abruptly brought to supine position with the head hanging down from the edge of the cot
- This position is maintained for at least a minute, while observing for reproduction of vertigo and nystagmus, with fast component towards the dependent, diseased ear. In contrast, geotropic nystagmus (fast component away from the ground) is seen with central nystagmus
- In BPPV, there is latency of 3-10 seconds before the symptoms and signs are elicited. They last 20-30 seconds and then abate (habituation or adaptation). In cupulolithiasis, adaptation does not occur because the adherent otoconia are in constant contact with the cupula
- This test is positive only if posterior semicircular canal is involved. It is negative with involvement of other canals.

- When the horizontal semicircular canal is diseased, symptoms and signs are reproduced by the roll test (rolling the head from one side to another).

Central Versus Peripheral Vertigo (Table 3.12)

Table 3.12: Difference between central and peripheral vertigo.

	Central	Peripheral
Severity	Mild	More severe
Associated neurological signs	Present	Absent
Autonomic symptoms (nausea, vomiting, sweating)	Absent	Present
Aural symptoms (tinnitus, deafness, fullness)	Absent	Present

Central Versus Peripheral Nystagmus (Table 3.13)

Table 3.13: Difference between central and peripheral nystagmus.

	Central	Peripheral
Latency	None	3–30 seconds
Direction	Gaze evoked/direction changing	Fixed
Consistency	Less	More
Fatigability	None	Present
Adaptation	None	Present
Axis of nystagmus	Pure horizontal/vertical	Usually rotary (fast phase towards the dependent diseased ear)
Suppression by visual fixation (most valuable clue)	No	Yes
Past pointing	Towards the slow phase of nystagmus, with either limb	In the direction of fast phase
Fukuda test	Rotation towards slow phase of nystagmus	Rotation towards fast phase of nystagmus

SOME PRACTICAL POINTS

- Aural fullness is nonspecific and can occur with external/middle/inner ear disease
- Autophony (reverberation of one's voice) is seen only with external or middle ear disease
- Tinnitus:
  - *High frequency:* Acoustic tumor/presbycusis
  - *Low frequency:* Meniere's disease
- *Pulsatile tinnitus:* Variety of vascular lesions, perilymphatic fistula and idiopathic intracranial hypertension (IIH). Reduced by Valsalva/head turning or pressure over jugular vein

- Lesions of SC canals cause rotatory sensations, those of utricle/saccule cause linear sensation of tilt/levitation
- Tullio's phenomenon in labyrinthine disease, acoustic stimuli produce vertigo and nystagmus perhaps by utricular stimulation
- *Hallpike maneuver:* Suspect central lesion if:
  - Positive test with head turned to either side
  - Direction changing nystagmus
  - Lack of habituation of nystagmus as long as head is positioned down
  - No accompanying nausea
  - Mild or no vertigo inspite of nystagmus. Vertigo that lasts < 60 second
- Vestibular nerve has 2 divisions—superior (saccule and horizontal canal) and inferior (posterior canal). Vestibular neuronitis involves superior division
- Tumarkin Otolithic catastrophe: Acute vertigo with loss of muscle tone and power
- Bilateral meniere's syndrome: Seen in congenital syphilis
- Central vertigo: Chronic (unlike short lived peripheral vertigo)
- Labyrinthine stroke (infarct or hemorrhage) (vestibular artery involvement)
- Tornado epilepsy: Severe vertiginous seizure mimicking labyrinthine disease
- Cogan's syndrome: Vasculitis with tinnitus, vertigo, deafness and interstitial keratitis
- Drug induced vertigo: Aspirin.

BIBLIOGRAPHY

1. Bagai A, Thavendiranathan P, Detsky AS. Does this patient have hearing impairment. JAMA. 2006;295:416-28.
2. Baloh RW. Approach to the evaluation of the dizzy patient. Otolaryngol Head Neck Surg. 1995; 112;3-7.
3. Baloh RW. Episodic vertigo: central nervous system causes. Curr Opin Neurol. 2002;15:17-21.
4. Baloh RW, Honrubia V, Jacobson K. Benign positional; vertigo: clinical and oculographic features in 240 cases. Neurology. 1987;37: 371-8.
5. Baloh RW. Vertigo. Lancet. 1998;352:1841-6.
6. Barraclough K, Bronstein A. Diagnosis in general practice: vertigo. BMJ. 2009;339: b3493.
7. Brazis PW, Masdeu JC, Biller J. Localization in clinical Neurology, 6th ed. Philadelphia: Wolters Kluwer/Lippincott Williams and Wilkins. 2011.
8. Fetter M. Assessing vestibular function: which test, when? J Neurol. 2000;247: 335-42.
9. William W. Campbell. DeJong's The neurologic examination, 7th edition. Wolters Kluwer/Lippincott Williams and Wilkins; 2013.

GLOSSOPHARYNGEAL NERVE (IX N)

GRK Sarma

PHYSIOLOGIC BASIS (FIGS. 3.61 AND 3.62)

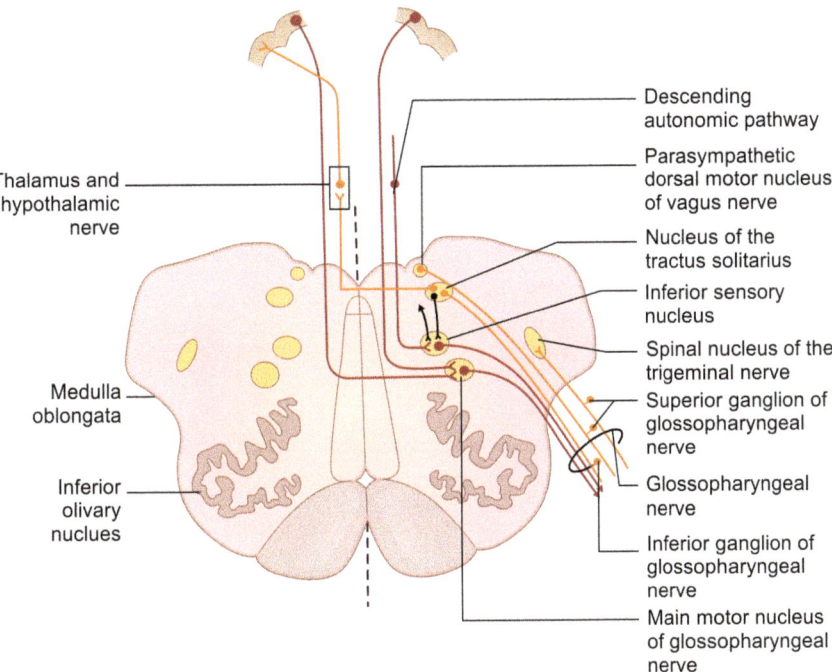

Fig. 3.61: Nuclei of glossopharyngeal nerve.

- The main components of the IX nerve, their nuclei and their functions are listed in the Table 3.14.

Table 3.14: Main components, nuclei and functions of IX nerve.

Component	Nuclei	Function
Motor	Nucleus ambiguus	Stylopharyngeus muscle, pharyngeal constrictors
Special visceral afferents	Nucleus of tractus solitarius	Taste from posterior 1/3 of tongue, pharynx
General visceral afferents	Nucleus tractus solitarius	• Posterior 1/3 of the tongue, pharynx, tonsils, • Chemoreceptor and baroreceptor afferents from carotid body and sinus
General somatic afferents	Spinal nucleus of trigeminal	Mucous membrane of tympanic cavity, mastoid air cells, auditory canal, pharynx, tonsils and posterior 1/3 of the tongue
Parasympathetic	Inferior salivatory nucleus	Parotid gland (secreto motor and vasomotor)

- The supranuclear innervations are bilateral. Therefore, unilateral palatal palsy does not occur with supranuclear lesions
- The nerve emerges from the brainstem in the groove between inferior olive and the inferior cerebellar peduncle. Cerebellopontine angle tumors can involve IX nerve at this level
- The nerve exits through the jugular foramen lateral to the X and XI nerves.
- Then, it enters the carotid sheath between the carotid artery and the jugular vein, descends down and passes between the external and internal carotid arteries
- Then it curves forward on the side of the neck to reach the pharyngeal wall, and terminates into its terminal branches

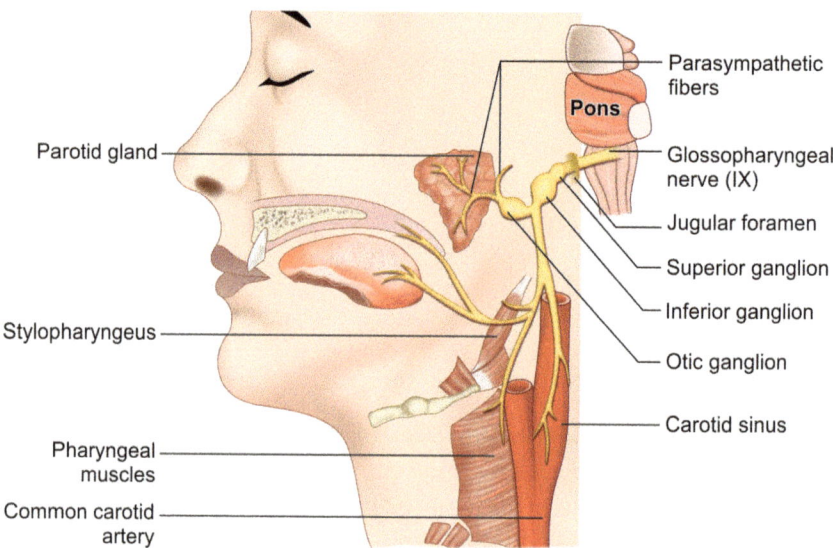

Fig. 3.62: Anatomy of glossopharyngeal nerve.

- The branches of IX nerve are: Tympanic, carotid, pharyngeal, lingual, tonsillar, muscular.

METHODOLOGY

For examination purposes, IX nerve is essentially a sensory nerve because other functions cannot be tested bedside.
- *Inspection:*
  - Slight palatal droop, mild dysphagia may be seen.
  - On vocalization, palate elevates symmetrically in isolated IX nerve lesions, but not if X is also involved.
  - Stylopharyngeus cannot be examined in isolation

- Sensory function is tested by assessing the taste on the posterior 1/3 of the tongue.
  - Ask pt to put out his tongue, hold with gloved hand or gauze piece.
  - Swab stick with a test item (sugar, salt, bitter and sour) is applied over the posterior tongue bilaterally
  - Patient is asked to indicate the taste by pointing to the taste name card.
- *Palatal reflex:*
  - Stimulate one side of soft palate with a swab stick
  - Look for elevation of the palate and ipsilateral deviation of the uvula in the normal person
  - If IX nerve is involved, this response is blunted
  - Afferent: IX; efferent IX and X
- *Pharyngeal reflex:*
  - Stimulate the posterior pharyngeal wall in the region of anterior faucial pillar with a swab stick
  - Note the elevation and constriction of the pharyngeal wall and elevation of the tongue
  - Afferent: IX, efferent IX and X
- *Autonomic:* Not tested bedside.

INTERPRETATION

As only limited functions are amenable to assessment, IX nerve lesions are localized by the associated deficits
- Exaggerated gag reflex (retching and vomiting on pharangeal stimulatin): UMN lesions of the coricobulbar fibers (pseudobulbar palsy)
- Long tract signs: Intrinsic brainstem lesion
- V, VIII associated lesion: Cerebellopontine angle (CPA) lesion
- IX, X, XI: Jugular foramen lesion
- IX, X, XI, XII: Retropharangeal or retroparotid space lesion
- Neuralgia in IX nerve distribution; idiopathic or compressive (tumors, infection,) and demyelination (occasionally multiple sclerosis)
- Unilateral weakness: Most likely LMN (UMN lesions have to be bilateral to produce deficits)
- Autonomic dysfunction in Guillain-Barre syndrome (GBS) is due to IX nerve involvement.

CAVEATS

- The gag reflex may be bilaterally absent in nearly 30% normal persons
- Hyperactive reflex may also be seen in some healthy persons
- The palatal sensation may be normal even in the presence of IX nerve lesion because of the contribution by the trigeminal nerve.

VAGUS NERVE (X N)

GRK Sarma

PHYSIOLOGIC BASIS

- The supranuclear control of the vagus is bilateral, but predominantly crossed
- Four nuclei contribute to the vagus nerve (Fig. 3.63):
    - **Nucleus ambiguus**: motor fibers to the skeletal muscles of pharynx and larynx. It also innervates the heart (parasympathetic fibers).
    - **Dorsal motor nucleus** of vagus: Fibers to the smooth muscles of pharynx, larynx, and parasympathetic fibers to thoracic (except the heart) and abdominal viscera
    - **Nucleus solitarius**: General visceral afferents from pharynx, larynx, viscera of thorax and abdomen, and the aortic receptors (baroreceptors and chemoreceptors).
    - **Nucleus of the spinal tract of the trigeminal** nerve: General somatic sensation from the pharynx, larynx, ear canal, external surface of the tympanic membrane and meninges of the posterior fossa

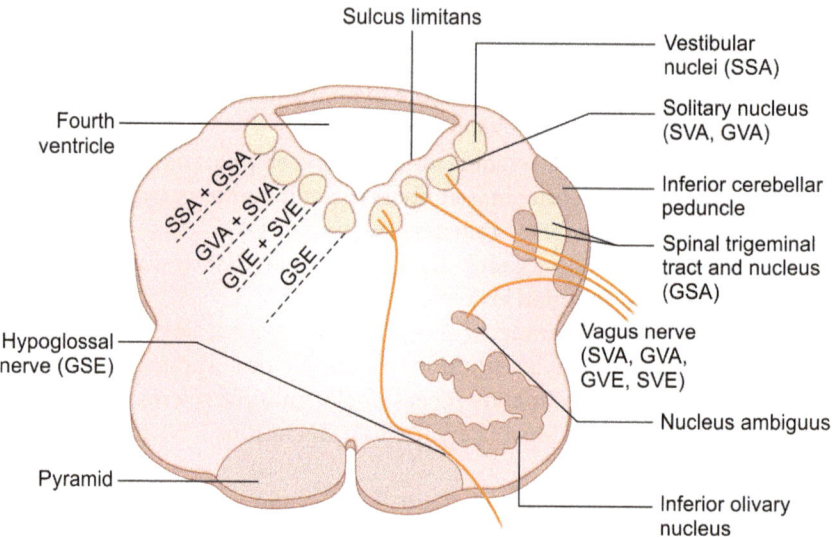

Fig. 3.63: Schematic cross-section of lower brainstem to show various cranial nerve nuclei and their functions.
(SSA: special somatic afferent; GSA: general somatic afferent; SVA: special visceral afferent; GVA: general visceral afferent; GVE: general visceral efferent; SVE: special visceral efferent; GSE: general somatic efferent)

- The more cephalad portion of the X nucleus represents pharyngeal and palatal muscles, while the more caudal region represents larynx. Lesions of the brainstem, thus, can cause selective weakness of pharynx and palate, sparing the larynx.
- The vagus nerve emerges from the medulla below the IX nerve, traverses the jugular foramen and enters the carotid sheath (Figs. 3.64 and 3.65)
- It travels between the carotid artery and the jugular vein to the base of the neck
- In the upper part of the neck, it gives off the **pharyngeal** and the **superior laryngeal** branches. In the lower part of the neck, it gives **recurrent laryngeal** nerves
- The **pharyngeal branches** innervate:
    - Uvular muscle (shortens and bends the uvula backwards to block nasal passage while swallowing)
    - Levator palatini (raises the soft palate while swallowing to block the nasal passages)
    - Palatopharyngeus (draws the pharyngopalatine arches together to close the faucial orifice, depress the soft palate and elevate the thyroid cartilage and pharynx)
    - Salpingopharyngeus (works along with palatopharyngeus)
    - Palatoglossus (elevates the posterior part of the tongue and depresses the soft palate)
    - Pharyngeal constrictors (force the food into esophagus while swallowing).
- The **superior laryngeal** nerve innervates the cricothyroid muscle (the chief tensor of the vocal cords). It is mainly a sensory nerve to the larynx.
- The recurrent laryngeal nerves arise from the lower part of the neck and take different course on each side. The right recurrent laryngeal nerve loops under the subclavian artery, while the left-sided one loops under the aortic arch.
- The **recurrent laryngeal** nerve innervates the laryngeal muscles except the cricothyroid:
    - *Posterior cricoarytenoid:* Abduct the vocal cords
    - *Lateral cricoarytenoids:* Adductors of vocal cords
    - *Thyroarytenoids:* Shorten and relax the vocal cords
    - *Arytenoid muscle:* Closes the glottic rim by approximating the arytenoids.
- The vagus continues into the thoracic and abdominal cavities to supply the viscera.

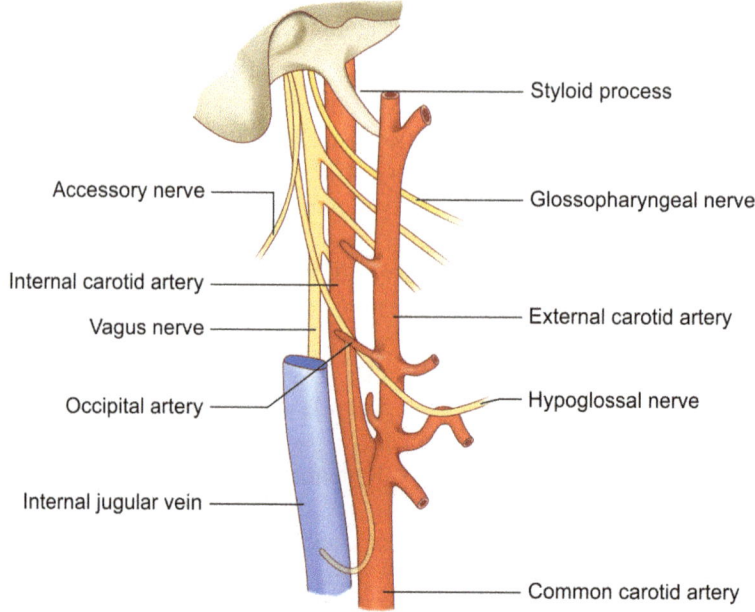

Fig. 3.64: Course and the branches of the vagus nerve.

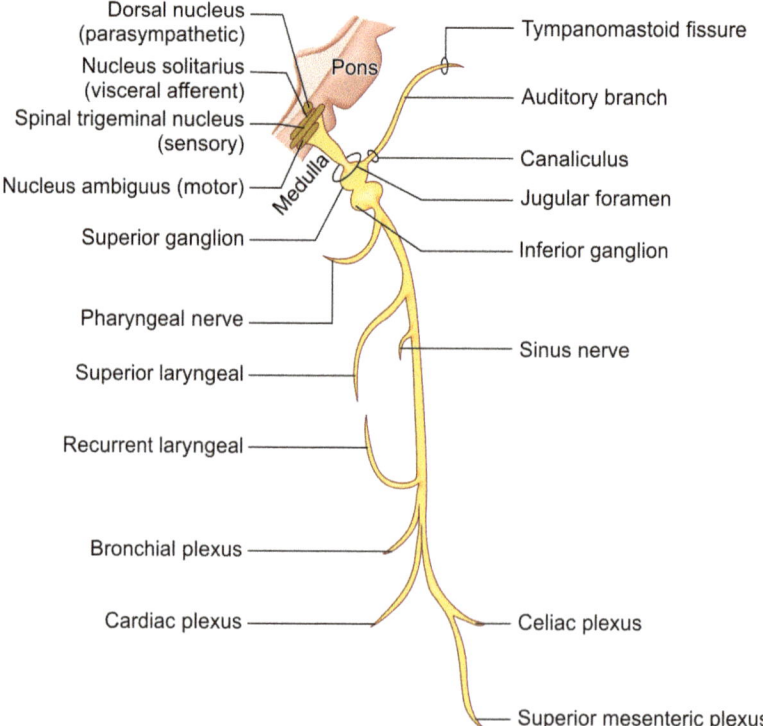

Fig. 3.65: The course and branches of the vagus nerve.

METHODOLOGY

Four components of vagus are available for testing:
1. *Sensory functions* are not routinely tested
2. *Autonomic functions* are discussed in a separate chapter
3. Motor functions
4. Reflexes.

Motor Functions

- Examine the uvula, palate, pharynx and the larynx
- *Uvula:*
  - Position of uvula at rest (midline or deviated)
  - Position of uvula on phonation (midline or deviated).
- *Palate and pharynx:*
  - Examine at rest for symmetry of the palatal arches
  - Examine the degree of elevation of palatal arches on phonation (patient says 'aah')
  - *Palatal and pharyngeal reflexes:* described in the section on IX nerve
  - Assess the voice for nasal quality
  - Assess for nasal regurgitation while swallowing.
- *Larynx:*
  - *Voice:*
    - Assess the voice quality while talking. Look for breathy voice in adductor palsy and diplophonia
    - If this is normal, ask patient to turn head to either side and re-assess for hoarseness of the voice
    - Laryngoscopy is required for more accurate assessment.
  - *Swallowing:*
    - Assess for choking while swallowing
    - Look for elevation of larynx on either side during swallowing.

Reflexes

- *Palatal reflex:* Described above
- *Pharyngeal reflex:* Described above
- *Nasal (sneeze or sternutatory) reflex:* Stimulation of the nasal mucosa with a cotton wisp produces forceful exhalation resembling a sneeze.
  - Afferents: V nerve,
  - Efferents: VII, IX and X nerve.
- Other reflexes (oculocardiac, carotid sinus, vomiting and hiccup) are not tested bedside routinely.

INTERPRETATION

- Deviation of uvula to one side suggests contralateral weakness

- The median raphe normally raises in the midline during phonation. A deviation to one side suggests contralateral weakness
- Flattening and drooping of the palatal arch on one side suggests weakness of the levator veli palatini on that side. It must be remembered that tensor veli palatine (trigeminal innervated) may prevent complete drooping
- Bilateral flattening, drooping and immobility suggest bilateral levator veli palatini weakness. Again, tensor veli palatini may prevent complete drooping
- Nasal twang to voice and nasal regurgitation indicate velopharyngeal insufficiency. In unilateral lesions, it may be transient, in bilateral lesions, it is more chronic
- Greater difficulty to swallow liquids is seen with palatal weakness because of nasal regurgitation. Equal difficulty for liquids and solids is seen with pharyngeal weakness
- Curtain movement (movement of pharyngeal wall to one side on pharyngeal stimulation) indicates contralateral pharyngeal weakness
- Hoarseness of voice indicates vocal cord adductor weakness due to recurrent laryngeal nerve palsy. Other findings in this lesion include low volume, short phrases and mild inspiratory stridor, diplophonia on vowel prolongation (due to unequal frequencies of the two vocal cords). On laryngoscopy, the paralyzed vocal cord is near the midline, while the healthy cord crosses the midline to meet it
- In mild cases, hoarseness is noted only when head is turned to one side
- Unilateral failure of laryngeal elevation during swallowing indicates ipsilateral pharyngeal muscle weakness
- Stridor indicates abductor paralysis. It is more severe in bilateral recurrent laryngeal nerve palsies
- *Localization of vagal nerve lesions is guided by the following findings:*
    - *Upper neck level:* Pharyngeal and laryngeal weakness
    - *Lower neck level/recurrent laryngeal nerve lesion:* Only laryngeal weakness
    - *Superior laryngeal nerve lesion:* Minimal hoarseness, laryngeal sensory loss
    - *Jugular foramen:* IX, X, XI palsy
    - *Retroparotid or retropharyngeal:* IX, X, XI, XII palsy
    - *Brainstem lesions:* Associated long tract signs. More cephalad lesions cause palatopharyngeal weakness, sparing larynx due to somatotopic organization
    - *Cortical lesions:* Mostly bilateral lesions are required to produce dysfunction, that manifests as 'pseudobulbar palsy'.

BIBLIOGRAPHY

1. Brazis PW, Masdeu JC, Biller J. Localization in clinical neurology, 6th edition. Philadelphia: Wolters Kluwer/Lippincott Williams and Wilkins; 2011.
2. Campbell WW. DeJong's. The Neurologic examination, 7th edition. Wolters Kluwer/Lippincott Williams and Wilkins.
3. Davies AE, Kidd D, Stone SP, et al. Pharyngeal sensation and gag reflex in healthy subjects. Lancet. 1995;345:487-8.
4. Drulias C, Tzinas S, Harlafatis N Jr, et al. The superior laryngeal nerve. Am surg. 1976;42:635-8.
5. Erman EB, Alexandra E, Kejner BS, et al. Disorders of cranial nerves IX and X. Semin Neurol. 2009;29: 85-92.
6. Hughes TA, Wiles CM. Palatal and pharyngeal reflexes in health and in motor neuron disease. J Neurol Neurosurg Psychiatry. 1996;61:96-8.

ACCESSORY CRANIAL NERVE (XI N)

GRK Sarma

PICTORIAL PRETEST

This 30-year-old man is admitted with acute stroke and right hemiplegia.

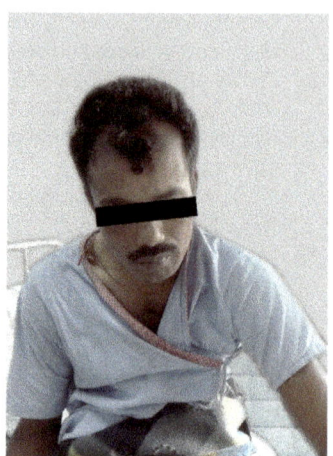

Questions

1. Comment on the direction of the head tilt.
2. Identify which muscle is weak and on which side.
3. Can you explain the head tilt in this patient with left hemispheric infarction and right-sided hemiplegia?

PHYSIOLOGICAL BASIS (FIGS. 3.66 AND 3.67)

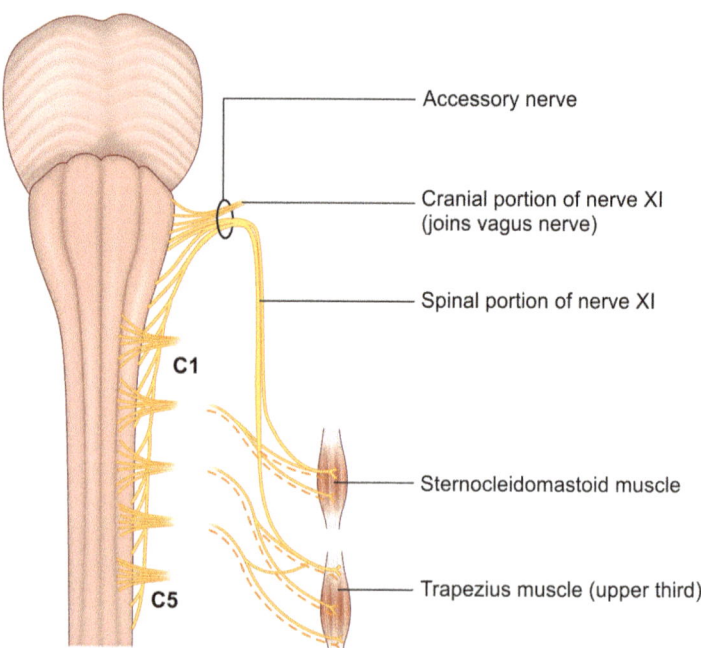

Fig. 3.66: Schematic diagram of XI cranial nerve and its branches.

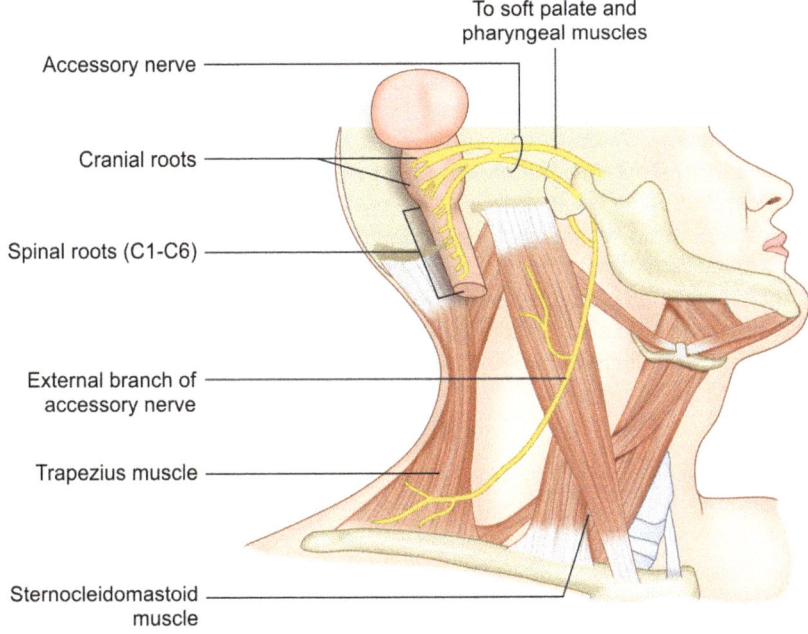

Fig. 3.67: Cranial and spinal branches of XI cranial nerve.

- *Cranial nerve XI comprises of two components:* Cranial and spinal
- The cranial component cannot be tested separately from the vagus nerve
- The spinal component is tested by examining two neck muscles; Sternocleidomastoid (SCM) anteriorly and trapezius posteriorly
- Cranial component arises in medulla from caudal portion of nucleus ambiguus and dorsal motor nucleus of vagus. It emerges from medulla below X nerve rootlets, joins the spinal component in the jugular foramen and leave it shortly, to join the X nerve. It innervates, through recurrent laryngeal nerve, all the intrinsic muscles of larynx except cricothyroid
- The spinal portion arises from ventral horn cells in C2-6 segments of cervical cord, which are in continuity with nucleus ambiguus (NA), emerges between anterior and posterior roots, ascends into cranium through foramen magnum to exit through jugular foramen. The spinal portion descends close to internal jugular vein to enter the posterior aspect of sternocleidomastoid. After innervating the SCM, it emerges from the middle of its posterior border, near the greater auricular nerve, passes through the posterior triangle of neck to enter the upper border of trapezius and supplies it
- The SCM is neck flexor and rotator of head to opposite side. Acting together, both SCM cause neck flexion, bring the head forward and downward
- Trapezius is a neck extensor. It also elevates, retracts and rotates the shoulder, causing abduction above 90°. Its lower fibers depress the scapula and stabilize it.

- Dissociation of weakness of SCM and trapezius can occur at supranuclear, nuclear and infranuclear levels (Figs. 3.68 A to C)
- The supranuclear innervation to both SCM and trapezius is bilateral, but predominantly ipsilateral for SCM and predominantly contralateral for trapezius. Theoretically, thus, dissociation of weakness of SCM and trapezius can occur, but is overshadowed by compensatory action of other neck muscles
- At nuclear level, SCM is represented in the proximal part and trapezius in the distal part of the nucleus. Here, dissociation of weakness of SCM and trapezius can occur with lesions involving either cell groups
- At infranuclear level dissociation of SCM and trapezius weakness can occur in lesions involving posterior triangle of neck, after the nerve exits SCM (which is spared).

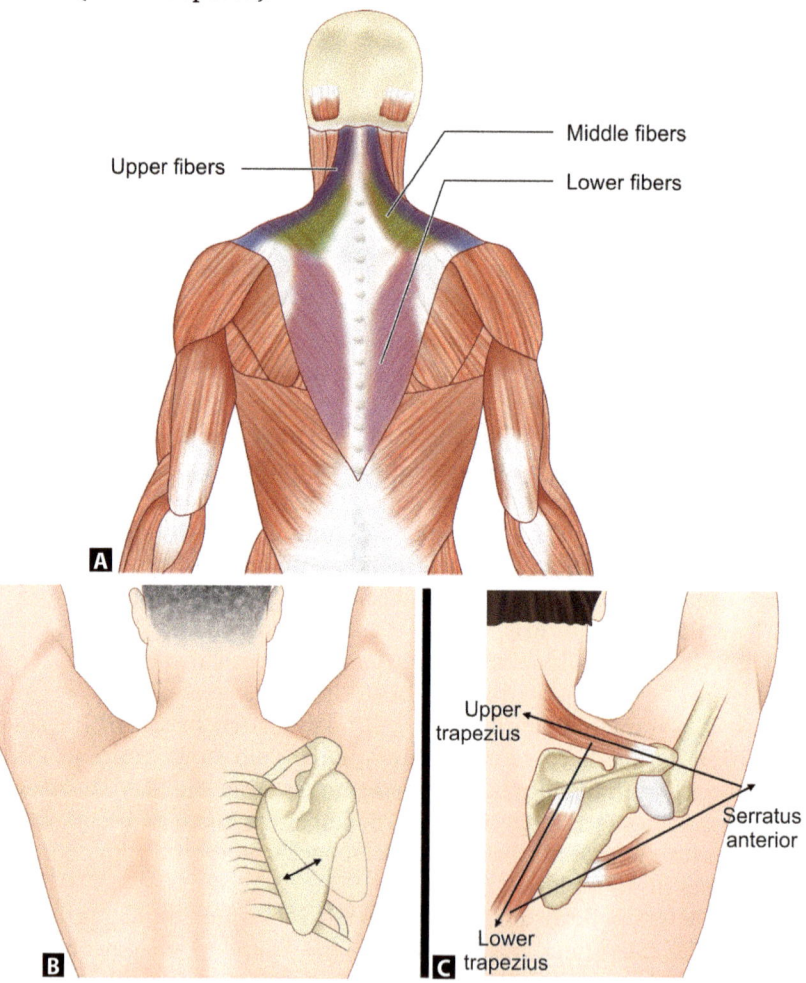

Figs. 3.68A to C: Upper and lower trapezius muscle fibers and their line of action on scapula contrasted with that of serratus anterior to understand different patterns of scapular winging.

METHODOLOGY

A. *Inspect for:*
   - Head tilt, deviation to one side
   - Head drop forward or backward
   - Winging of scapula; assess if it changes with arm abduction or shoulder protrusion
   - Squaring of shoulder
   - Drooping of shoulder
   - Flattening of trapezius ridge
   - Wasting, fasciculations of SCM, trapezius
   - Head lag on sitting from supine.
B. *Palpation and power* assessment: Palpate the muscles for assessing the bulk and tone.

Testing Sternocleidomastoid

- Ask the patient to turn his head to opposite side against your resistance. Feel and observe the muscle during this action
- Assess neck flexion against resistance (Both SCM required).

Testing Trapezius

- Ask the patient to shrug his shoulder against your resistance (upper fibers)
- Assess shoulder abduction above 90° against your resistance (upper fibers)
- Ask the patient to abduct his arm horizontally with palm facing upwards Then attempt to push his elbow forward (Lower and middle fibers required for this action)
- Assess neck extension in prone position (Both trapezii required).

INTERPRETATION

- *Thin elongated neck:* Sternomastoid wasting
- *Head drop backwards:* Bilateral SCM weakness
- *Head tilt and deviation to one side:* Ipsilateral SCM weakness (head turns to the weak side)
- Inability to flex neck against resistance indicates SCM weakness bilaterally
- Head lag when patient arises from supine suggests bilateral SCM weakness. Compensatory platysma over action may be visible
- *Head drop forward:* bilateral trapezius weakness
- *Shoulder drooping:* ipsilateral trapezius weakness
- *Loss of trapezius contour and squaring of shoulder:* trapezius weakness
- Winging of scapula suggests trapezius weakness. Here, the winging becomes more prominent on abduction of shoulder and decreases on protrusion.

- In trapezius weakness, the scapula is displaced downward and laterally and the inferior angle of scapula typically juts out (Compare with winging in serratus anterior weakness).

CAVEATS

- Winging of scapula is also seen in weakness of serratus anterior. However, here, the winging increases on forward movement of the shoulder as in pushing against a wall.
- Neck flop in parkinsonism may be mistaken as neck extensor weakness. But on formal testing, the strength of trapezii will be normal.
- Abnormal head position is also common in cervical dystonia. This is identified by the fact that the involved muscles are often hypertrophied and taut, rather than atrophic and flaccid as in LMN weakness.
- Trapezius weakness can cause chronic shoulder drooping, traction and muscular pain, secondary adhesive capsulitis. Thus, patients with painful shoulder conditions must be examined carefully for trapezius weakness, lest the original cause of painful shoulder is left untreated.

Causes of Dropped Head Syndrome

- Inflammatory myopathies
- Myasthenia gravis
- Motor neuron disease
- Isolated neck extensor myopathy
- Adult onset acid maltase deficiency
- Chronic inflammatory demyelinating polyneuropathy (CIDP)
- Desmin myopathy
- Nemaline myopathy
- Lambert-Eaton myasthenic syndrome (LEMS)
- Myotonic dystrophy
- Hypothyroidism
- Hypoparathyroidism
- Syringomyelia

ANSWERS TO THE PRETEST

- The head is rotated and tilted to the left.
- This suggests left sternocleidomastoid weakness.
- This patient has right hemiplegia, but his left sternocleidomastoid is weak. This is because, the motor cortex stores "movement information" and not "individual muscle information". Thus, the left hemisphere controls head turning to the right (i.e. the left sternocleidomastoid) and the right hemisphere controls head turning to the left (i.e. the right sternocleidomastoid). Thus, the left hemispheric stroke in this patient weakened the ipsilateral sternocleidomastoid and caused head turning to the left side.

BIBLIOGRAPHY

1. Al-Shaklee A, Katirji B. Spinal accessory neuropathy, droopy shoulder and thoracic outlet syndrome. Muscle Nerve. 2003;28:383-5.
2. Berardelli A, Prior A. corticobulbar and corticospinal projections to neck muscles motoneurons in man. A functional study with magnetic and electrical transcranial brain stimulation. Exp Brain Res. 1991;87:402-6.
3. Berry H, Ea M, Mrazek AC. Accessory nerve palsy: a review of 23 cases. Can J Neurosci. 1991;18:337.
4. Brazis PW, Masdeu JC, Biller J. Localization in clinical neurology, 6th edition. Philadelphia: Wolters Kluwer/Lippincott Williams and Wilkins; 2011.
5. Campbell WW. DeJong's The neurologic examination, 7th edition. Wolters Kluwer/Lippincott Williams and Wilkins; 2013.
6. Fitzgerald T. Sternomastoid paradox. Clin Anat. 2001;14:330-1.
7. Massey EW. Spinal accessory nerve lesions. Semin Neurol. 2009;29: 82-4.
8. Nalini A, Ravishankar S. Dropped head syndrome in syringomyelia: report of 2 cases. J Neurol Neurosurg Psychiatry. 2005;76:290-91.

HYPOGLOSSAL NERVE (XII N)

GRK Sarma

PICTORIAL PRETEST

Both the pictures belong to the same patient.

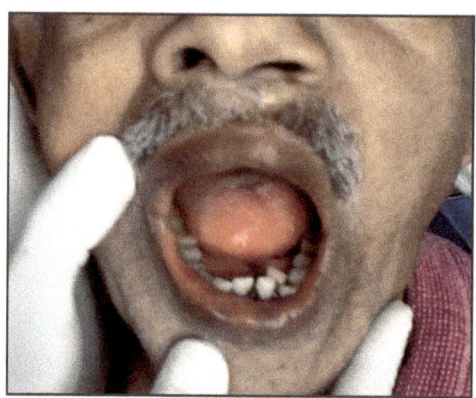

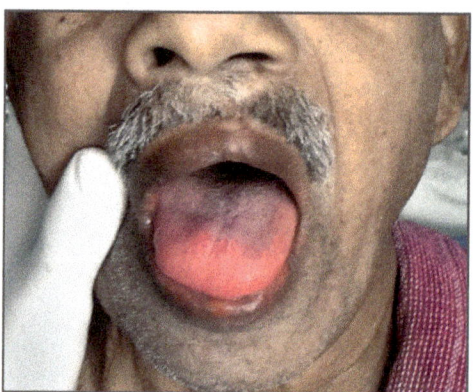

Question

1. Explain the variable tongue deviation and identify the correct side of tongue weakness.

Cranial Nerves

Anatomical and Physiological Basis (Figs. 3.69 and 3.70)

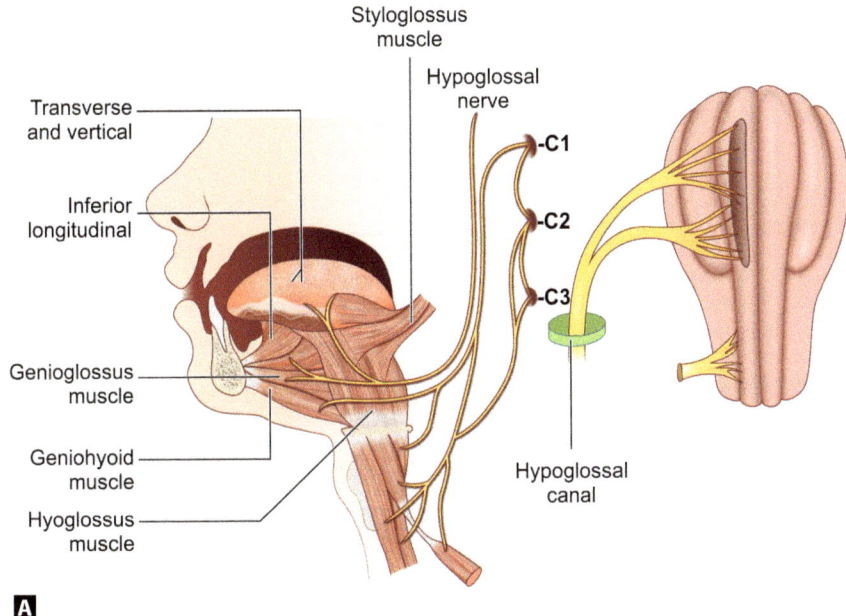

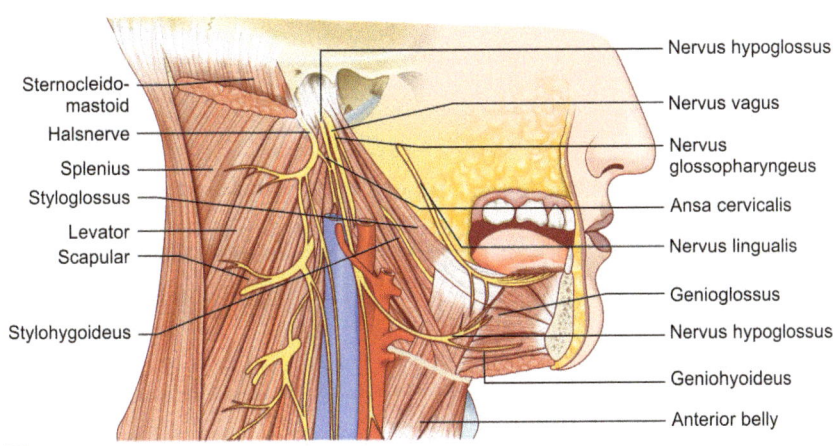

Figs. 3.69A and B

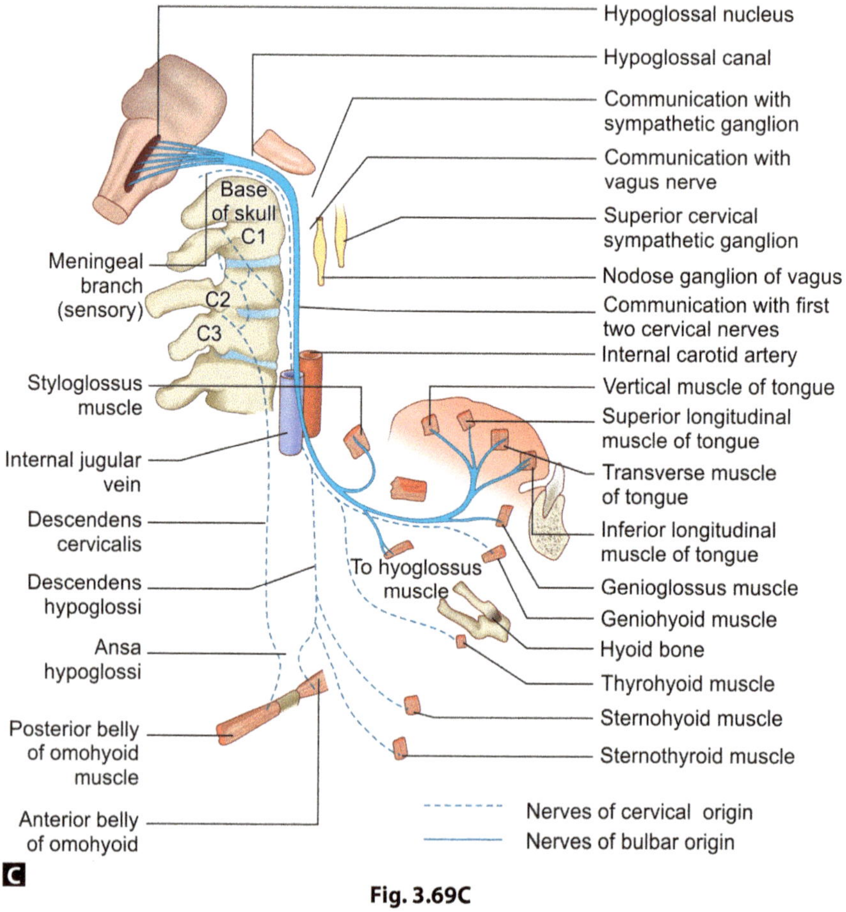

Fig. 3.69C

Figs. 3.69A to C: Course and branches of XII cranial nerve.

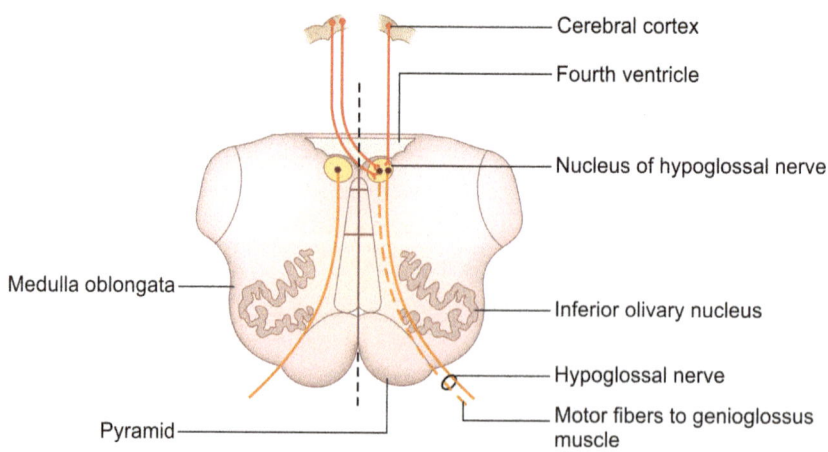

Fig. 3.70: Anatomy and course of XII cranial nerve in the brainstem.

- It is a pure motor nerve that supplies all **the intrinsic and extrinsic muscles** of the tongue. These are longitudinal, transverse and vertical (intrinsic) muscles, genioglossus, geniohyoid, hyoglossus and styloglossus (extrinsic muscles)
- The longitudinal column of hypoglossal nucleus lies at the floor of the 4th ventricle in the paramedian region. The nuclei of both the sides lie in close proximity here so that a lesion in this area can cause bilateral lower motor neuron palsy of the hypoglossal nerve
- The fibers from the nucleus travel lateral to the medial lemniscus, medial longitudinal fasciculus and the pyramid. A lesion at this level can produce the combination of deficits including ipsilateral 12th nerve palsy, INO, contralateral hemiparesis, and hemianesthesia
- The hypoglossal nerve emerges from the medulla between the pyramid and the inferior olive and then pass through the anterior occipital condylar foramen to begin the extracranial course. Lesions (usually metastases) at the occipital condyle, thus produce occipital pain and tongue weakness (occipital condyle syndrome)
- At the base of the skull, the XII nerve is in close proximity to IX, X, XI nerves. Lesions at the skull base can cause variable combination of these cranial nerve deficits
- In the extracranial region, the nerve descends vertically close to the internal carotid artery and internal jugular vein, along with IX and X nerves and the sympathetic chain
- Below the angle of the mandible, it turns anteriorly and reaches the tongue to supply all the extrinsic and intrinsic muscles
- Supranuclear control of the XII nerve is by corticobulbar fibers originating from the lower portion of the precentral gyrus. These pass through the internal capsule and descend to pontomedullary junction where they decussate. Genioglossus has only contralateral innervations, while other tongue muscles have bilateral representation
- The longitudinal intrinsic muscle on each side helps to retract the tongue backwards and ipsilaterally. This is opposite to the action of genioglossus that protrudes and pushes the tongue to the other side. Therefore, in unilateral XII nerve palsy, the unprotruded tongue is deviated to the contralateral (healthy side), but on protrusion, it is deviated to the ipsilateral (weaker) side.

Methodology

- *Inspection:* Ask the patient to open his mouth, with tongue placed inside. Note the size, shape, position of the tongue, tremors, chorea, dyskinesias and fasciculations, if any. Ask the patient to protrude the tongue and observe for any deviation from the midline.
- *Palpation:* After wearing the gloves, feel the tone of the tongue. Ask the patient to press one cheek at a time with his tongue tip against your finger placed on the cheek (outer aspect) and assess the power.

- *Percussion:* Tap the tongue with a blunt point (for example, tongue depressor blade) and watch for myotonia (this test is needed only in patients suspected to have myotonia).

Observations

- Note increased furrowing in atrophy
- Hypertrophy
- Fasciculations
- On protrusion, note any deviation of tip of the tongue to one side
- Note spasticity/hypotonia
- Note decreased force of tongue pressure against resistance
- Note myotonia.

Interpretation

- Enlarged tongue may be seen in some myopathies like Duchenne's, and in amyloidosis, hypothyroidism, Down's syndrome
- Atrophic tongue indicates lower motor neuron lesion involving the hypoglossal nerve, including motor neuron disease
- Atrophy on one half of the tongue indicates ipsilateral hypoglossal nerve lesion
- On protrusion of tongue, deviation of its tip to one side indicates weakness of ipsilateral genioglossus or contralateral upper motor neuron lesion. These are differentiated by the tone of the tongue and presence of fasciculations
- On percussion, persistent dimpling suggests myotonia, which is classically seen in myotonic dystrophy.

Caveats

- Some normal tongues have corrugated edges and deep furrows and should be differentiated from true atrophy by associated signs
- The tongue normally shows little movements, especially on protrusion. This can be minimized by observing it at complete rest
- Patients with buccolingual apraxia find it difficult to protrude the tongue on command. This can be differentiated from true pseudobulbar palsy by the fact that spontaneous tongue movements like smacking of lips and speech may be preserved
- In patients with unilateral facial palsy, the protruded tongue may appear to be deviated because of the facial asymmetry. This can be overcome by drawing the angle of the mouth towards the paralyzed side
- The deviation of the tongue tip at rest and on protrusion may be in opposite directions and mislead the examiner. It must be understood that, on protrusion, the intact genioglossus **pushes** the tip of the tongue **towards the paralyzed side**. But, at rest, the intact intrinsic muscles of the tongue on normal side **pull** the tongue **towards the normal side**.

ANSWER TO THE PRETEST

In first figure, the tongue appears deviated to left as indicated by the median furrow. In second figure, the tongue appears deviated to the right. These deviations in opposite directions can be understood by the differences in the anatomy of intrinsic and extrinsic muscles of the tongue.

On protrusion, the intact genioglossus pushes the tip of the tongue towards the paralyzed side. But, at rest, the intact intrinsic muscles of the tongue on normal side pull the tongue towards the normal side. Hence, it can be concluded that in this patient, there is right hypoglossal nerve palsy.

BIBLIOGRAPHY

1. Brazis PW, Masdeu JC, Biller J. Localization in clinical neurology, 6th edition. Philadelphia: Wolters Kluwer/Lippincott Williams and Wilkins; 2011.
2. Campbell WW. DeJong's the neurologic examination, 7th edition. Wolters Kluwer/Lippincott Williams and Wilkins; 2013
3. Capobianco DJ, Brazis PW, Rubino FA, et al. Occipital condyle syndrome. Headache. 2002;42:142-6.
4. Keane JR. Twelfth nerve palsy: analysis of 100 cases. Arch Neurol. 1996;53:561-6.
5. Lance JW, Anthony M. Neck tongue syndrome on sudden turning of head. J Neurol Neurosurg Psychiatry. 1980;43:97-101.
6. Lin HC, Barkhaus PE. Cranial nerve XII: the hypoglossal nerve. Semin Neurol. 2009;29: 45-52.
7. Riggs JE. Distinguishing between extrinsic and intrinsic tongue muscle weakness in unilateral hypoglossal palsy. Neurology. 1984;34:1367.
8. Umapathi T, Venkatasubramanian N, Leck KJ, et al. Tongue deviation in acute ischemic stroke: a study of supranuclear twelfth cranial nerve palsy in 300 stroke patients. Cerebrovasc Dis. 2000;10:462-5.

CHAPTER 4

Motor System

GRK Sarma

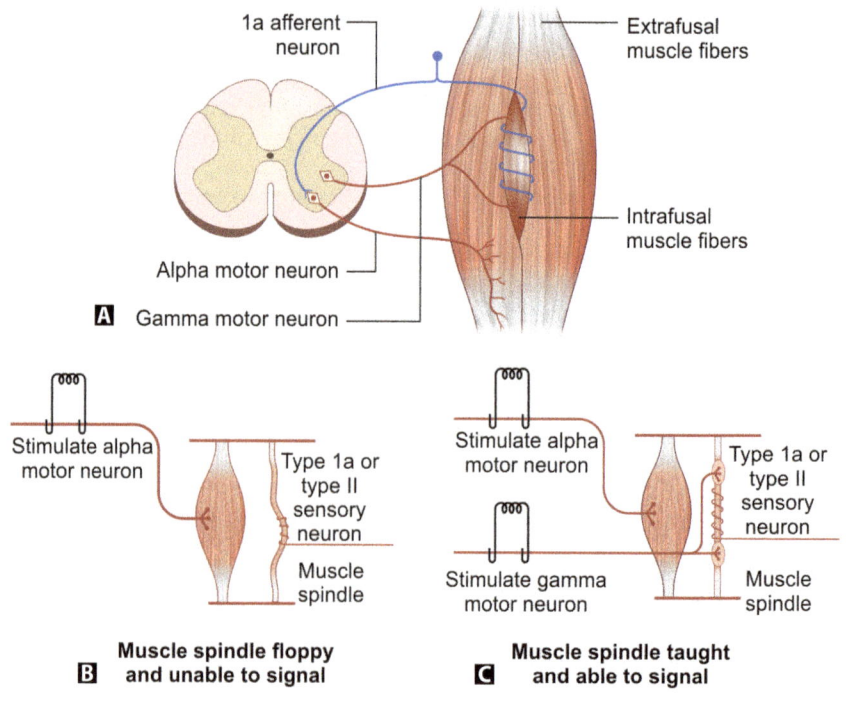

Figs. 4.1A to C: Spinal segmental control of muscle tone and the alpha-gamma coactivation.

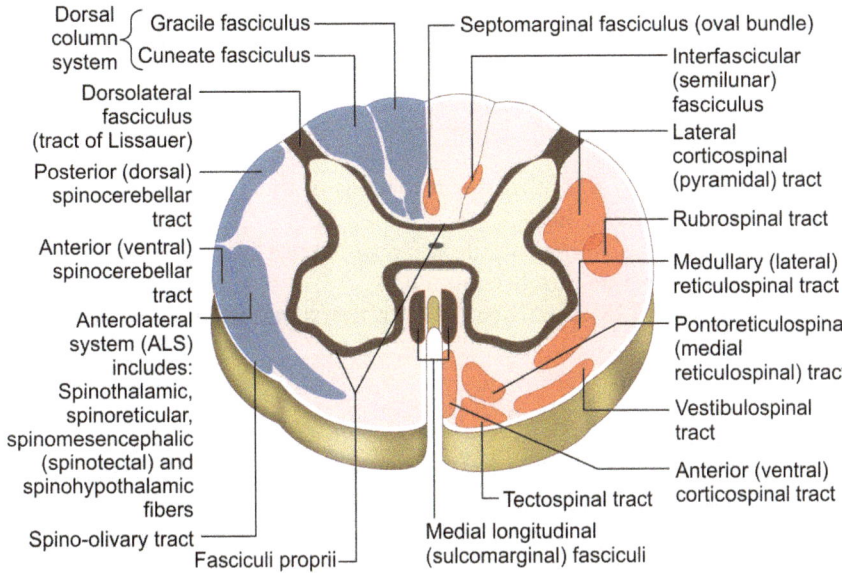

Fig. 4.2: Descending influences that modulate muscle tone.

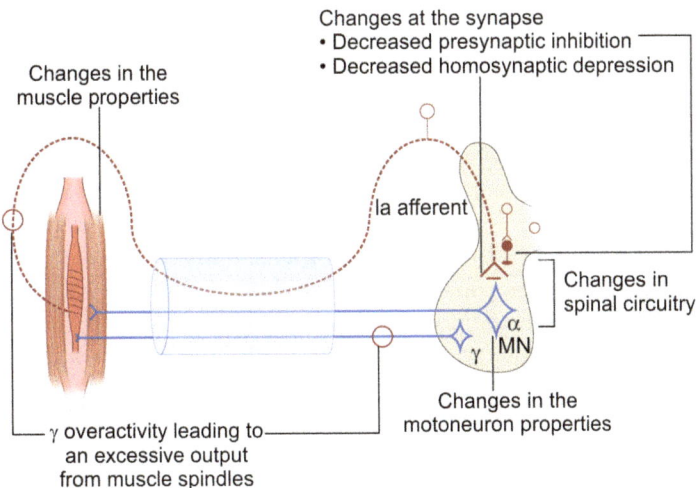

Fig. 4.3: Pathogenesis of spasticity.

MUSCLE TONE

Physiologic Basis

- Muscle tone is defined as the resistance of a relaxed muscle to passive movement
- It is produced by the inherent properties of the muscle like viscosity, elasticity, and extensibility
- It determines the resting attitude and position of a limb. It also determines the efficiency of the muscle contraction
- It is maintained by spinal segmental reflexes and modulated by supraspinal influences.

Spinal Segmental Control

- Skeletal muscles contain **extrafusal** fibers (contractile units) and **intrafusal** fibers (muscle spindles)
- The muscle spindles are supplied by the efferent gamma motor neurons and the afferent **Group Ia fibers** (that discharge in **phasic** manner) and **Group II** (A Beta) fibers (that discharge in **tonic** manner)
- When a muscle is passively stretched while testing muscle tone, essentially **the spindles** are stretched, their afferents fire repetitively and activate the alpha motor neurons of the same muscle, causing contraction
- The same afferents activate the inter-neurons which release inhibitory transmitters to the alpha motor neurons of the various other muscles causing their relaxation. These include **presynaptic, reciprocal and recurrent inhibitory interneurons**. Impaired activation of these interneurons by corticospinal, reticulospinal and rubrospinal tracts plays a major role in development of **spasticity**. Some of these tracts also play a role in **rigidity** (see below)
- The gamma motor neurons cause muscle spindle contraction during voluntary action. In the absence of this activity, the spindles become lax when the muscle contracts and lose their ability to activate the alpha motor neurons. During **normal voluntary action**, therefore, both alpha and gamma motor neurons are activated (**alpha-gamma coactivation**).

Supraspinal Influences

Rubrospinal Tract

- Originates from the caudal part of red nucleus in the midbrain and immediately crosses to the opposite side. Red nucleus is in turn influenced by corticospinal tract and cerebellum (globose and emboliform nuclei)
- It descends in the spinal cord, just anterior to the lateral corticospinal tract and terminates mostly over the anterior horn cells and to some extent over the inhibitory and excitatory interneurons
- The predominant pattern of rubrospinal activation is excitation of **limb flexors** and inhibition of limb extensors

- It also backs up the lateral corticospinal tract in control of **distal fine activities**. Therefore, the disability is greater if both these tracts are damaged.

Reticulospinal Tracts

These are important **regulators of basic tone and posture**
- The **medial (pontine)** reticulospinal tract terminates on the ipsilateral alpha and gamma motor neurons directly to favor **axial trunk muscle extensor** action. It is driven by **somatosensory input** and its dysfunction is responsible for exaggerated cutaneous reflexes in myelopathies.
- The **lateral (medullary)** reticulospinal tract terminates bilaterally on anterior horn cells as well as interneurons and favors **predominantly flexor** action. It is driven heavily by inputs from motor, premotor and supplementary motor cortical inputs.

Vestibulospinal Tracts

These are also important, along with reticulospinal tracts, in controlling the tone and posture.
- The **lateral vestibulospinal** tract arises from the lateral vestibular nucleus and terminates on **ipsilateral** alpha and gamma motor neurons associated with **extensor muscles, especially proximal muscles**
- The **medial vestibulospinal** tract arises from medial vestibular nucleus, terminates mainly on **the interneurons** and **inhibits** the alpha and gamma motor neurons of **axial** and neck musculature.

Corticospinal Tracts

- Arise from motor, premotor and supplementary motor cortices (layer V)
- Those fibers that decussate in the medulla descend as **lateral corticospinal** tracts and terminate on alpha and gamma motor neurons of the contralateral side. These control the **distal, especially skilled**, movements
- The uncrossed fibers descend as **anterior corticospinal** tracts and finally decussate at the segmental level in the spinal cord anterior commissure to terminate on alpha and gamma motor neurons. Few axons of this uncrossed tract terminate on ipsilateral motor neurons. This tract controls **the axial musculature**

The following Table 4.1 summarizes the major descending tracts and their effects on various muscles

Table 4.1: Major descending tracts and their effects on various muscles.

Flexor, distal musculature	Extensor, proximal musculature
• Lateral corticospinal	• Anterior corticospinal
• Lateral reticulospinal	• Medial reticulospinal
• Rubrospinal	• Medial vestibulospinal

Extrapyramidal System

- Ib inhibitory system in the spinal cord normally determines the muscle length-tension relationship
- This system is inhibited by the nucleus gigantocellularis of the dorsal reticulospinal tract
- Overactivity of the nucleus gigantocellularis in Parkinson's disease may account for the rigidity
- Alternate mechanisms of extrapyramidal rigidity include: increased cortical excitability, impaired corticospinal and rubrospinal inhibition of the Ib inhibitory interneurons and enhanced tonic stretch reflex activity of the muscle
- The core defect may be the loss of dopaminergic modulation of basal ganglia function rather than loss of any specific neural pathways, unlike dystonia (which develops after a focal lesion in the lentiform nucleus).

Methods and Observation

- Bedside examination of tone is often subjective and qualitative
- Correct assessment requires a relaxed and cooperative patient
- The objectives of the examination are to assess:
    - If the tone is normal, decreased or increased
    - If it is increased, is it rigidity or spasticity?
    - Is there any pattern to the increased tone to suggest a particular tract involvement?

Inspection

- Inspect the position and attitude of the limbs and trunk in supine, sitting and standing postures
- Common patterns of motor dysfunction in spastic conditions are tabulated and summarized in Box 4.1

Box 4.1: Common patterns seen in spastic disorders.

- Striatal toe
- Pes valgus
- Pes equinovarus
- Extended knee
- Flexed knee
- Adducted thigh
- Flexed hip
- Thumb in palm
- Clenched fist
- Flexed wrist
- Pronated forearm
- Flexed elbow
- Adducted, internally rotated shoulder

- In hemiplegia due to stroke, the upper limb is flexed at elbow and pronated at forearm, wrist is flexed, and fingers are flexed. The lower limb is held in extension. This is due to the over-action of antigravity muscles
- In paraplegia due to spinal lesions, the lower limbs are typically held in flexion

- In hypotonia in chorea, when the upper limb is outstretched, the wrist flexes and the fingers hyperextend, resulting in "spooning"
- In Parkinsonism, there is a stoop or lateral trunk flexion (Pisa sign) due to rigidity of axial and truncal muscles.

Palpation

- Ensure patient relaxation (the most important pre-requisite for tone assessment)
- Feel the consistency of the muscles: Normally muscles are firm on palpation. Hypotonic muscles feel flabby and hypertonic muscles feel taut.
- Look for excessive laxity at individual joints.

Passive Stretching at Individual Joints

- Move the muscle through its entire range of motion first slowly and then rapidly
- To evaluate rigidity, the joint is moved to and fro at a rate of 0.5 to 2 cycles per second. For spasticity, it is moved at increasing speed
- If this assessment at different speeds is not performed, one may miss mild spasticity
- If the tone is increased, assess if it is present at low velocity stretch (rigidity) or at high velocity stretch, associated with a catch at a particular angle (spasticity)
- If there is rigidity, assess if it is uniform throughout the range (lead pipe like), or interrupted by tremor (cog wheel-like).

Other Tests: From Proximal to Distal

- **Neck** (Head dropping test): Place the patient supine, keeping your hand under his head, on the bed. With the other hand, lift the head briskly and allow it to drop. Normally, the head drops quickly into the examiner's hand. In neck flexor rigidity, this is delayed
- **Shoulder** (Babinski tonus test): Abduct the shoulder and flex the forearm. In hypotonia, the elbow can be flexed to a more acute angle than normal. In hypertonia, the angle is much reduced
- **Shoulder** (Shoulder shaking test): Place your hand on patient's shoulders and shake them back and forth briskly. Look for reciprocal movement of the shoulders. A decrease in the range of arm swing suggests extrapyramidal rigidity. Increased range of movement occurs with hypotonia
- **Arm** (Arm dropping test): raise the patient's arm to the shoulder level and release. Look for the speed of the arm dropping down. It is increased in hypotonia and decreased in hypertonia
- **Froment's maneuver**: Ask the patient to perform a repetitive movement of the contralateral limb (like opening and closing the fist or supination pronation of forearm) while examining the tone of one upper limb. In extrapyramidal disease, rigidity is activated or reinforced by this maneuver

- **Leg rolling:** With the patient is supine position, gently roll the leg internally and externally. The ease with which this can be done depends on the tone of the rotators of the hip and also the integrity of the hip joint
- **Knee (Wartenberg pendulum test):** Patient sits at the edge of the cot, with legs hanging freely. Give both legs a backward equal push and release. Normally, the leg oscillates 6–7 times before halting. If the response is increased in range and duration, it suggests hypotonia. If the movements are jerky, irregular, it suggests spasticity. If the swing time is reduced, it is suggestive of extrapyramidal rigidity
- **Ankle:** Move the ankle in full range of dorsiflexion and extension while assessing the tone.

Look for all components of the "UMN syndrome"
- Look for associated positive signs: Inappropriate co-contraction of antagonistic muscles, hyperactive tendon reflexes, exaggerated cutaneous reflexes including the Babinski sign
- Look for associated negative signs: Weakness, fatigue, loss of dexterity (spastic paresis).

Interpretation

- Hypotonia: Implies a lesion involving the motor unit (anterior horn cell, nerve roots, peripheral nerves or the muscles) or an acute central lesion like a stroke or spinal cord lesion. Rarely, the tone remains low in chronic lesion involving the primary motor cortex. Central and peripheral hypotonia in an infant are discussed further in pediatric neurology section.
- Hypertonia can be due to:
  - Pyramidal tract disease (spasticity)
  - Diffuse frontal lobe disease (paratonia)
  - Extrapyramidal disease (rigidity)
  - Spinal cord lesions (spasticity, tetanus, strychnine poisoning, stiff person syndrome)
  - Muscle diseases (myotonia, McArdle syndrome, tetany)
  - Mechanical alterations in muscle can mimic hypertonia (e.g. contracture).

Spasticity
- Increased muscle tone in certain groups of muscles, that is velocity dependent, usually with a catch and release, is the hallmark of spasticity.
- It is graded by modified Ashworth scale as below:
  - Grade 0: No increase in muscle tone
  - Grade 1: Catch and release or a minimal resistance at the end of range of movement
  - Grade 1+: catch followed by minimal resistance throughout the range of remainder (less than half) of movement.

- Grade 2: marked increase in tone through most of the range of movement, but the affected body part is easily moved
- Grade 3: Considerable increase in tone, passive movement difficult
- Grade 4: Affected body part rigid in flexion or extension
- Another scale used in therapeutic trials is the Spasm Frequency Scale.

Score	Criteria
0	No spasms
1	No spontaneous spasms
2	Occasional (≤1/ hour) spontaneous spasms and easily induced spasms
3	2–10 spontaneous spasms per hour
4	> 10 spontaneous spasms per hour

- Spasticity of cerebral and spinal origin differ in some aspects, but **there are exceptions** to each of these features:

	Cerebral spasticity	Spinal spasticity
Laterality	Often unilateral/asymmetric	Often bilateral, symmetric
Limb posture	Extension of lower limb with upper limb flexed (hemiplegic posture)	Flexion of all involved limbs is typical (paraplegic/tetraplegic posture)
Exaggerated cutaneous reflexes and spasms	Less frequent (other than Babinski sign)	Typical (triple flexion of hip, knee, ankle on slight touch)
Initial hyporeflexia after acute insult	Few days	Weeks

Paratonia/Gegenhalten (German: to hold against)
- Variably increased muscle tone that is not direction-specific, but proportional to the force and velocity of stretch, and persists inspite of instructions to relax, is the hallmark of gegenhalten.
- Is a form of hypertonia of diffuse frontal lobe disease as in dementias.
- It may mimic spasticity by its velocity dependence and rigidity by involving agonists and antagonists
- In contrast to spasticity, clasp knife phenomenon is absent (it increases, instead of relaxing, as the applied force is increased)
- In contrast to rigidity, it is not increased by contralateral limb movement (no reinforcement).

Rigidity
- Increased muscle tone that uniformly involves both agonists and antagonists, and increased by activity of contralateral muscles, but is uninfluenced by velocity of stretch, is the hallmark of rigidity
- It is differentiated from other disorders of increased muscle tone by the phenomenon of co-activation or reinforcement

- Unless this phenomenon is elicited, a diagnosis of extrapyramidal rigidity cannot be made
- It is a manifestation of extrapyramidal disease, but is non-localizing by itself
- It is graded as a part of the Unified Parkinson's disease rating scale as follows:

Score	Criteria
0	Non
1	Detectable rigidity in the neck, shoulder. Activation phenomenon is present. One or both arms show mild, negative, resting rigidity
2	Moderate rigidity in neck and shoulders; resting rigidity is present if patient is not on medications
3	Rigidity severe in neck and shoulders; resting rigidity cannot be reversed by medication

- Rigidity is differentiated from spasticity as follows:

	Spasticity	Rigidity
Muscle groups	Not uniformly involved (antigravity muscles preferentially affected)	Uniformly involves agonists and antagonists
Relation to range of movement	Not uniform (initial free interval and then a catch)	Uniform throughout the range of movement
Clasp knife phenomenon (catch followed by release)	May be present	Absent
Stimulus dependence	Velocity dependent (Develops at fast stretch)	Length dependent (Felt at slow or fast stretch)
Deep tendon reflexes	Exaggerated	Normal
Babinski sign	Often positive	Negative
Negative motor sign	True weakness	Bradykinesia

Tetanus
- Clinically manifests as generalized stiffness of muscles of jaw (trismus), facial muscles (risus sardonicus), abdomen, respiratory and limbs muscles
- The **hallmark** is intermittent, spontaneous and reflex **spasms** of the involved muscles (due to failure of inhibitory interneurons to suppress these reflexes)
- It is caused by the neurotoxin of *Clostridium tetani* which inhibits release of inhibitory neurotransmitters (GABA, glycine) from the inhibitory interneurons of the spinal cord. Strychnine, another neurotoxin, blocks the receptors of these neurotransmitters and produces similar clinical effects
- Electrophysiological manifestation of this alteration is a decreased or absent silent period after paired stimulation during H reflex recording.

Stiff person syndrome
- Is a subacute or chronic autoimmune disorder caused by antibodies against GABA, produced as an idiopathic or paraneoplastic syndrome.

- There is rigidity of muscles of the trunk, neck, abdomen, back and proximal limbs
- There are painful spasms of these muscles.

Myotonia
- Is a disorder of muscle membrane (channelopathy) caused by an inability of a contracted muscle to relax.
- The resting tone of the muscles is normal.
- It can be elicited either by contracting a muscle or by percussion of the muscle.
- It can be elicited in the following regions from above downwards:
  - Eyelids: Ask the patient to close his eyes tightly and then open
  - Tongue: Place a tongue blade transversely across the tongue and percuss
  - Forearm: Percuss the extensor digitorum communis and observe the delay in relaxation of the extended fingers
  - Thenar eminence: Percuss the eminence with a hammer to produce a dimple that relaxes slowly
  - Hand grip: Ask the patient to grip his hand for a few seconds and then try to relax
  - Other muscles: Observe during spontaneous activities and by percussion over the muscles of interest
- Once myotonia is noted, ask patient to exercise the muscle several times and observe if myotonia improves (most myotonic disorders) or worsens (paramyotonia).
- Look for muscle hypertrophy (myotonia congenita), weakness, and eyelid myokimia that give a clue to the diagnosis.

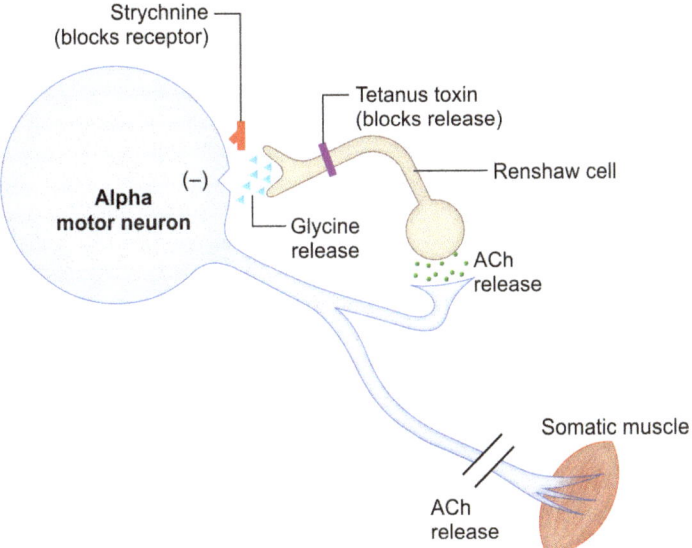

Fig. 4.4: Site of action of tetanus toxin and strychnine.

Caveats

- If the patient is not relaxed, the muscle tone may appear increased, tendon reflexes may be exaggerated and even clonus may appear.
- The pendulum test may be falsely positive due to mechanical changes of the muscle even in the absence of spasticity.
- Parkinsonism can initially present with shoulder pain due to rigidity, which can be mistaken for periarthritis of shoulder.

BIBLIOGRAPHY

1. Gelber DA, Jeffery DR (Eds). Clinical evaluation and management of spasticity. 2010. (Humana Press)
2. Mayer NH, Esquenazi A, Childers MK. Common patterns of clinical motor dysfunction. Muscle Nerve. 1997;(suppl 6):S21-S35.
3. Pedersen E, Klemar B, Torring J. Counting of flexor spasms. Acta Neurol Scand. 1979; 60: 164-9.

ASSESSMENT OF MUSCLE POWER—GENERAL PRINCIPLES

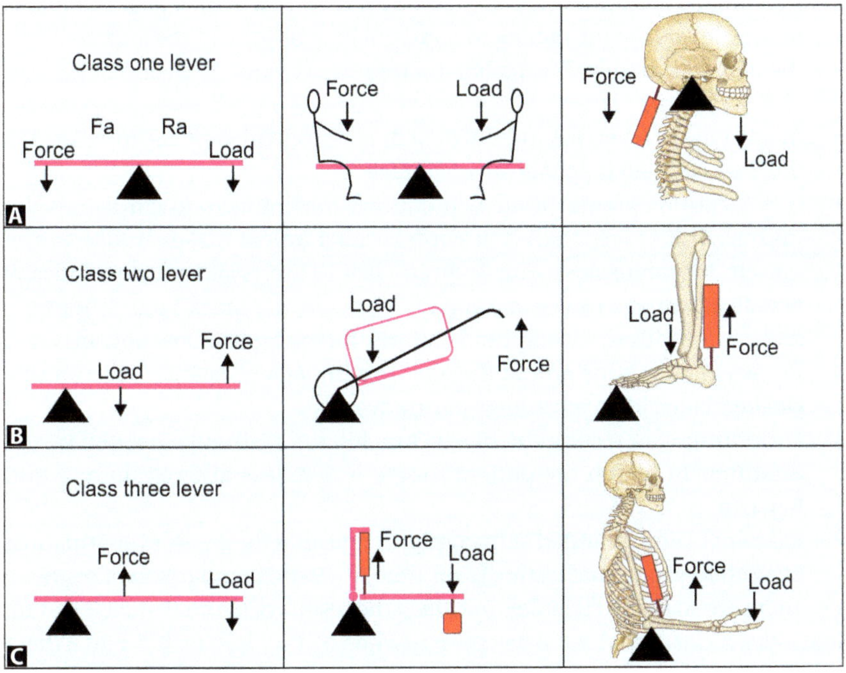

Figs. 4.5A to C: Different classes of levers and their general examples (2nd column) and specific examples in human musculoskeletal system (3rd column).

Fa: The perpendicular distance between the fulcrum and the moving force (patient's muscle force)
Ra: The perpendicular distance between the fulcrum and the resistance force (examiner's force)

Concept of Levers Applied to Muscle Testing

- Studying the basic mechanics of lever systems helps in a more rational and systematic muscle power examination
- A lever is a simple machine that has a rigid bar that rotates around an axis (fulcrum).

There are three classes of levers (Figs. 4.5A to C):
- Class I levers have the fulcrum (F) at the center and the effort (E) and the load (L) on either side of the fulcrum. An example of this type of lever is the simple balance. In the human body, head flexion and extensions involve class I lever action (L-F-E system)
- Class II levers have both the effort and the load on the same side of the fulcrum but the arm of the effort is longer than that of the load. (An example of this type of lever is a nut cracker or a wheel barrow). In the human body, ankle plantar flexion involves class II lever action by the gastrosoleus muscles (F-L-E system)

- In class III levers, the effort and the load are again on the same side of the fulcrum, but the arm of the load is longer than that of the effort. Examples of such levers are the fishing rod and the long broom. In the human body, the elbow flexion by biceps brachii represents class III lever mechanism (F-E-L system)
- In any type of lever, the force arm of the effort divided by the force arm of the load is called mechanical advantage.
- If this ratio is greater than 1, it confers mechanical advantage to the muscle. If it is less than 1, it confers mechanical disadvantage to the muscle. Most muscles in our body are class III levers and are mechanically at a disadvantage (this is a trade off for achieving quick large amplitude movement with small amplitude efforts; for example elbow flexion)
- By varying the force arm of the load (examiner's resistance), the muscle can be placed at an advantage or disadvantage.
- For example, in testing the biceps brachii, the resistance needed by the examiner to match the patient's force is 50% less at wrist than at mid forearm
- Examiners are reminded of the test principle that the same lever arm must be used in sequential testing (over time) for valid comparison of results.

There are so many variables that affect the results of manual muscle testing that a clear consensus has not yet been reached on the "best technique" if there is one. However, some general principles must be understood to minimize intra and inter observer variability.

The General Rules of Muscle Power Testing

- **Decide on what is to be tested**: It is not necessary to test each muscle in every patient. In a patient with myositis on treatment and follow up, it suffices to examine the muscle groups (e.g., shoulder abductors, adductors etc.). In a patient with brachial plexus lesion, it is essential to examine the individual muscles.
- **Explain the patient** and make him comfortable: an uncooperative or apprehensive patient is likely to yield more variable results.
- **Place the patient in appropriate position:** For example, hip flexion and knee extension are tested in sitting position, knee flexion in prone position, neck flexion in supine and neck extension in prone positions. There are no short cuts to proper positioning.
- **Place the body part appropriately:** the part has to be positioned in such a way that the line of action is perpendicular to gravity and the muscle has to work against the gravity. If this fails, then gravity is minimized (never "eliminated"), by placing the line of action of muscle parallel to gravity on a flat, smooth table or cot minimizing the frictional resistance.
- **Expose the muscle and feel:** if this is possible. Feeling muscle contraction through clothing is unreliable

- **Assess the passive range** of movement of the joint before muscle testing
- **Stabilize** the segment proximal to the joint being tested to avoid substitutions/trick movements.

Specific Rules of Muscle Testing

Now, more specific issues in muscle testing will be discussed, namely:
1. What should be the patient's joint position (flexion, extension or mid position)?
2. Where should the examiner apply the resistance (proximal/ distal/ mid level)?
3. How long does the patient have to sustain the effort?

Patient's Limb Position: There are two variations

1. **"Break test":** The limb is kept in the end position of the muscle being tested (for example: full elbow flexion). Patient is asked to resist the examiner's efforts to overcome the muscle action (e.g. examiner attempts to extend the elbow). If the patient's biceps is weak, the examiner breaks his effort and the elbow extends.
2. **"Make test":** The limb is partially moved in the direction of muscle action and the examiner applies resistance to it. (for example, elbow is partially flexed as the examiner tries to prevent full flexion).
3. Using the break test will give a higher grade to a muscle than the make test. Moreover, the results of make test are more variable than the break test. Therefore, **break test is recommended** by authoritative books on muscle examination.
4. An exception that favors make test is a muscle that crosses two joints (e.g. hamstrings, gastrocnemius). Such a muscle is mechanically disadvantaged. Hence, it is placed in mid position which result in a favorable length-tension relationship.

Examiner's Resistance

1. In general, the examiner has to apply his resistance as far **distal** as possible from the fulcrum **without crossing another joint**.
2. An exception is hip abductors, against which, the resistance is applied at the ankle to match the physiological forces that this muscle works against. Similarly, for the scapular muscles the resistance is applied on the arm and not scapula (again, the physiological forces faced by this muscle justify the long lever testing)
3. Another exception to this rule is when a joint is unstable or painful. For example, if the knee is unstable/painful, a more distal force may be applied, but recorder so that the next examination of the patient can be done in the identical fashion.

How Long Should the Patient Sustain the Effort

1. The examiner's resistance has to be increased gradually (over few seconds) and not abruptly
2. The patient has to sustain the effort for 3-5 seconds (no clear consensus exists).

How Can the Examination be Modified In Individual Case

1. Examiner must adapt his technique to the patient's muscular developmental level.
2. This adaptation can be achieved by varying the following:
   i. Moment arm of the load (examiner's force)
   ii. Length of the muscle at the moment of testing
3. For example, while examining a frail patient, advantage may be given to the patient by applying a more proximal resistance than usual, first on the healthier limb. Then the weak limb may be examined with resistance at the same level.

Grading of Muscle Strength

There are 2 ways to grade the muscle weakness:
1. Using validated scales
2. Using functional capabilities.

The Medical Research Council (MRC) scale is commonly used to grade the muscle strength (see table below). There are two main concerns with this scale: (i) The change in grades is not linear. For example, a change from grade 4 to 3 is not the same as 2 to 1. (ii) Grade 4 encompasses a wide range of powers clubbed into one grade. The modified MRC scale is a 10 point scale which attempts to address the second concern (Table 4.2).

The MRC scale:
- Grade 5: Muscle contracts normally against full resistance.
- Grade 4: Muscle strength is reduced but muscle contraction can still move joint against resistance.
- Grade 3: Muscle strength is further reduced such that the joint can be moved only against gravity with the examiner's resistance completely removed. As an example, the elbow can be moved from full extension to full flexion starting with the arm hanging down at the side.
- Grade 2: Muscle can move only if the resistance of gravity is removed. As an example, the elbow can be fully flexed only if the arm is maintained in a horizontal plane.
- Grade 1: Only a trace or flicker of movement is seen or felt in the muscle or fasciculations are observed in the muscle.
- Grade 0: No movement is observed.

Rule of Thumb

Whenever uncertainty exists, give the lower MRC grade.

Table 4.2: Expanded Medical Research Council (MRC) scale for manual muscle testing.

Modified MRC grade	Criteria
5	Normal power
5−	Equivocal, barely detectable weakness
4+	Definite, but slight weakness
4	Able to move the joint against combination of gravity and some resistance
4−	Capable of minimal resistance
3+	Capable of transient resistance, but collapses abruptly
3	Active movement against gravity
3−	Able to move against gravity, but not through full range
2	Able to move with gravity eliminated
1	Trace contraction
0	No contraction

Table 4.3: Functional assessment of muscle weakness.

Location	Signs or symptoms of weakness
Facial	Inability to bury eyelashes, horizontal smile, inability to whistle
Ocular	Double vision, ptosis, disconjugate eye movements
Bulbar	Nasal speech, weak cry, nasal regurgitation of liquids, poor suck, difficulty swallowing, recurrent aspiration pneumonia, cough during meals
Neck	Poor head control
Trunk	Scoliosis, lumbar lordosis, protuberant abdomen, difficulty sitting up
Shoulder girdle	Difficulty lifting objects overhead, scapular winging
Forearm/Hand	Inability to make a tight fist, finger or wrist drop, inability to prevent escape from hand grip
Pelvic girdle	Difficulty climbing stairs, waddling gait, Gower's sign
Leg/Foot	Foot drop, inability to walk on heels or toes
Respiratory	Use of accessory muscles

In the subsequent sections, individual muscle testing is described using the above discussed principles.

BIBLIOGRAPHY

1. Campbell WW. DeJong's the Neurologic examination, 7th edition. Wolters Kluwer/Lippincott Williams & Wilkins; 2013.
2. Hislop H. Daniels and Worthingham's Muscle Testing: Techniques of Manual Examination. Elsevier India; 2013.
3. Houglum PA, Bertoti DB. Brunnstrom's Clinical Kinesiology, 6th edition. FA Davis publications; 2012.
4. Kendall FP, McCreary EK. Muscle testing and function. 4th edition, BaltimoreMD: Williams and Wilkins; 1993.

SCAPULAR MOVEMENTS

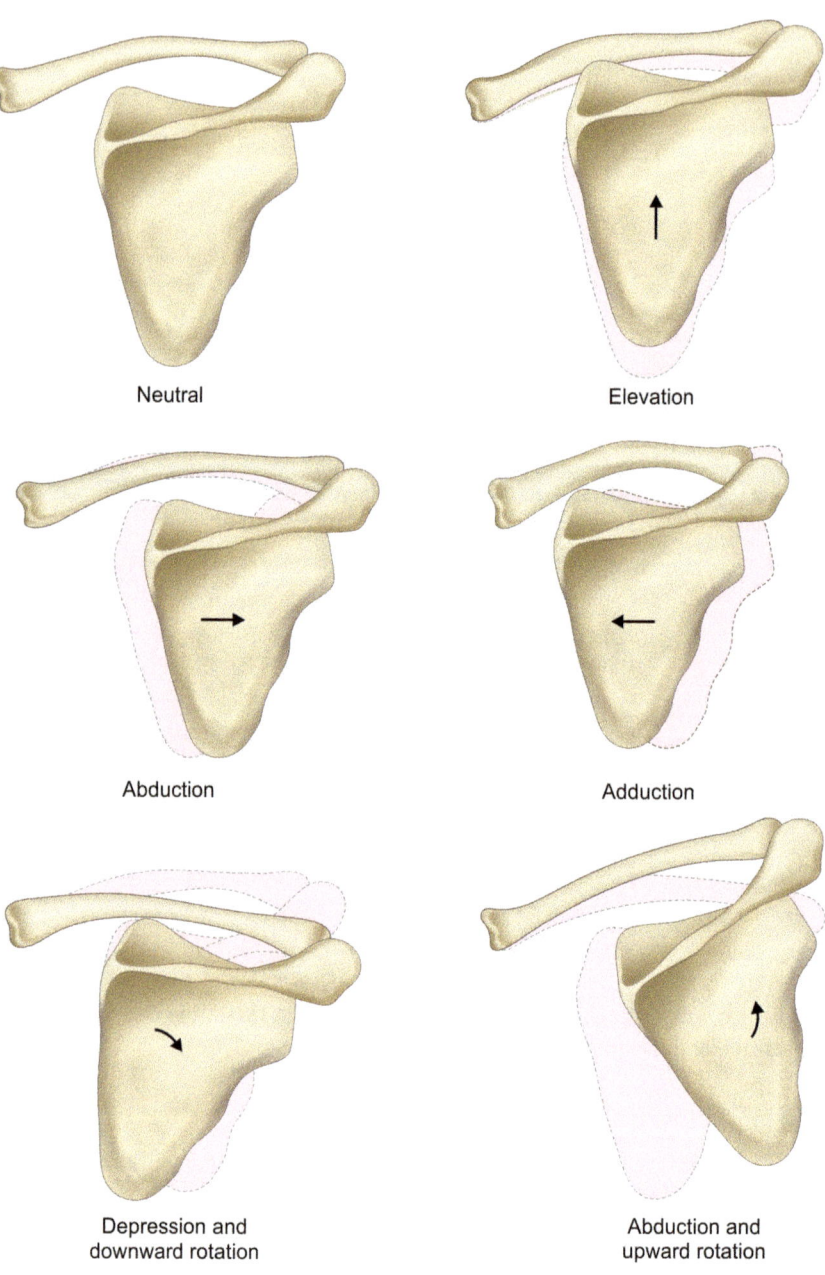

Fig. 4.6: Scapular motions.

SCAPULAR ABDUCTION AND FORWARD ROTATION

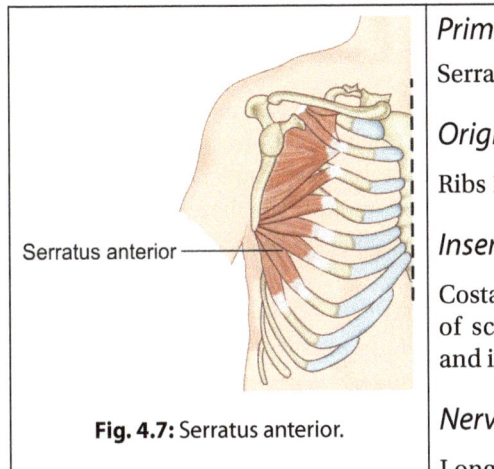 **Fig. 4.7:** Serratus anterior.	*Prime Mover* Serratus anterior *Origin* Ribs 1-8 *Insertion* Costal margin of the ventral surface of scapula including the superior and inferior angle. *Nerve Supply* Long thoracic nerve (C5, 6, 7 roots).

Methodology

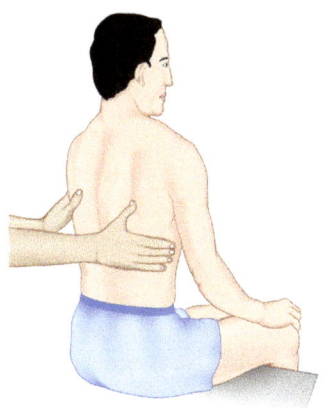

Fig. 4.8: Examination for symmetry of scapular position.

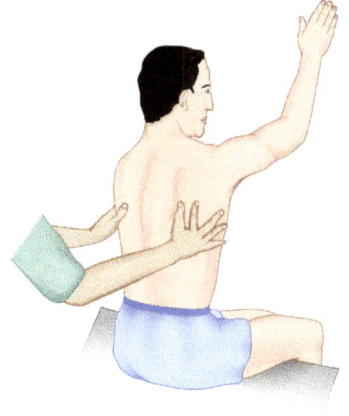

Fig. 4.9: Assessing the range of movement of scapula.

- Patient in sitting position, examine from behind
- Place the hands holding the angle of scapula in the angle between the stretched thumb and the index finger
- Compare the symmetry of scapula in vertical and horizontal planes
- Normally, both the scapular tips are at level and tucked in. If they are tilted away, it indicates trapezius weakness or shortening of pectoralis minor

- The degree of separation of thumbs from the spinous processes is normally 1–3 inches. An asymmetry in this separation suggests that the farther scapula is rotated forward, indicating serratus weakness (winging).
- Range of movement: Passively raise the arm in forward flexion above the head, while observing the scapula. Normally, the scapula remains stable up to 60° of elevation of the arm. Beyond this, the scapula and glenohumeral joint move in synchronous motion to complete the flexion. If the scapula starts to move at an angle less than 60°, it suggests limitation of glenohumeral joint mobility.
- Assessing the strength of serratus anterior:
    - If the scapular position is normal at rest and patient can flex the shoulder forward through full range in a smooth fashion, the power is at least grade 3/5
    - If there is scapular winging and patient cannot flex the arm overhead in a smooth fashion, the power is less than grade 3/5
- Serratus can be palpated anterior to the inferior angle of scapula near the axillary border for grade 1 contractions.
- For grade 2/5 power, scapula can be felt to be abducted during attempted flexion, though actual flexion movement is not visible.
- In grade 3/5, the arm can be flexed through complete range, but does not overcome even minimal force by the examiner

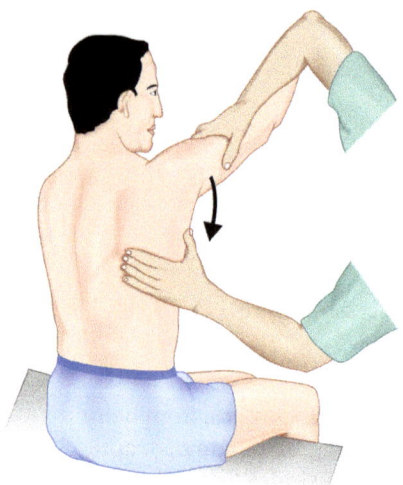

Fig. 4.10: Assessing the power of serratus anterior.

SCAPULAR ELEVATION

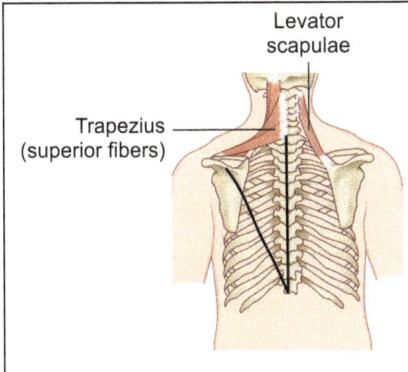

Fig. 4.11: Elevators of scapula.

Muscle

Trapezius (upper fibers), rhomboideus.

Origin (Trapezius)

External occipital protuberance and medial 1/3 of superior nuchal line.

Insertion (Trapezius)

Posterior border of lateral 1/3 of clavicle.

Nerve Supply (Trapezius)

Spinal accessory nerve.

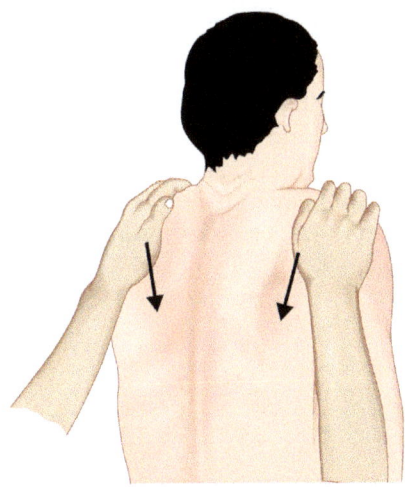

Fig. 4.12: Assessment of power of trapezius against gravity.

Assessment

- Patient sitting, examiner standing behind the patient
- Place the hands over the shoulders
- Ask patient to raise (shrug) both shoulders simultaneously as if trying to touch the ears. Examiner tries to push the shoulders down to assess the power.
- Grade 2 and 1 can be assessed with patient supine or prone, with gravity eliminated.

SCAPULAR ADDUCTION

Muscles

Trapezius (middle fibers) and Rhomboideus.

Origin

T1-T5 spinous processes and inter-spinous ligaments.

Examination

- Patient in prone position, shoulder abducted 90°, elbow flexed and dangling down from the edge of the cot
- Examiner stands on the test side with hand placed just proximal to elbow.
- Patient attempts to raise the elbow towards the ceiling while examiner pushes the elbow downwards to the floor

By the rhomboids: The rhomboids can substitute for the trapezius in adduction of the scapula. They cannot, however, substitute for the upward rotation component. When substitution by the rhomboids occurs, the scapula will adduct and rotate downward.

When the posterior deltoid muscle is weak, support the patient's shoulder with the palm of one hand, and allow the patient's elbow to flex. Passively move the scapula into adduction via horizontal abduction of the arm. Have the patient hold the scapula in adduction as the examiner slowly releases the shoulder support. Observe whether the scapula maintains its adducted position. If it does, it is Grade 3.

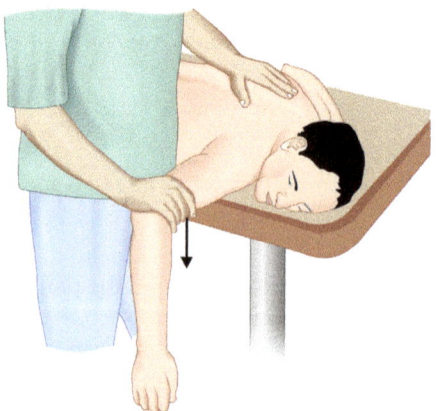

Fig. 4.13: Assessment of middle fibers of trapezius.

SCAPULAR DEPRESSION AND ADDUCTION

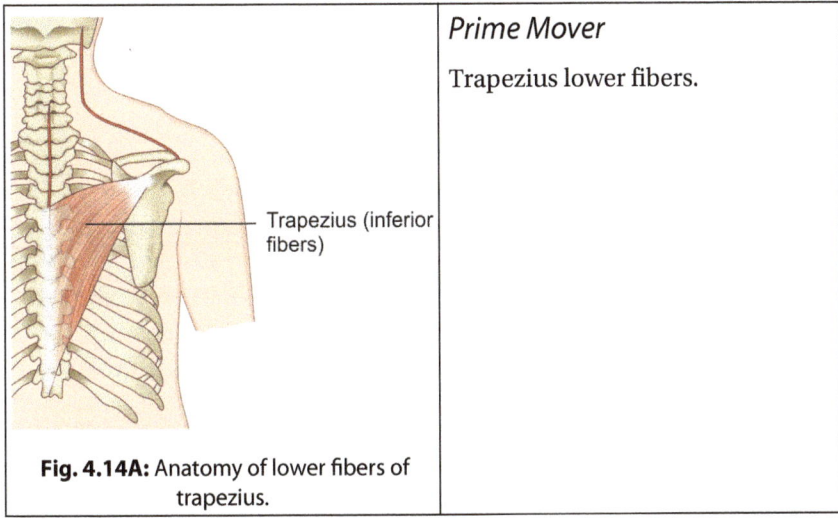

	Prime Mover
Fig. 4.14A: Anatomy of lower fibers of trapezius.	Trapezius lower fibers.

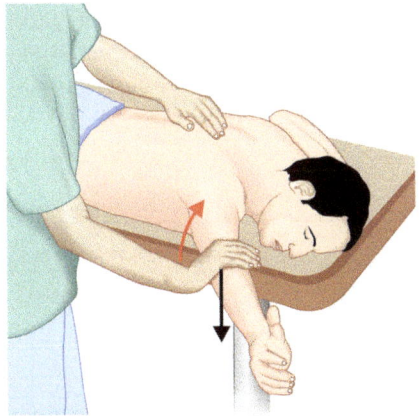

Fig. 4.14B: Examinations of lower fibers of trapezius.

Examination Technique

Patient Position

Prone, arm abducted to nearly 145° (in line of action of lower trapezius fibers), thumb pointing towards the ceiling.

Examiner

- On the test side, keeps hand over at midarm and tries to push towards the floor while the patient tries to raise it towards the ceiling.
- Palpate the trapezius with the other hand.

SCAPULAR ADDUCTION AND DOWNWARD ROTATION

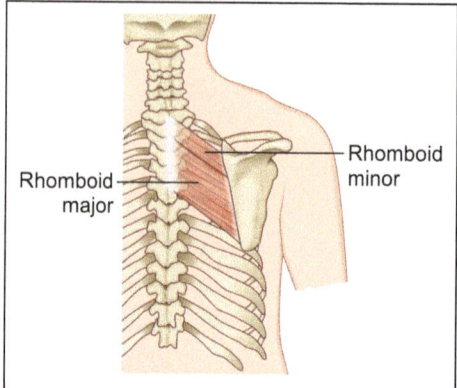

Fig. 4.15: Anatomy of rhomboid muscles.

Prime Mover

Rhomboideus major and minor.

Origin

Rhomboid major:
- T2-T5 vertebrae (spinous processes)
- Supraspinous ligaments.

Rhomboid minor:
- C7-T1 vertebrae (spinous processes)
- Ligamentum nuchae.

Insertion

Scapula (vertebral border between root of spine and inferior angle).

Nerve Supply

Dorsal scapular nerve (C5).

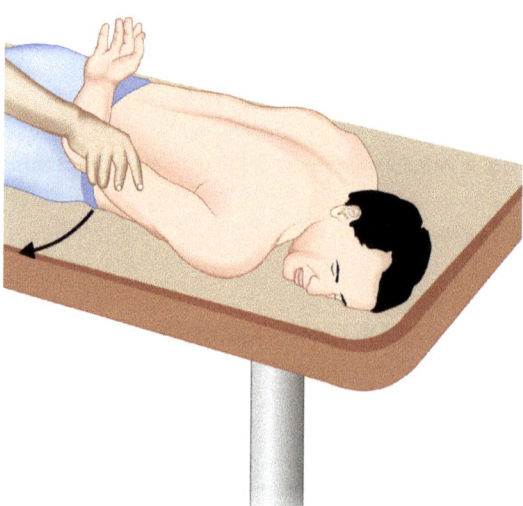

Fig. 4.16: Testing of rhomboid muscles.

Methodology

Patient: Prone, head turned to either side, shoulder adducted, internally rotated, elbow flexed with forearm resting over the back.
Examiner: Standing by the test side, holds the arm above elbow, giving outward and downward force. Patient is asked to resist this force. Rhomboids can be felt medial to the scapula.

Caveat

The middle fibers of the trapezius can substitute for the adduction component of the rhomboids.

The middle trapezius cannot, however, substitute for the downward rotation component. When substitution occurs, the patient's scapula will adduct with no downward rotation.

SHOULDER FLEXION

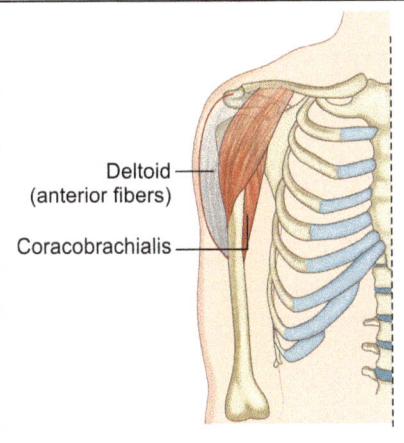

Prime Mover

Deltoid, anterior fibers.

Origin

Clavicle (anterior superior border of lateral 1/3 of shaft).

Insertion

Humerus (deltoid tuberosity on shaft).

Nerve Supply

Axillary nerve (C5, 6).

Fig. 4.17A: Anatomy of shoulder flexors.

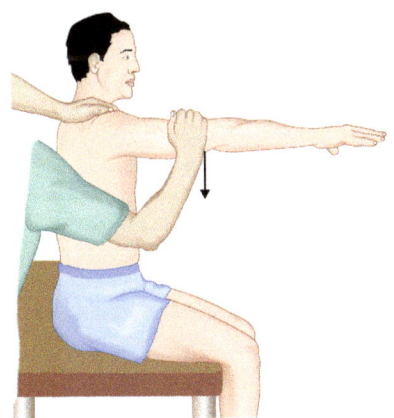

Fig. 4.17B: Testing of shoulder flexion.

Methodology

Patient: Sitting, arms by the side with forearm pronated, raises the arm to 90°.
Examiner: On the test side, one hand placed over the distal arm just above elbow, giving downward force, which the patient has to resist. The other hand stabilizes the shoulder.

Caveat

- Biceps brachii can flex the shoulder when the arm is externally rotated (forearm is supinated). Hence, it is important to avoid this trick movement by keeping the forearm pronated
- Pectoralis major can also be substituted during flexion, but results in adduction. This can be avoided by preventing adduction
- Trick movements by using trapezius causes shoulder elevation. Examiner therefore needs to stabilize the shoulder during the test.

SHOULDER EXTENSION

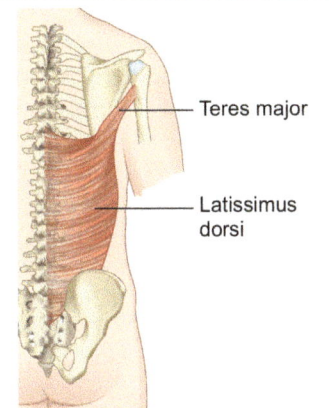

Fig. 4.18A: Anatomy of latissimus dorsi.

Prime Mover

Latissimus dorsi, teres major, deltoid posterior fibers.

Latissimus Dorsi

Origin: T6-T12, L1-L5, and sacral vertebrae (spinous processes, supraspinous ligaments, ribs 9-12 by slips interdigitating with obliquus abdominis externus) Ilium (crest, posterior) thoracolumbar fascia.
Insertion: Humerus (intertubercular sulcus, floor).
Nerve supply: Thoracodorsal nerve (C6, 7, 8).

Teres Major

Origin: Scapula (dorsal surface of inferior angle).
Insertion: Humerus (intertubercular sulcus, medial lip).
Nerve supply: Lower subscapular nerve and thoracodorsal nerve (C 5-8).

Deltoid

Origin: Scapula (spine on lower lip of lateral and posterior borders).
Insertion: Humerus (deltoid tuberosity on midshaft via humeral tendon).
Nerve supply: Axillary neve (C5,6).

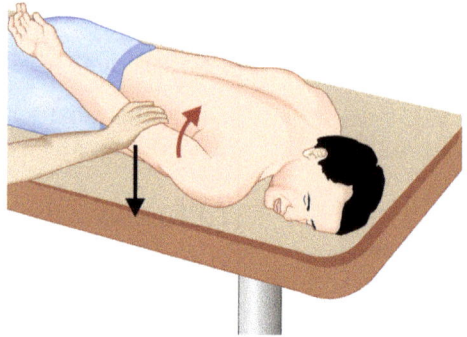

Fig. 4.18B: Testing of latissimus dorsi.

Position of patient: Prone with arms at sides and shoulder internally rotated (palm up).

Position of examiner: Stand at test side. Hand used for resistance is contoured over the posterior arm just above the elbow.

Method: Patient raises arm off the table, keeping the elbow straight.

Isolation of Latissimus Dorsi

Position of patient: Prone with head turned to test side, arms are at sides and shoulder is internally rotated (palm up). Test shoulder is raised to the level of the chin.

Position of examiner: Stand at test side. Grasp forearm above patient's wrist with both hands.

Test: Patient depresses arm caudally attempting to reach his feet. In so doing, he approximates the rib cage to the pelvis, while the examiner attempts to push in opposite direction (towards the head).

If the patient is able to perform the above test, perform the following test to confirm the grade as 5/5.

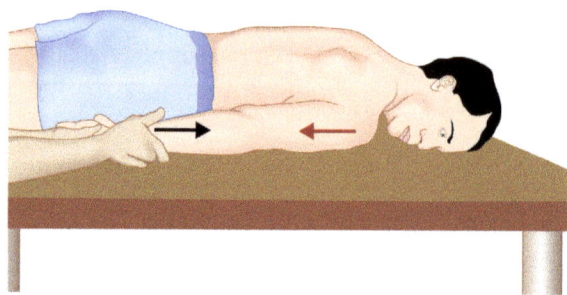

Fig. 4.19: Testing of latissimus dorsi with gravity eliminated.

Position of patient: sitting, with hands flat on table adjacent to hips.
Position of examiner: Stand behind patient. Fingers are used to palpate fibers of the latissimus dorsi on the lateral aspects of the thoracic wall just above the waist.
Test: Patient pushes down on hands and lifts buttocks from table.

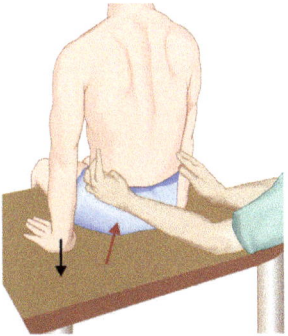

Fig. 4.20: Testing of latissimus dorsi against gravity.

SHOULDER ABDUCTION

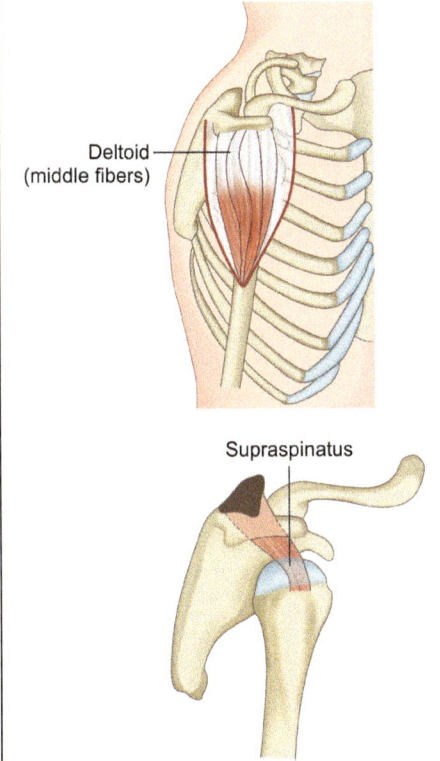

Fig. 4.21: Anatomy of shoulder abductors.

Prime Movers
Deltoid middle fibers, supraspinatus.

Origin
Deltoid (middle fibers): Scapula (acromion, lateral margin, superior surface, and crest of spine).
Supraspinatus: Scapula (supraspinous fossa, medial 2/3).

Insertion
Deltoid: Humerus (deltoid tuberosity on shaft via humeral tendon)
Supraspinatus: Greater tubercle of humerus.

Nerve Supply
Deltoid: Axillary nerve (C5,6)
Supraspinatus: Suprascapular nerve (C5,6)

Position of patient: Sitting with arm at side and elbow slightly flexed and forearm pronated. Head may be turned to opposite side to make supraspinatus accessible for palpation.

Position of examiner: Stand behind patient. Hand giving resistance is placed over arm just above elbow. The other hand stabilizes the shoulder.

Test: Patient abducts arm to 90° against downward force of the examiner.

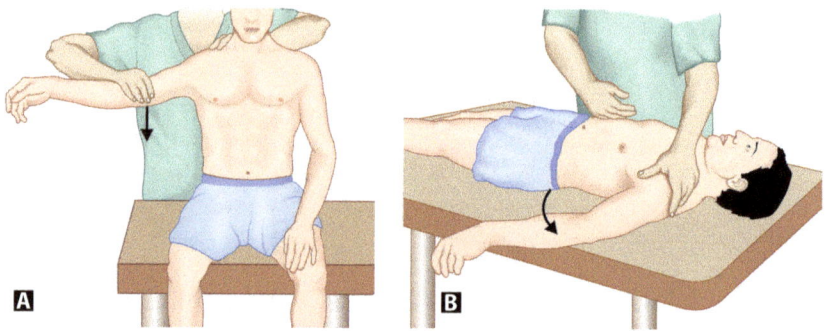

Figs. 4.22A and B: (A) Testing of shoulder abduction against gravity; (B) with gravity eliminated.

Caveats

- Trick movement by shoulder elevation can mimic shoulder abduction. So it is necessary to stabilize the shoulder from being elevated
- Trick movement by trunk lateral flexion to opposite side needs to be avoided by instructing the patient to keep his trunk straight
- Trick movement by biceps brachii can mimic shoulder abduction, when the forearm is supinated. Hence, the test has to be done with forearm pronated and elbow slightly flexed.

SHOULDER ADDUCTION

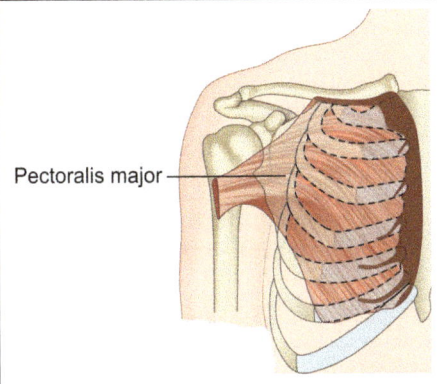

Fig. 4.23: Anatomy of pectoralis major.

Pectoralis Major

Origin:
Clavicular part: Clavicle (sternal 1/2 of anterior surface)
Sternal part: Sternum (anterior surface down to rib 6), Ribs 2–7 (costal cartilages).

Insertion:
- Humerus (intertubercular sulcus, lateral lip)
- Both parts converge on a bilaminar common tendon

Nerve supply:
- Sternal head: Medial pectoral nerve (C7,8 T1)
- Pectoral head: Lateral pectoral nerve (C5,6).

Methodology

Patient: Supine, elbow flexed, shoulder abducted to 90° (whole muscle)/ 60 (clavicular head) or 120° (sternal head).

Examiner: By the test side, hand placed over distal forearm. Patient is asked to bring the arm across the chest towards the clavicle (up and inwards) for clavicular head. For testing sternal head, patient is asked to bring the arm across towards opposite pelvis (down and in).

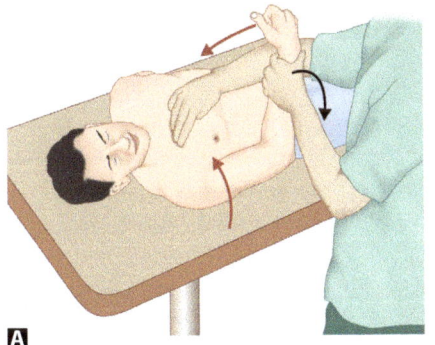 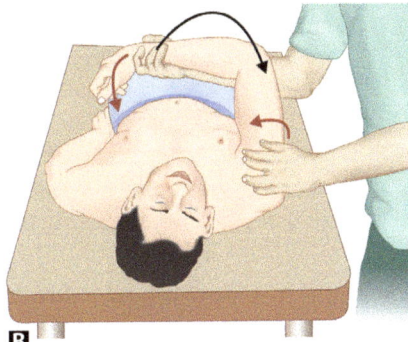

Figs. 4.24A and B: (A) Testing of pectoralis major clavicular head and (B) sternal head.

SHOULDER EXTERNAL ROTATION

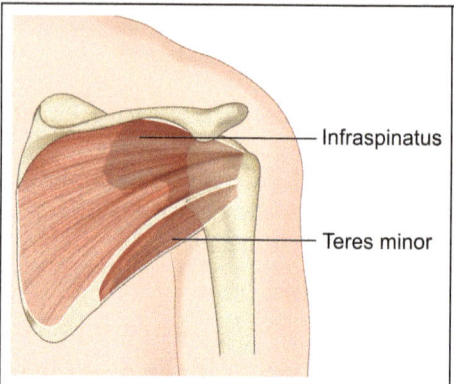

Infraspinatus

Origin: Scapula (infraspinous fossa, medial 2/3).

Insertion: Humerus (greater tubercle, middle facet).

Nerve supply: Suprascapular nerve (C5,6).

Teres Minor

Origin: Scapula (lateral border, superior 2/3).

Insertion: Humerus (greater tubercle, lowest facet) humerus (shaft, distal to lowest facet).

Nerve supply: Axillary nerve (C5,6).

Fig. 4.25: Anatomy of external rotators of the shoulder.

Methodology

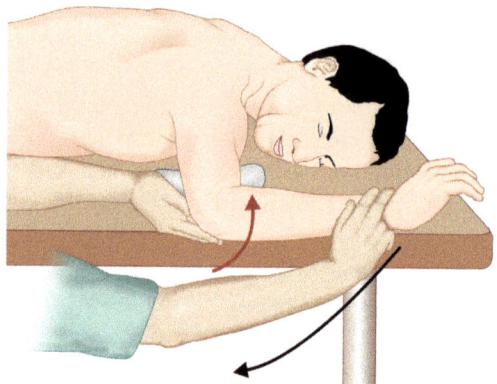

Fig. 4.26: Examination of shoulder external rotation against gravity (in sitting position, the same muscles can be tested having eliminated the gravity).

Patient: Prone, head turned to the test side. Shoulder abducted to 90°, elbow flexed.

Examiner: On test side, one hand supporting the elbow, the other hand 2 fingers placed over the wrist, giving downward pressure.

Patient tries to lift the forearm against examiner's resistance.

SHOULDER INTERNAL ROTATION

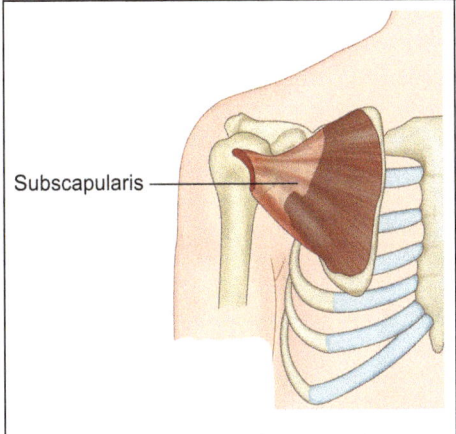

Fig. 4.27: Anatomy of subscapularis.

Prime Movers

Subscapularis, latissimus dorsi, pectoralis major, teres major.

Origin

Scapula (fills fossa on costal surface).

Insertion

Humerus (lesser tubercle).

Nerve Supply

Upper and lower subscapular nerves [branches of posterior cord of brachial plexus (C5, 6)].

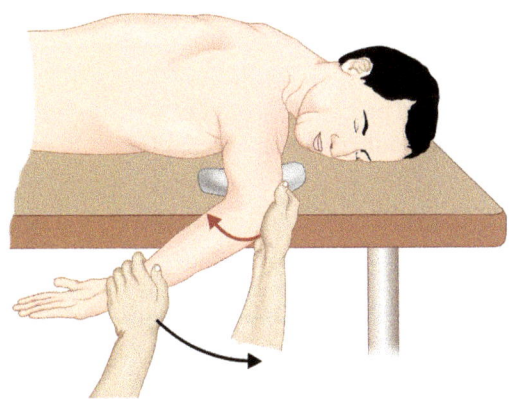

Fig. 4.28: Testing of shoulder internal rotation.

Patient: Prone, head turned to test side, arm abducted 90°, elbow flexed and hanging by the side.

Examiner: On the test side, one hand stabilizing the elbow. The other hand placed over the distal forearm on volar aspect, tries to push the forearm anteriorly and upward.

Patient is asked to bring his forearm backwards and rotate upwards.

Caveat: Forearm pronation can mimic shoulder internal rotation.

EXAMINATION OF FOREARM AND HAND

ELBOW FLEXION

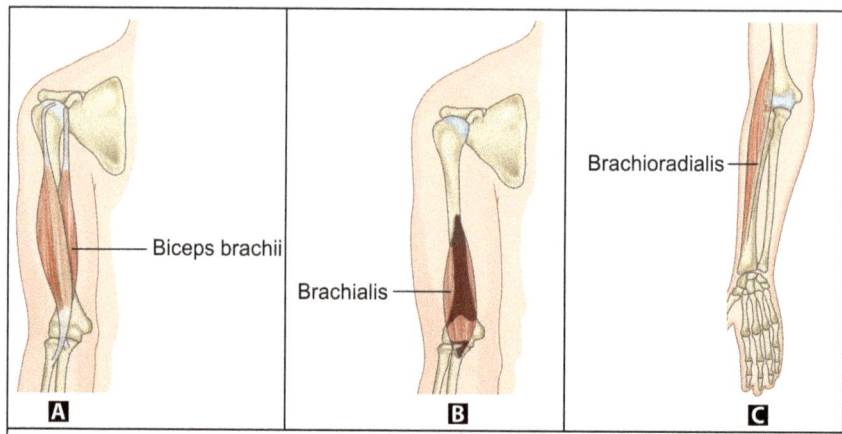

Figs. 4.29A to C: (A) Anatomy of biceps brachii, (B) brachialis and (C) brachioradialis.

Biceps Brachii

Origin:
- Short head: Coracoid process of scapula
- Long head: Supraglenoid tubercle of scapula.

Insertion:
- Short head: Radius
- Long head: Bicipital aponeurosis.

Nerve supply: Musculocutaneous nerve (C5,6).

Brachialis

Origin: Distal half of shaft of humerus, anterior surface.
Insertion: Ulna- coronoid process and tuberosity.
Nerve supply: Musculocutaneous nerve (C 5,6).

Brachioradialis

Origin: Lateral supracondylar ridge.
Insertion: Distal radius, just proximal to styloid process.
Nerve supply: Radial nerve (C5,6).

Patient: Sitting with arms at his sides. If sitting is not possible, the same can be tested in supine position. Elbow kept in mid-flexion (90°) and wrist and fingers relaxed (do not allow gripping which activates these flexors).

Elbow rotation position varies with the muscle being tested as follows:
- Supination: For biceps brachii
- Semipronation: For brachioradialis
- Pronation: For brachialis

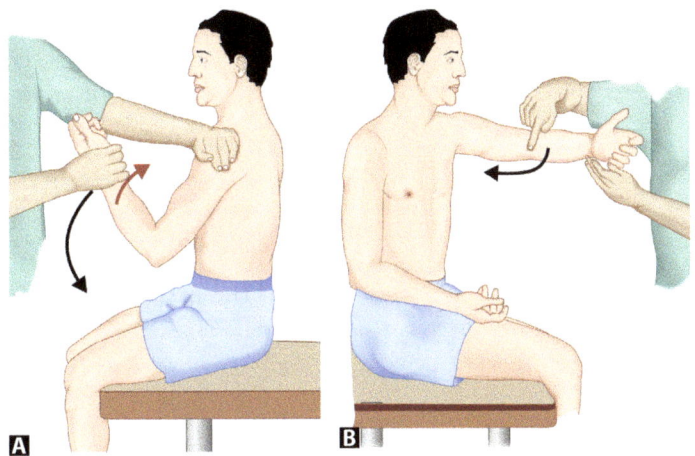

Figs. 4.30A and B: (A) Elbow flexion with forearm in supination to test biceps brachii against gravity; (B) Examination of elbow flexion with gravity eliminated.

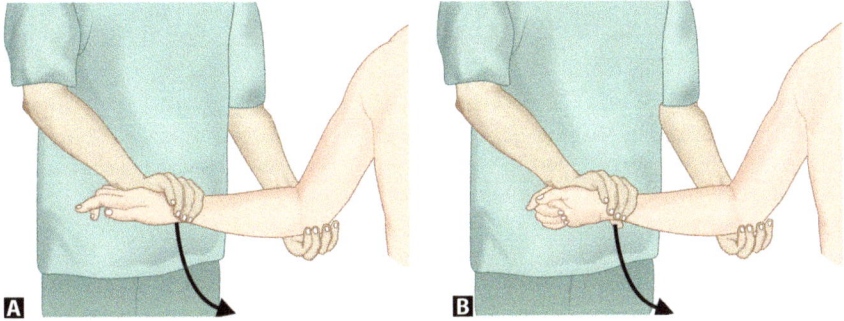

Figs. 4.31A and B: Elbow flexion with forearm fully pronated (brachialis) and semipronated (brachioradialis).

Examiner: Standing in front of the patient, one hand stabilizing the elbow, other hand placed over the flexor aspect of the forearm proximal to the wrist. Patient tries to pull and bend the elbow against examiner's resistance.

For testing grade 2 power, eliminate gravity by abducting the shoulder to 90° in sitting position or in supine position.

Caveats: Wrist flexors can compensate to some extent in elbow flexion. Therefore, wrist and finger flexors must be kept relaxed in all test positions.

ELBOW EXTENSION

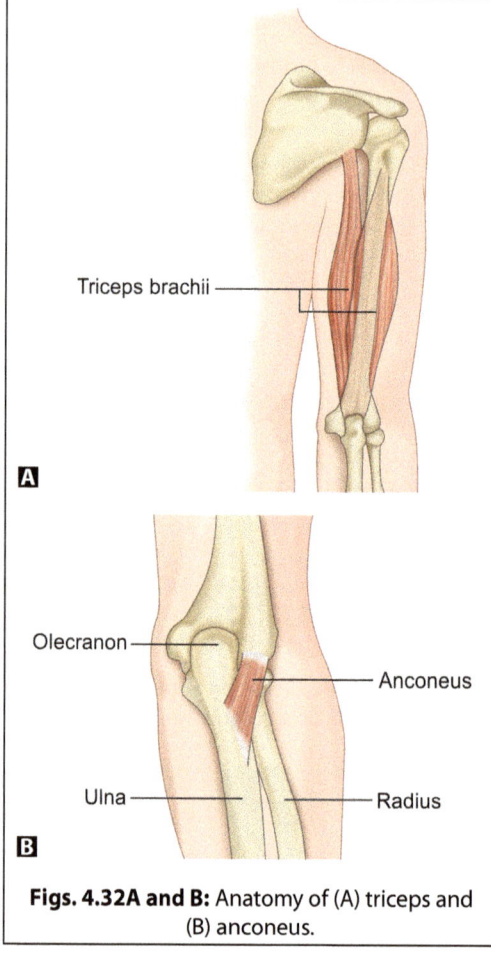

Triceps

Origin:
- Long head: Infraglenoid tuberosity of scapula
- Medial head: Posterior surface of shaft of humerus
- Lateral head: Posterior surface of shaft of humerus.

Insertion: All heads by common tendon on to the olecranon process of ulna.

Nerve supply: Radial nerve (C 7).

Figs. 4.32A and B: Anatomy of (A) triceps and (B) anconeus.

Methodology

Patient: Prone, arm abducted to 90 with forearm hanging freely from the edge of the cot.

Examiner: On the test side, supports the arm just proximal to elbow with one hand. The other hand is placed over the dorsum of the forearm, applying resistance to patients attempts to straighten the elbow.

Alternately, patient is in sitting position, arm abducted and elbow flexed. Examiner supports the arm from behind with one hand. Patient attempts to straighten the elbow against examiner's resistance.

For assessing grade 2 weakness, patient is placed in sitting position, with arm abducted to 90°. Examiner supports the elbow with one hand and observes if patient can straighten the elbow.

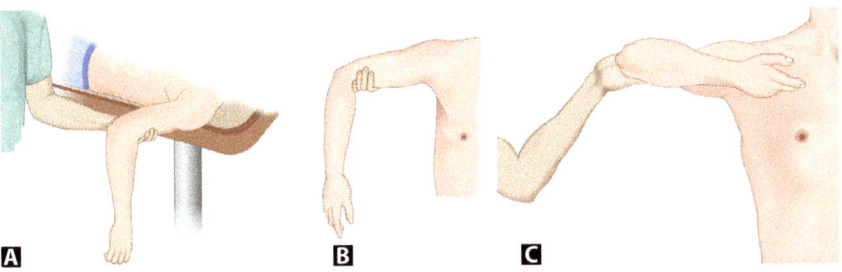

Figs. 4.33A to C: (A) Testing of triceps against gravity in prone position; (B) Sitting position; (C) Testing of triceps with gravity eliminated (the forearm movement must be parallel to the ground).

FOREARM SUPINATION

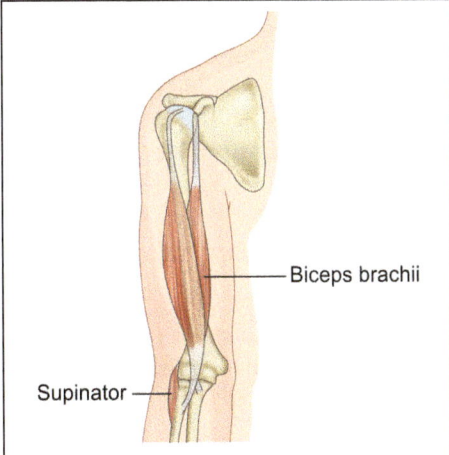

Fig. 4.34A: Anatomy of forearm supinators.

Prime Movers

Supinator, biceps brachii.

Supinator

Origin: Humerus (lateral epicondyle), Ulna (supinator crest).
Insertion: Proximal: 1/3 of shaft of radius.
Nerve supply: Supinator: Radial nerve (C6,7,8).

Biceps Brachii

See in elbow flexion.

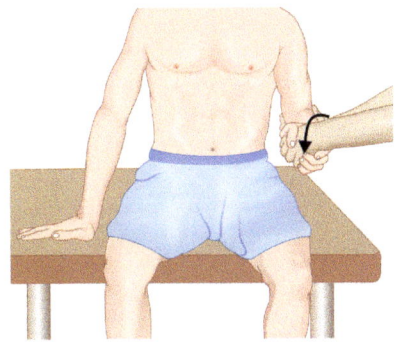

Fig. 4.34B: Testing of supinators of forearm.

Methodology

Patient: Sitting, elbow flexed 90°, forearm in pronation.

Examiner: Stands in front of the patient, supports the elbow with one hand. The other hand grasps the patient's hand as in a hand shake.

Test: Patient attempts to supinate (palm up) against examiner's resistance.
 For grade 2 weakness, patient fully flexes the elbow and then attempts supination, having eliminated gravity.

FOREARM PRONATION

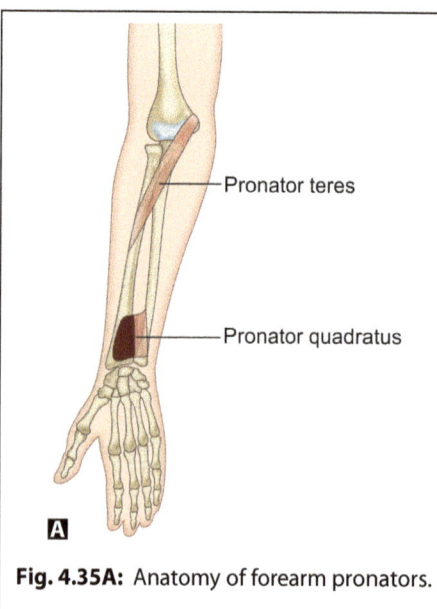

Pronator Teres

Origin: Shaft of humerus proximal to medial epicondyle, coronoid process of ulna.
Insertion: Radius (lateral aspect of midshaft).
Nerve supply: Median nerve (C6,7).

Pronator Quadratus

Origin: Ulna (oblique ridge on distal ¼ of anterior surface)
Insertion: Radius (shaft, anterior surface distally; also area above ulnar notch)
Nerve supply: Anterior interosseous branch of median nerve (C8, T1).

Fig. 4.35A: Anatomy of forearm pronators.

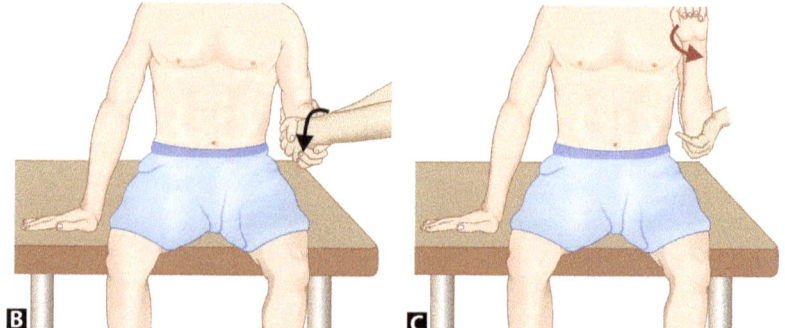

Figs. 4.35B and C: (B) Testing of forearm pronation against gravity and (C) with gravity eliminated.

Methodology

Patient: Sitting, elbow flexed 90° and close to the trunk, forearm in supination (Fig. 4.36B). Wrist and fingers must be relaxed.

Examiner: In front of the patient, supports elbow with one hand. Examiner's other hand grasps patient's corresponding hand (right for right and left for left) grasps patient's hand as if in a hand shake.

Test: Patient tries to pronate (palm down) against examiner's resistance.

Modification: For testing grade 2 or less power (Method in Fig. 4.35C), patient fully flexes the elbow with forearm in supination (palm facing the patient) and attempts to pronate (palm facing away from him). This eliminates gravity and brings out grade 2 power.

Caveats

- Patients usually recruit shoulder internal rotation to overcome examiner's resistance to pronation. This must be avoided by fixing the shoulder tucked close to the trunk.
- If the wrist and fingers are not relaxed, the flexor carpi radialis and finger flexors can produce some amount of pronation, even if pronators are very weak.

WRIST FLEXION

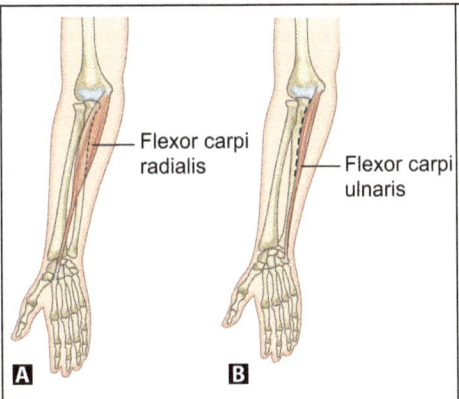

Figs. 4.36A and B: (A) Anatomy of flexor carpi radialis and (B) flexor carpi ulnaris.

Flexor Carpi Radialis

Origin: Humerus (medial epicondyle via common flexor tendon).
Insertion: 2nd and 3rd metacarpals (base, palmar surface).
Nerve supply: Median nerve (C6, 7).

Flexor Carpi Ulnaris

Origin: Humeral head (medial epicondyle via common flexor tendon).
Ulnar head (olecranon, medial margin; shaft, proximal 2/3 posterior via an aponeurosis)
Insertion: Pisiform bone, Hamate bone, 5th metacarpal base
Nerve supply: Ulnar nerve (C8, T1).

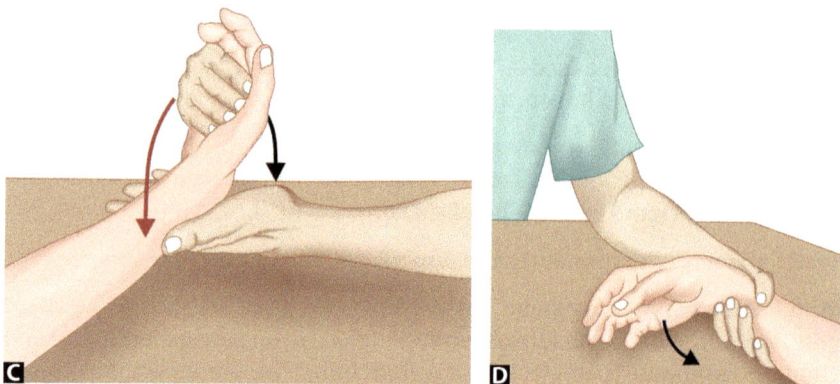

Figs. 4.36C and D: (C) Examination of wrist flexion against gravity; (D) with gravity eliminated.

Methodology

Patient: Sitting, forearm resting on the table in supination (Fig. 4.36C), wrist in neutral position. Fingers relaxed.

Examiner: Supports the forearm with one hand underneath it. His other hand offers resistance to wrist flexion by placing over the palm.

Test: To test the FCR, resistance is directed towards the 2nd metacarpal, with examiner attempting ulnar deviation of the hand. To test FCU, resistance is directed towards the 5th metacarpal with examiner attempting radial deviation of the hand. Patient tries to flex the wrist.

Modifications: To test for power grade 2 or 1/5, the position is similar except the forearm is semipronated with ulnar border resting on the table (Fig. 4.36D). Patient attempts wrist flexion in this position having eliminated the gravity.

WRIST EXTENSION

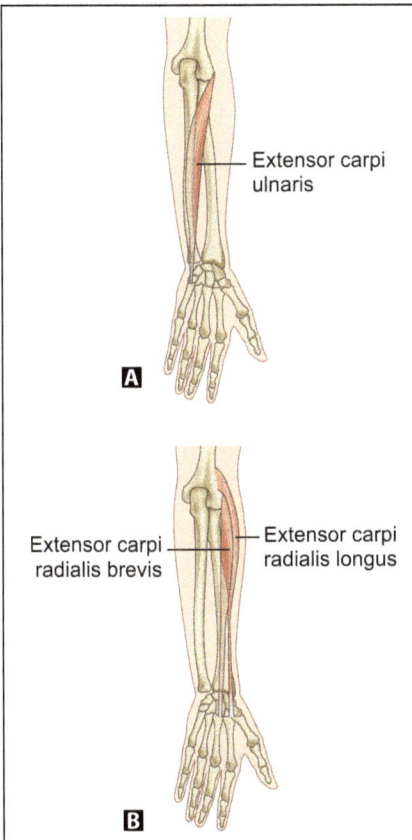

Figs. 4.37A and B: Anatomy of (A) extensor carpi ulnaris and (B) extensor carpi radialis longus and brevis.

Extensor Carpi Radialis Longus

Origin: Humerus (lateral supracondylar ridge, distal 1/3), common forearm extensor tendon.

Insertion: 2nd metacarpal bone (base on radial side of dorsal aspect).

Nerve supply: Radial nerve (C6,7).

Extensor Carpi Radialis Brevis

Origin: Humerus (lateral epicondyle via common forearm extensor tendon).

Insertion: 3rd metacarpal bone (base of dorsal surface on radial side).

Nerve supply: Posterior interosseous nerve (C6,7).

Extensor Carpi Ulnaris

Origin: Humerus (lateral epicondyle via common extensor tendon), Ulna (posterior border).

Insertion: 5th metacarpal bone (tubercle on medial side of base).

Nerve supply: Posterior interosseous nerve (C7, 8).

Methodology

Patient: Sitting, with elbow flexed, forearm pronated and resting on the table. Fingers relaxed.

Examiner: Supports the distal forearm with one hand on its volar aspect. Offers resistance with his other hand placed over the dorsal aspect of the metacarpals.

To test all the three extensors, patient is asked to extend the wrist straight without any deviation, while resistance is applied uniformly over the dorsum.

To test extensor carpi radialis longus and brevis, resistance is applied over the 2nd and 3rd metacarpals in the direction of flexion and ulnar deviation.

To test extensor carpi ulnaris, resistance is applied over the 5th metacarpal in the direction of wrist flexion and ulnar deviation.

For testing grade 2 or 1/5 power, forearm is placed as in the above test except that the forearm is semipronated to eliminate gravity.

Caveats:

If fingers are not relaxed, substitution occurs and wrist extension is produced even if the extensor muscles are weak.

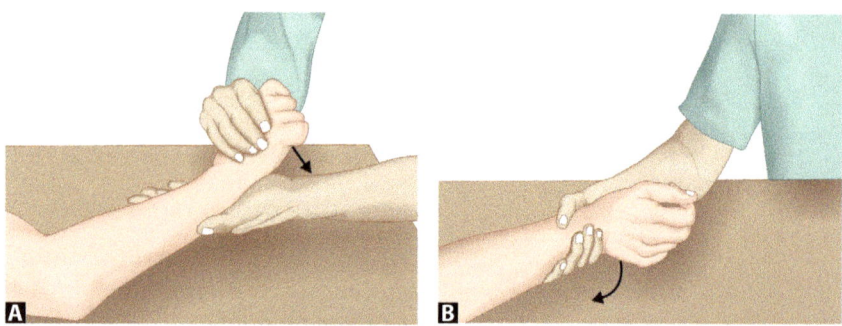

Figs. 4.38A and B: (A) Examination of wrist extension; (B) Examination of wrist extension with gravity eliminated.

METACARPOPHALANGEAL EXTENSION

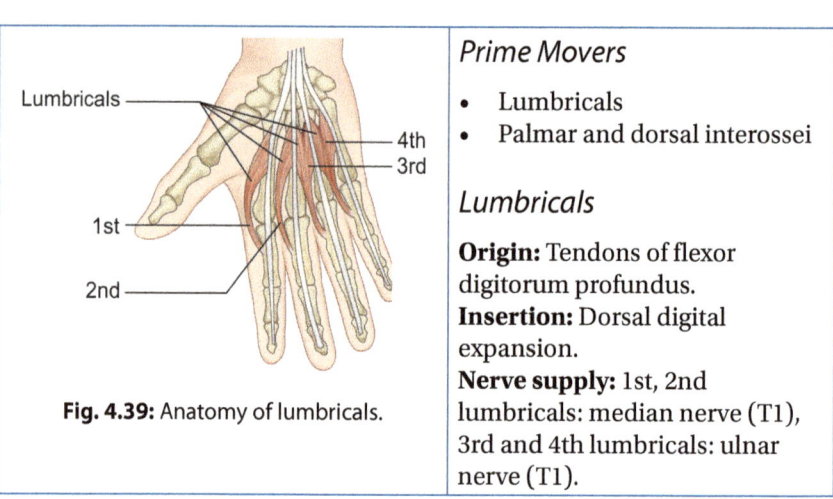

Fig. 4.39: Anatomy of lumbricals.

Prime Movers
- Lumbricals
- Palmar and dorsal interossei

Lumbricals

Origin: Tendons of flexor digitorum profundus.
Insertion: Dorsal digital expansion.
Nerve supply: 1st, 2nd lumbricals: median nerve (T1), 3rd and 4th lumbricals: ulnar nerve (T1).

Methodology

Patient: Sitting, forearm in supination, hand resting on the table. Flexes the metacarpophalangeal joint to 90° keeping the fingers extended.

Examiner: Stabilizes the metacarpals proximal to MCP joints with one hand. The other hand is placed over the palmar aspect of the proximal row of phalanges. He resists patient's attempt to flex MCP joints beyond 90.

For assessing grade 2 or 1/5 power, forearm is semipronated and test is repeated without examiner's resistance.

Caveats

Flexor digitorum profundus (EDP) can substitute for lumbrical action. Therefore, fingers must be kept in full extension throughout the test to minimize the FDP component.

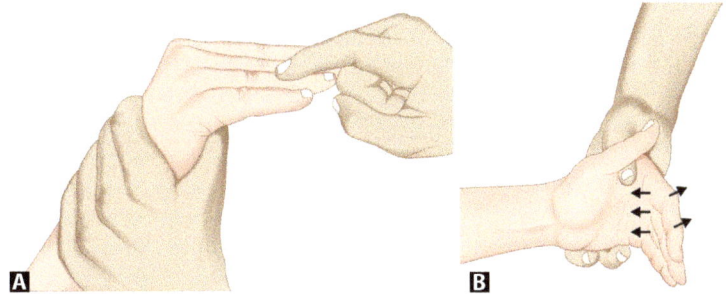

Figs. 4.40A and B: (A) Testing of lumbricals against gravity and (B) Testing of metacarpophalangeal extension with gravity eliminated.

FINGER FLEXION AT PROXIMAL AND DISTAL INTERPHALANGEAL JOINTS

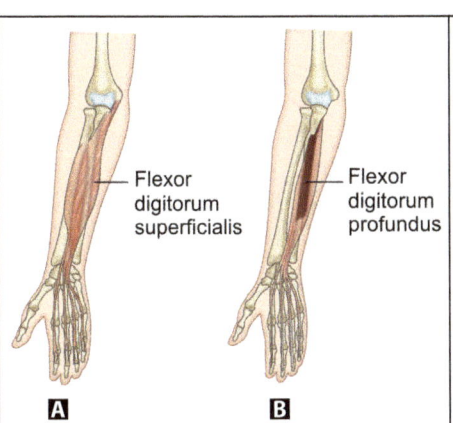

Figs. 4.41A and B: Anatomy of (A) flexor digitorum superficialis and (B) flexor digitorum profundus.

Prime Movers

- Flexor digitorum superficialis
- Flexor digitorum profundus

Flexor Digitorum Superficialis

Origin: Medial epicondyle of humerus, coronoid process of ulna, anterior aspect of radial shaft.

Insertion: Sides of middle phalanges of digits 2 to 5.

Nerve supply: Median nerve (C7, 8, T1)

Flexor Digitorum Profundus

Origin: Proximal ¾ of ulna (anterior and medial aspect).

Insertion: Palmar aspect of base of distal phalanges 2 to 5.

Nerve supply: Lateral part of the muscle (supplying 4th and 5th digits) is by anterior interosseous nerve (C8, T1); medial part (supplying 2nd and 3rd digits) by ulnar nerve (C8, T1).

Methodology for Testing Flexor Digitorum Superficialis

Patient: Forearm supinated, resting on the table, hand resting on the table. Fingers extended.

Examiner: With one hand, holds all the fingers other than the one being tested in extension. With the other hand, applies resistance over the middle phalanx (distal end) in a direction of extension, while the patient attempts to flex the proximal interphalangeal (PIP) joint.

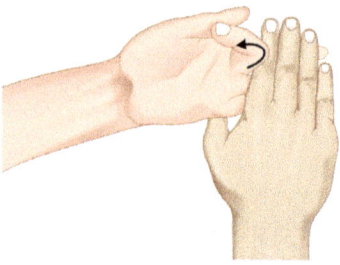

Fig. 4.42: Testing of flexor digitorum superficialis (FDS).

Caveats

- Flexor digitorum profundus can achieve flexion at MCP. This can be avoided by preventing flexion of DIP throughout the test
- If the wrist is allowed to extend instead of remaining in neutral position, passive flexion of MCP joints can occur due to stretching of the FDS tendon (Tenodesis action). Therefore, examiner has to ensure that the wrist remains neutral throughout the test
- If a patient cannot isolate one finger to produce MCP flexion, he may be allowed to flex two adjacent fingers.

TESTING OF DISTAL INTERPHALANGEAL FLEXION

Patient: Sitting with forearm supinated and resting on the table. Extends fingers at all joints.

Examiner: Stabilizes the middle phalanx by holding it on either side. With other hand, offers resistance to the palmar aspect of distal phalanx while patient attempts to flex it. Each finger must be tested separately.

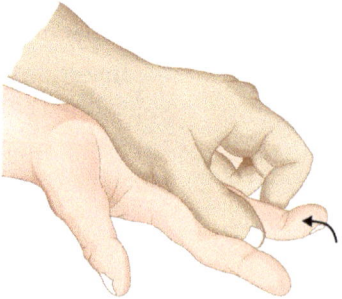

Fig. 4.43: Testing of flexor digitorum profundus.

Caveats: If wrist is allowed to extend instead of remaining in neutral position, tenodesis effect can produce DIP flexion.

FINGER METACARPOPHALANGEAL EXTENSION

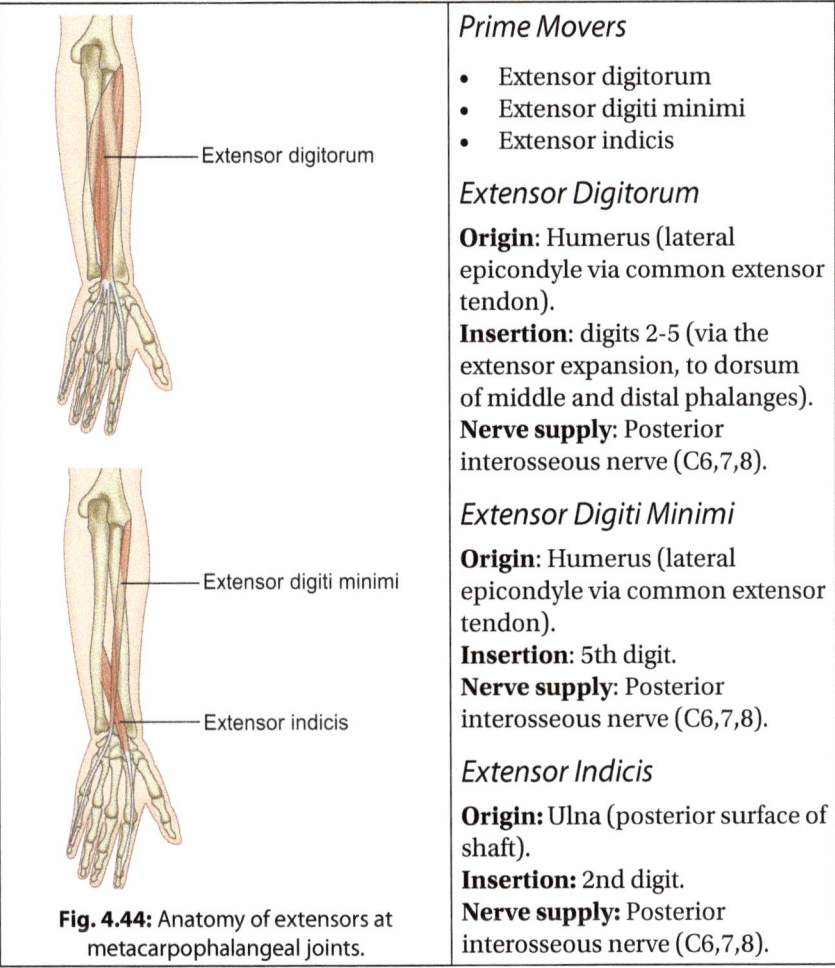

Prime Movers

- Extensor digitorum
- Extensor digiti minimi
- Extensor indicis

Extensor Digitorum

Origin: Humerus (lateral epicondyle via common extensor tendon).
Insertion: digits 2-5 (via the extensor expansion, to dorsum of middle and distal phalanges).
Nerve supply: Posterior interosseous nerve (C6,7,8).

Extensor Digiti Minimi

Origin: Humerus (lateral epicondyle via common extensor tendon).
Insertion: 5th digit.
Nerve supply: Posterior interosseous nerve (C6,7,8).

Extensor Indicis

Origin: Ulna (posterior surface of shaft).
Insertion: 2nd digit.
Nerve supply: Posterior interosseous nerve (C6,7,8).

Fig. 4.44: Anatomy of extensors at metacarpophalangeal joints.

Methodology

Patient: Position of Patient: Forearm in pronation, wrist in neutral. MP joints and IP joints are in relaxed flexion posture.

Examiner: stabilizes the wrist with one hand. Place the index finger of the other hand across the dorsum of all proximal phalanges. Patient attempts to extend the MCP against the resistance of examiner's index finger

For extensor digiti minimi and extensor indicis, the 5th and 2nd digits are selectively examined in the same way as above.

Caveat: Flexion of wrist can produce MCP extension by tenodesis action.

FINGER ABDUCTION

	Prime Movers
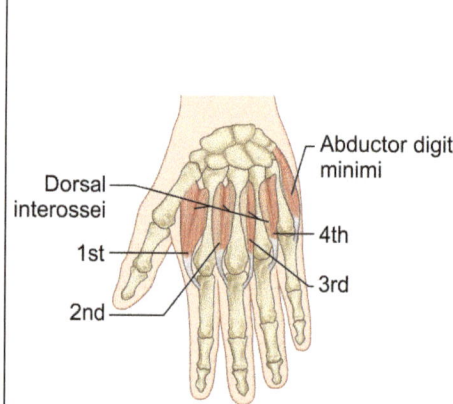 **Fig. 4.45:** Anatomy of finger abductors.	• Dorsal interossei • Abductor digiti minimi *Dorsal Interossei* **Origin:** Each muscle arises by 2 heads from adjacent sides of metacarpals • 1st dorsal: Between thumb and index finger • 2nd dorsal: Between index and long fingers • 3rd dorsal: Between long and ring fingers • 4th dorsal: Between ring and little fingers **Insertion:** • 1st dorsal: Index finger (radial side) • 2nd dorsal: Long finger (radial side) • 3rd dorsal: Long finger (ulnar side) • 4th dorsal: Ring finger (ulnar side) **Abductor digiti minimi:** **Origin:** Pisiform bone. **Insertion:** 5th digit (base of proximal phalanx, ulnar side). **Nerve supply:** Ulnar nerve (T1).

Methodology

Patient: Forearm pronated, wrist in neutral position, fingers extended (but not hyperextended).

Examiner: Supports the wrist with one hand. With other hand, gives resistance to two adjacent fingers, one on radial side and the other on ulnar side, so as to squeeze the two fingers together.

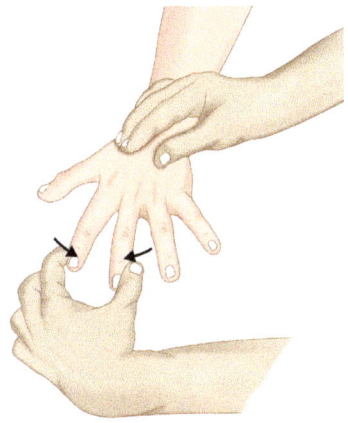

Fig. 4.46: Testing of finger abductors.

FINGER ADDUCTION

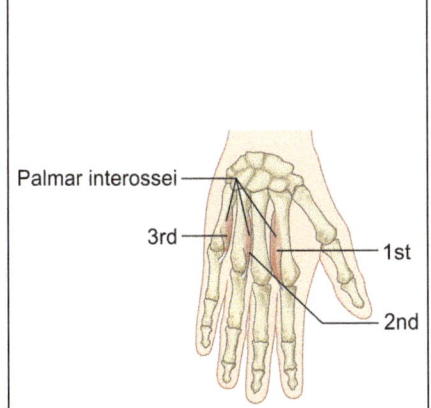

Fig. 4.47: Anatomy of finger adductors.

Prime Movers: Palmar Interossei

Origin: Metacarpal bones 2, 4, and 5
- 1st palmar: 2nd metacarpal (ulnar side)
- 2nd palmar: 4th metacarpal (radial side)
- 3rd palmar: 5th metacarpal (Radial side)

Insertion: Dorsal extensor expansion
- 1st palmar: Index finger (proximal phalanx, ulnar side)
- 2nd palmar: Ring finger (proximal phalanx, radial side)
- 3rd palmar: Little finger (proximal phalanx, radial side)

Nerve supply: Ulnar nerve T1.

Methodology

Patient: Sitting, forearm pronated and resting on the table. Wrist and MCP joints neutral, fingers extended and adducted.

Examiner: Holds the middle phalanx of each of the two adjacent fingers and tries to pull apart.
   Patient resists this movement of abduction.

It is difficult to differentiate grade 4 and 5 for small muscles of the hand like interossei. They must be graded in comparison to the other hand or based on examiner's experience with normal persons.

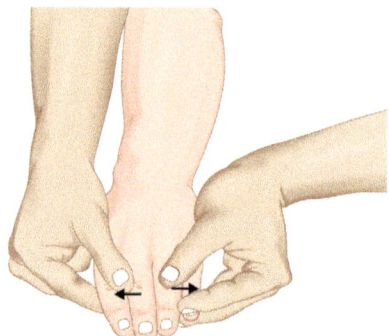

Fig. 4.48: Testing of finger adductors.

Caveats

Long finger flexors can substitute for adduction of fingers. Hence flexion of fingers must be avoided.

THUMB MOVEMENTS

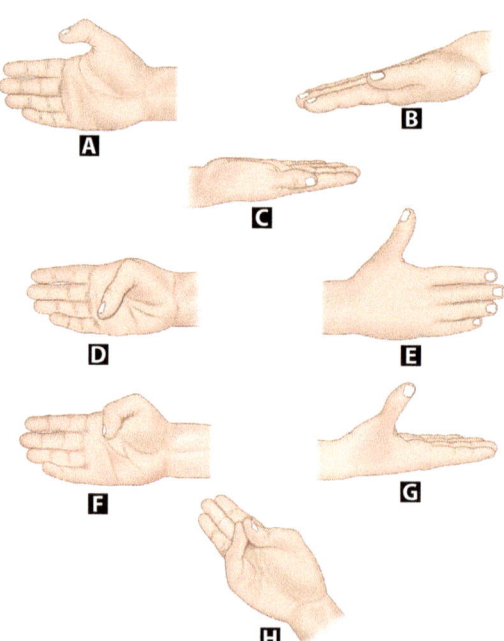

Figs. 4.49A to H: Motions of the thumb. (A) IP flexion; (B) MP and IP extension; (C) Neutral; (D) MP flexion; (E) Abduction in plane of hand (fingers); (F) MP and IP flexion; (G) Abduction 90° from plane of hand; (H) Opposition.

THUMB FLEXION

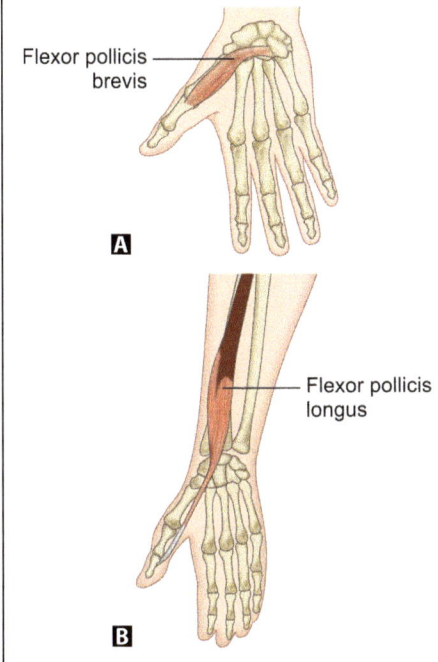

Figs. 4.50A and B: Anatomy of (A) flexor pollicis brevis and (B) flexor pollicis longus.

Flexor Pollicis Brevis

Origin: Flexor retinaculum (distal), trapezium bone.
Insertion: Thumb (base of proximal phalanx).
Nerve supply: Median nerve (C8,T1).

Flexor Pollicis Longus

Origin: Radius (anterior surface of middle 1/2) and adjacent interosseous membrane. Ulna [coronoid process, lateral border (variable)]. Humerus (medial epicondyle).
Insertion: Thumb (base of distal phalanx, palmar surface).
Nerve supply: Median nerve (C8,T1).

Flexor Pollicis Brevis

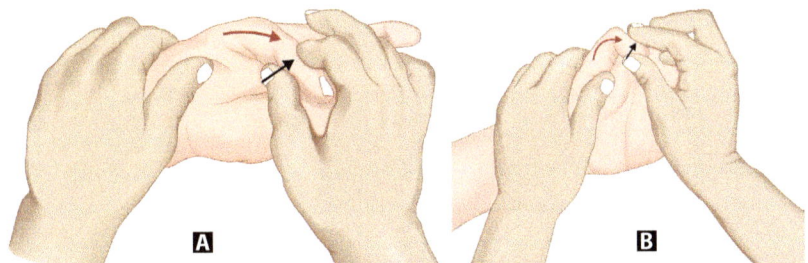

Figs. 4.51A and B: (A) Testing of flexor pollicis brevis and (B) flexor pollicis longus.

Methodology

Patient: Sitting, forearm in supination, wrist, MCP, thumb relaxed and in neutral position, thumb lying close to the 2nd metacarpal.

Examiner: Holds the metacarpal bone of the thumb with one hand and also stabilizes the wrist. With the other hand, offer one-finger resistance to the proximal phalanx of the thumb while the patient attempts to bring the thumb across the palm in the direction of flexion. Insist on keeping the distal interphalangeal joint in extension.

Caveat: Flexor pollicis longus can produce flexion of the MCP joint if the DIP joint is flexed. Hence, avoid DIP joint during the test.

Flexor Pollicis Longus

Test position is same as above, except that examiner's resistance is offered to the distal phalanx of the thumb.

THUMB EXTENSION

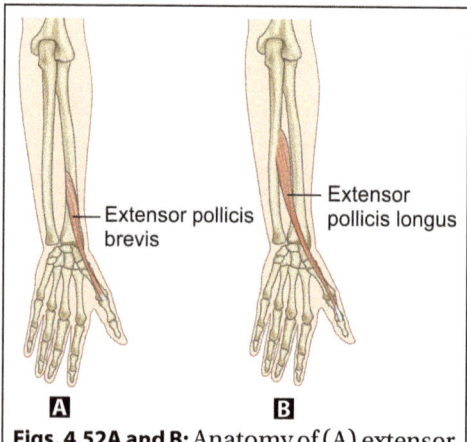

Extensor Pollicis Brevis

Origin: Posterior surface of radius.

Insertion: Proximal phalanx of thumb.

Nerve supply: Deep branch of radial nerve (C7, 8).

Extensor Pollicis Longus

Origin: Posterior surface of middle 1/3 of shaft of ulna.

Insertion: Base of distal phalanx of thumb.

Nerve supply: Deep branch of radial nerve (C7, 8).

Figs. 4.52A and B: Anatomy of (A) extensor pollicis brevis and (B) extensor pollicis longus.

Extensor Pollicis Brevis

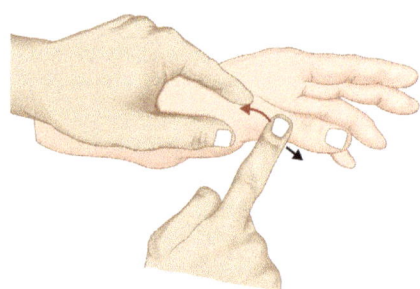

Fig. 4.53: Testing of extensor pollicis brevis.

Methodology

Patient: Forearm in midposition and wrist in neutral; carpometacarpal and IP joints of the thumb are relaxed.

Examiner: Stabilizes MCP joint by firmly holding the 1st metacarpal. With other hand, offers one finger resistance on the proximal phalanx of thumb, while the patient tries to extend the MCP joint (as if pointing to the ceiling).

Caveat

Extensor pollicis longus can flex the MCP joint. The clue to this substitution is extension of the interphalangeal joint during the test. This can be minimized by not allowing extension of interphalangeal joint while testing.

Extensor Pollicis Longus

Test position is same as above, except that the examiner's resistance is applied over the dorsum of distal phalanx so as to flex the interphalangeal joint.

Caveats

The muscles of the thenar eminence (abductor pollicis brevis, flexor pollicis brevis, and adductor pollicis) can extend the IP joint by flexing the CMC joint (an extensor tenodesis).

THUMB ABDUCTION

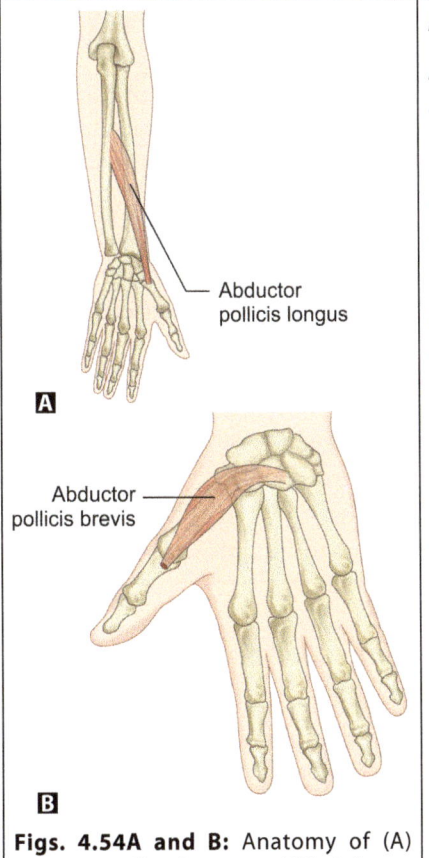

Figs. 4.54A and B: Anatomy of (A) abductor pollicis longus and (B) abductor pollicis brevis

Prime Movers

Abductor pollicis longus:
- Origin: Ulna (posterior surface laterally). Radius (shaft, middle 1/3 of posterior aspect
- Insertion: Thumb: 1st metacarpal
- Nerve supply: Posterior interosseous nerve (C7,8).

Abductor pollicis brevis:
- Origin: Flexor retinaculum, scaphoid bone, trapezium bone
- Insertion: Thumb (base of proximal phalanx, radial side). Lateral fibers: Extensor expansion of thumb
- Nerve supply: Median nerve (T1).

Abductor Pollicis Longus

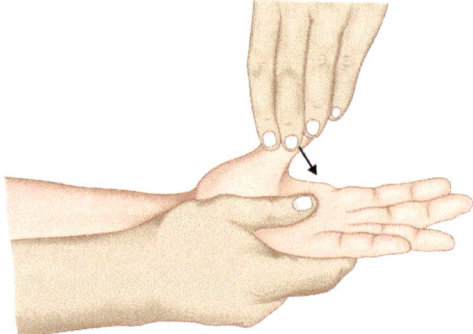

Fig. 4.55: Testing of abductor pollicis longus.

Methodology

Position of patient: Forearm supinated and wrist in neutral; thumb relaxed in adduction.

Examiner: Stabilize the metacarpals of the four fingers and the wrist. Resistance is given on the distal end of the 1st metacarpal in the direction of adduction. Patient abducts the thumb away from the hand in a plane parallel to the finger metacarpals.

Caveat

1. The extensor pollicis brevis can substitute for APB. In this case, the line of pull will be in the dorsal direction.
2. If the abductor pollicis longus is stronger than the brevis, the thumb will deviate toward the radial side of the hand.
3. If the abductor pollicis brevis is stronger, deviation will be toward the ulnar side.

Abductor Pollicis Brevis

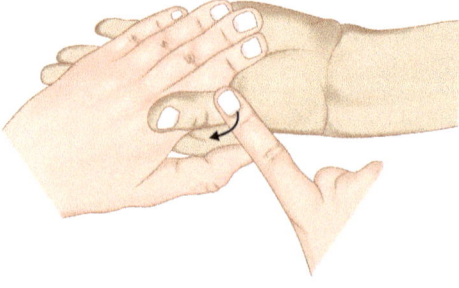

Fig. 4.56: Testing of abductor pollicis brevis.

Methodology

Position of patient: Forearm in supination, wrist in neutral, and thumb relaxed in adduction.

Examiner: Stabilize the metacarpals by placing the examiner's hand across the patient's palm with the thumb on the dorsal surface of the patient's hand.

Apply resistance to the lateral aspect of the proximal phalanx of the thumb in the direction of adduction.

Test: Patient abducts the thumb in a plane perpendicular to the palm, as in pointing to the ceiling.

Caveat

If the plane of motion is not perpendicular, but toward the radial side of the hand, the substitution may be by the abductor pollicis longus.

THUMB ADDUCTION

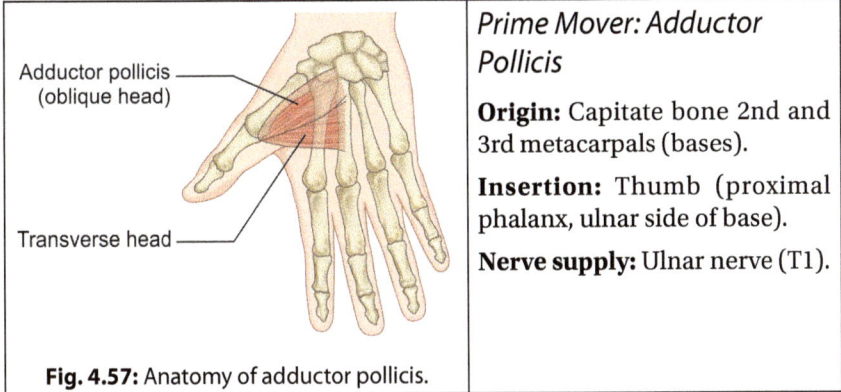

Prime Mover: Adductor Pollicis

Origin: Capitate bone 2nd and 3rd metacarpals (bases).

Insertion: Thumb (proximal phalanx, ulnar side of base).

Nerve supply: Ulnar nerve (T1).

Fig. 4.57: Anatomy of adductor pollicis.

Methodology

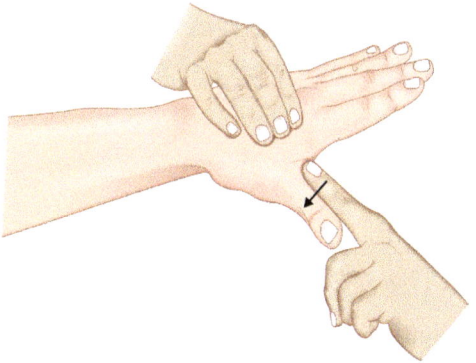

Fig. 4.58: Testing of adductor pollicis.

Patient: Forearm in pronation, wrist in neutral, and thumb relaxed and hanging down in abduction.

Examiner: Stabilize the metacarpals of the four fingers. Resistance is given on the medial side of the proximal phalanx of the thumb in the direction of abduction.

Patient adducts the thumb by bringing the 1st metacarpal up to the 2nd metacarpal.

Caveats

The flexor pollicis longus and brevis muscles can substitute for thumb adduction and must be kept inactive during testing.

THUMB OPPOSITION

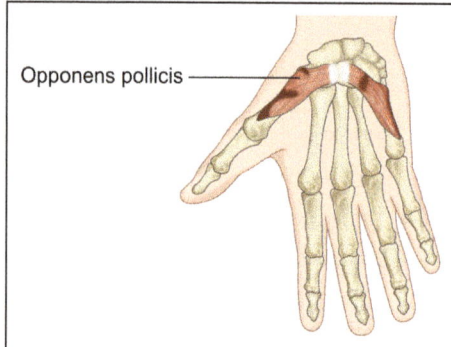

Prime Mover: Opponens Pollicis

Origin: Trapezium bone (tubercle). Flexor retinaculum.

Insertion: 1st metacarpal.

Nerve supply: Median nerve (recurrent thenar branch) (C8, T1).

Fig. 4.59: Anatomy of opponens pollicis.

Methodology

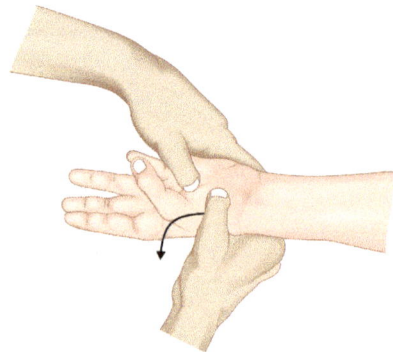

Fig. 4.60: Testing of opponens pollicis.

Position of patient: Forearm is supinated, wrist in neutral, and thumb in adduction with MP and IP flexion.

Examiner: Stabilize the hand by holding the wrist on the dorsal surface. Apply resistance for the opponens pollicis at the head of the 1st metacarpal in the direction of lateral rotation, extension, and adduction.

Patient raises the thumb away from the palm and rotates it so that its distal phalanx opposes the distal phalanx of the little finger forming the letter 'O' with thumb and little finger. Such apposition must be pad to pad and not tip to tip.

Caveats

If the patient opposes the tips of the thumb and little finger instead of the pads, the flexor pollicis longus will substitute for the action of opponens pollicis.

LITTLE FINGER OPPOSITION

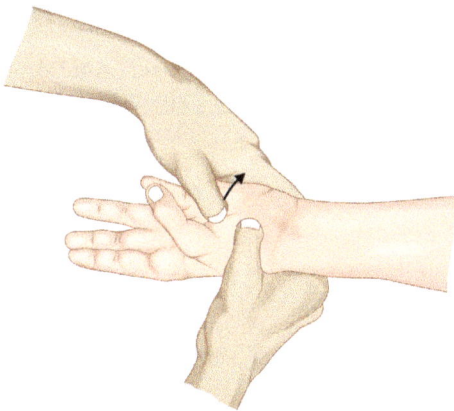

Fig. 4.61: Testing of opponens digiti minimi.

The methodology is same as above except that the resistance is given on the palmar surface of the 5th metacarpal in the direction of medial rotation (flattening the palm).

EXAMINATION OF POWER OF LOWER LIMB MUSCLES

HIP FLEXION

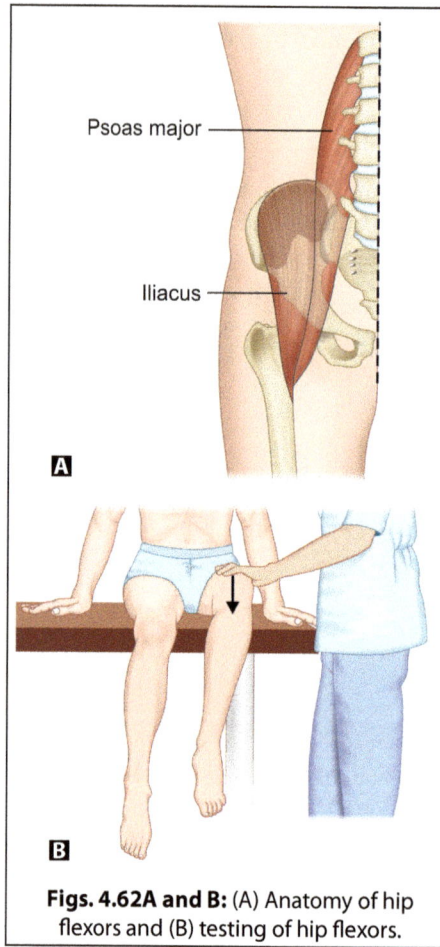

Psoas Major

Origin: Transverse processes of L1-5.
Insertion: Lesser trochanter (femur).
Nerve supply: L2, 3, 4 roots.

Iliacus

Origin: Sacrum, iliac fossa and crest.
Insertion: Lesser trochanter and shaft (femur).
Nerve supply: Femoral nerve (L2, 3).

Figs. 4.62A and B: (A) Anatomy of hip flexors and (B) testing of hip flexors.

Methodology

Patient: Sitting with legs freely hanging down the edge of the cot (or supine).

Examiner: By the test side, with hand placed over distal thigh above knee, giving downward force.

Test: Patient attempts to lift the leg upwards against resistance.

Modification: For testing grade 2 power, patient is in side lying position, attempting to flex the hip.

Caveats

- Sartorius can produce hip flexion. This is associated with external rotation and abduction of hip. Thus, examiner must ensure that hip is in neutral rotation during the test
- Tensor fascia latae can also cause hip flexion, but is associated with hip internal rotation and abduction. These deviations must be avoided during the test.

HIP EXTENSION

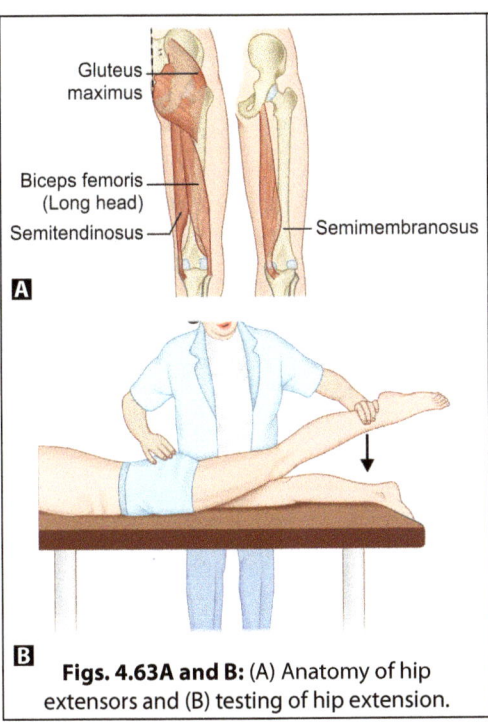

Gluteus Maximus

Origin: Posterior gluteal line, sacrum, coccyx.
Insertion: Gluteal tuberosity of femur and iliotibial band.
Hamstrings: See later sections
Nerve supply: Inferior gluteal nerve (L5-S2).

Figs. 4.63A and B: (A) Anatomy of hip extensors and (B) testing of hip extension.

Methodology

Patient: Prone, with arms placed comfortably overhead. To test all hip extensors together, the knee is kept in extension. To test gluteus maximus alone, knee is flexed to 90°.

Examiner: On the test side, one hand stabilizing the pelvis. The other hand is placed over the distal leg, just proximal to the ankle and downward force is applied. For an easier test, the resistance may be applied just proximal to the knee. This modification is required while testing thinly built frail individuals. While testing the gluteus maximus alone, resistance is applied just proximal to the flexed knee.

Test: Patient attempts to raise the leg off the bed against resistance, keeping the knee extended.

Modifications: For testing grade 2 power, patient is placed in side-lying position and is asked to extend the thigh without examiner's resistance.

HIP ADDUCTION

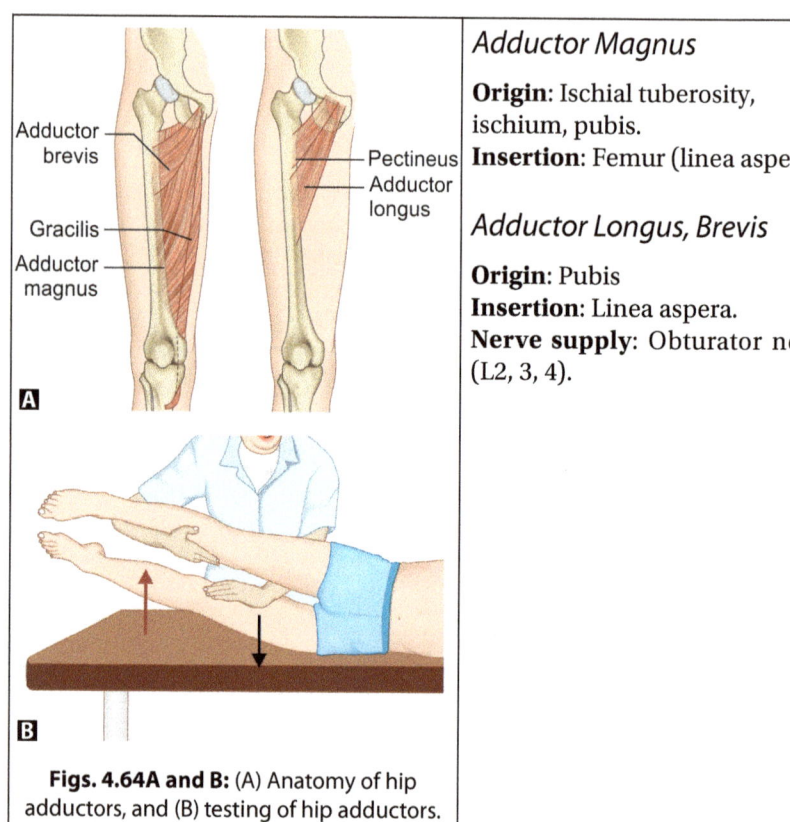

Adductor Magnus

Origin: Ischial tuberosity, ischium, pubis.
Insertion: Femur (linea aspera).

Adductor Longus, Brevis

Origin: Pubis
Insertion: Linea aspera.
Nerve supply: Obturator nerve (L2, 3, 4).

Figs. 4.64A and B: (A) Anatomy of hip adductors, and (B) testing of hip adductors.

Methodology

Patient: Side-lying with the limb to tested being the lower most. The other limb is abducted to 25° and supported by the examiner.

Examiner: Stands behind the patient. One hand supports the abducted limb. The other hand is paced over the medial aspect of the thigh just proximal to the knee, giving downward resistance to patient's attempt to adduct it.

Test: Patient is asked to raise the lower most thigh off the bed until it touches the abducted leg.

Modifications: To test grade 2 power, patient is supine and attempts adduction of thigh without examiner's resistance.

Caveats

- If the patient slightly turns prone, hamstrings will lift the thigh off the bed, mimicking adduction
- If the patient slightly turns supine, hip flexors will produce adduction like movement
- Therefore, true side-lying position is required to eliminate these substitutions.

HIP ABDUCTION

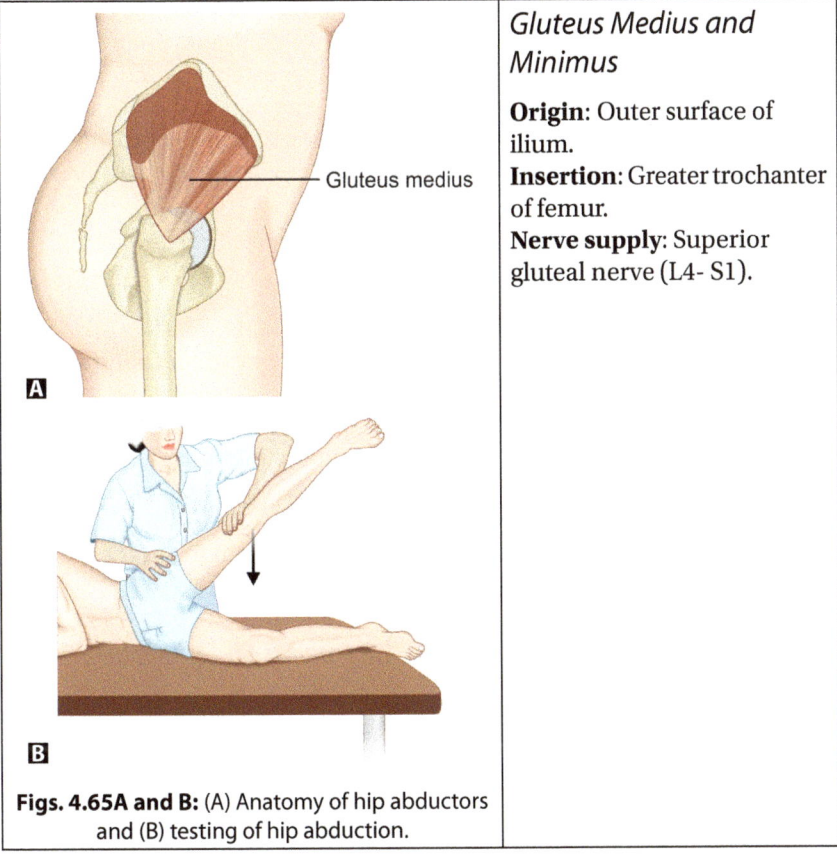

Gluteus Medius and Minimus

Origin: Outer surface of ilium.
Insertion: Greater trochanter of femur.
Nerve supply: Superior gluteal nerve (L4- S1).

Figs. 4.65A and B: (A) Anatomy of hip abductors and (B) testing of hip abduction.

Methodology

Patient: Side-lying with test leg uppermost. Place the limb slightly extended beyond the midline and the pelvis rotated slightly forward. Lowermost leg is flexed for stability.

Examiner: Standing behind patient. Hand used to give resistance is placed on the lateral surface of the knee. With the other hand, palpate the gluteus medius proximal to the greater trochanter.

Test: Patient abducts hip through without flexing the hip or rotating it in either direction.

Modifications: For testing grade 2 power, patient lies in supine position and abducts the hip while the examiner supports the ankle with one hand to reduce the friction.

Caveats

- Patient may use lateral trunk muscles and lift the pelvis, mimicking hip abduction. This can be identified by absence of gluteus medius contraction with the palpating hand
- Patient may externally rotate the hip and use hip flexors to lift the thigh, mimicking abduction. This can be avoided by testing abduction without allowing external rotation
- If the hip is slightly flexed, tensor fascia latae may achieve hip abduction like movement. Therefore, hip needs to be kept in slight extension while testing hip abduction.

HIP EXTERNAL ROTATION

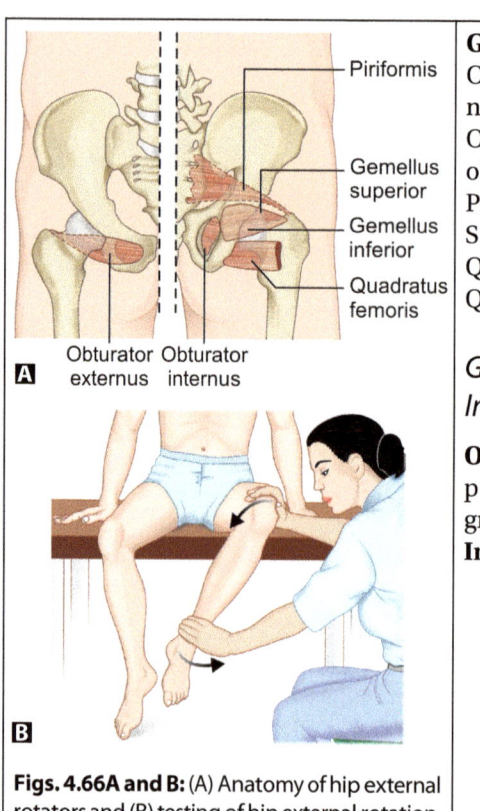

Gluteus maximus: See above
Obturator externus (obturator nerve/ L3, 4).
Obturator internus (nerve to obturator internus/ L5, S1).
Piriformis (nerve to piriformis/ S1, 2).
Quadratus femoris (nerve to Quadratus femoris, L5, S1).

Gemellus Superior and Inferior

Origin: Pelvis (sacrum/ischium/pubis/obturator membrane/greater sciatic foramen.
Insertion: Femur, medial aspect.

Figs. 4.66A and B: (A) Anatomy of hip external rotators and (B) testing of hip external rotation.

Methodology

Patient: Sitting, legs hanging down freely from the edge of the cot. Thigh is placed in externally rotated position to start with.

Examiner: On the test side, holds the ankle just above the malleoli with one hand. The other hand is placed on the lateral aspect of the thigh just above the knee. The two hands apply forces in opposite directions in attempting to produce a rotatory force of internal rotation against patient's efforts of external rotation.

Test: patient attempts to bring his heel towards the opposite knee against examiner's resistance.

Modifications: For testing grade 2 power, patient is in supine position, limb placed in internal rotation. Patient attempts to externally rotate the limb. Only gluteus maximus is palpable among the external rotators.

Caveats

Patient may produce trick movement by tilting the pelvis/ leaning to one side/ abducting the hip. This must be avoided.

HIP INTERNAL ROTATION

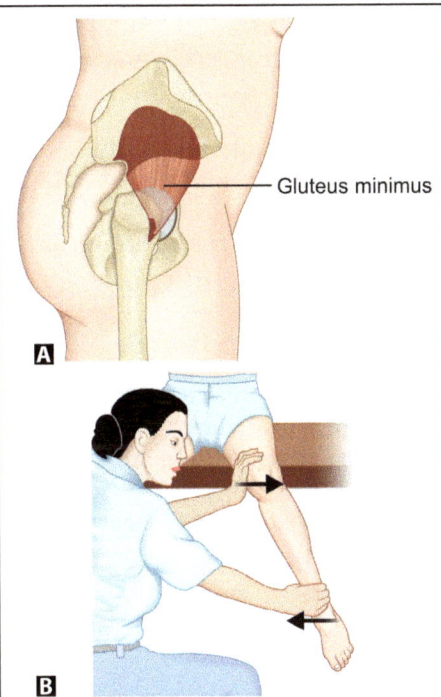

Gluteus Minimus and Medius

Origin: Outer surface of ilium.
Insertion: Greater trochanter of femur.
Nerve supply: Superior gluteal nerve (L4–S1).

Tensor Fascia Latae

Origin: Iliac crest, anterior superior iliac spine, fascia lata.
Insertion: Iliotibial band.
Nerve supply: Superior gluteal nerve (L4–S1).

Figs. 4.67A and B: (A) Anatomy of internal rotators of hip and (B) testing of hip internal rotation

Methodology

Patient: Sitting, legs hanging freely from the edge of the cot. The thigh may be placed in full internal rotation to start with. Patient has to maintain the limb in this position against examiner's resistance.

Examiner: In front of the patient. One hand grasps the ankle just above the malleoli and applies an inward pulling force. The other hand is placed on the medial aspect of the thigh just above the knee joint and applies as outward pushing force.

Test: Patient attempts to roll his leg as if reaching the cot with his foot.

Modifications: For assessing grade 2 power, patient is placed is supine position and tries to roll the test limb inward, without examiner's resistance.

Caveat

Patient may produce trick movements by tilting the pelvis/leaning to one side/adducting the hip. These must be avoided.

KNEE FLEXION

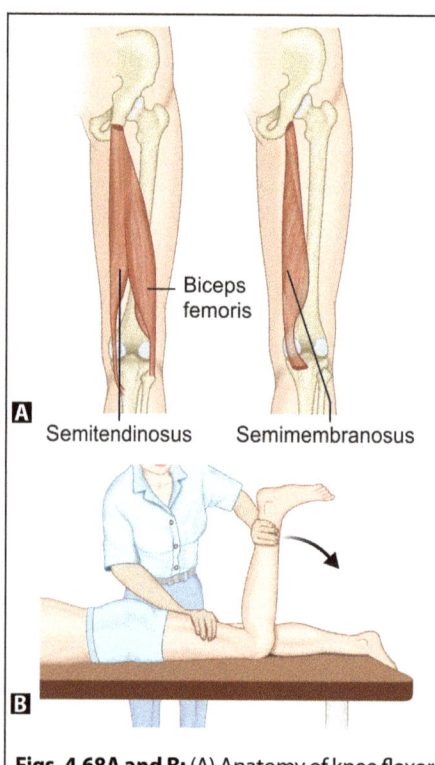

Semimembranosus and Semitendinosus

Origin: Ischial tuberosity
Insertion: Tibia (medial condyle and shaft)
Nerve supply: Tibial component of sciatic nerve (L5-S2).

Biceps Femoris

Origin: Ischial tuberosity, linea aspera of femur
Insertion: Fibula and lateral condyle of tibia
Nerve supply: Peroneal nerve/L5-S2.

Figs. 4.68A and B: (A) Anatomy of knee flexors and (B) testing of knee flexion against gravity.

Methodology

Patient: Prone with knee flexed to $30°$. Foot in the midline (avoiding rotation at knee).

Examiner: On the test side. Holds the leg just above the malleoli, applies downward direction towards the cot. The other hand is placed over the hamstrings for palpation.

Test: patient is asked to flex his knee against resistance.

Modifications:
- To test biceps femoris alone, foot needs to be externally rotated (toes pointing outward). Examiner applies downward and inward force along the line of action of biceps femoris
- To test medial hamstrings, foot has to be internally rotated (toes pointing towards midline). Examiner applies downward and outward force in the line of action of medial hamstrings
- To test grade 2 power, patient is in side-lying position attempting to flex the knee. Examiner supports the knee to reduce friction.

Caveats

- If during knee flexion, the foot rotates outward, it suggests biceps femoris is stronger than medial hamstrings
- If the foot rotates inwards, it suggests that medial hamstrings are stronger (this selectivity is explained by the different nerve supply of these two muscle groups).
- Sartorius may substitute in knee flexion, but this is associated with hip flexion and external rotation
- Patient may strongly dorsiflex the ankle to cause tenodesis effect of gastrocnemius to cause knee flexion.

KNEE EXTENSION

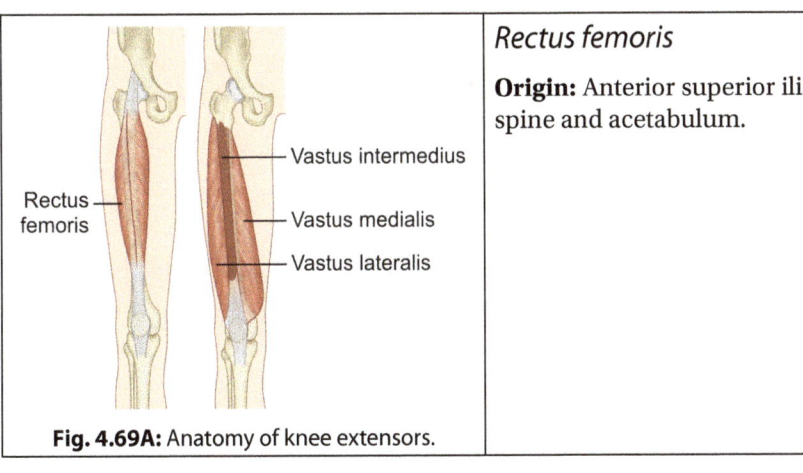

Rectus femoris

Origin: Anterior superior iliac spine and acetabulum.

Fig. 4.69A: Anatomy of knee extensors.

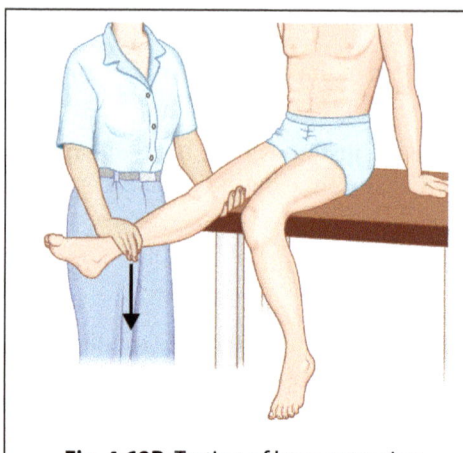

Fig. 4.69B: Testing of knee extension.

Vastus (Lateralis, Intermedius, Medialis)

Origin: Linea aspera, shaft of femur, greater trochanter.
Insertion (all muscles): Tibial tuberosity via ligamentum patellae.
Nerve supply: Femoral nerve (L2, 3, 4).

Methodology

Patient: Sitting, knee flexed, leg hanging freely at the edge of the table. Place a pad (or examiner's hand) under the distal thigh to keep the femur in horizontal position.

Examiner: On the test side, one hand placed over the distal leg just above the ankle applying downward and backward force.

Test: Patient is asked to straighten the knee against resistance, but not beyond 0 degrees.

Modifications: To assess grade 2 power, patient is side-lying, test side being upper most, supported by the examiner to reduce friction. Patient attempts knee extension.

Caveats

- Avoid hyperextension of the knee as this will lock the knee which appears like grade 5 power
- If a patient has limited SLR, knee extension will be limited to that angle. Hence, test the SLR before testing quadriceps and limit the movement to that angle to avoid discomfort.

ANKLE PLANTAR FLEXION

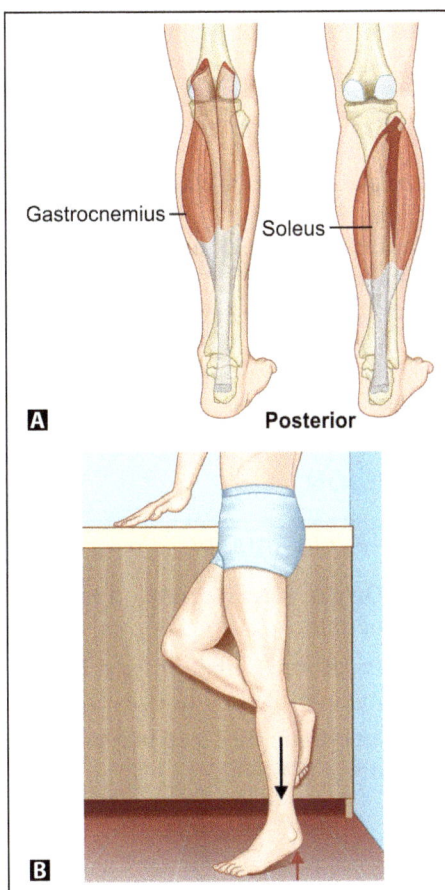

Figs. 4.70A and B: (A) Anatomy of ankle plantar flexors and (B) testing of ankle plantar flexion against gravity.

Gastrocnemius

Origin: Posterior aspect of femoral medial and lateral condyles.
Insertion: Calcaneus via tendocalcalneus.
Nerve supply: Tibial nerve (S1, 2).

Soleus

Origin: Posterior aspect of tibia and fibula
Insertion: Calcaneus via tendocalcaneus
Nerve supply: Tibial nerve (S1, 2).

Methodology

Patient: Standing, knee straight (extended). Other leg is raised off the ground. He can take minimal support with hands to maintain balance.

Examiner: Standing or sitting to get a lateral view of the test limb.

Test: Patient raises the heel through full range of motion to stand on toe tips. This is repeated 25 times without break. If patient completes 25 full range movements, it is graded 5. Between 10–25 times is graded 4, between 1–9 times is graded 3.

Modifications:
- To isolate soleus, same test is done with knee slightly flexed
- To test grade 2 power, patient is in prone position and plantar flexes ankle without examiner's resistance.

Caveats

- Tibialis posterior can produce ankle plantar flexion and simultaneous inversion. Avoiding inversion eliminates this action
- Peronei can also produce ankle plantar flexion and simultaneous foot eversion. Avoiding eversion eliminates this muscle
- Toe flexors can produce ankle plantar flexion, but this involves more of forefoot flexion
- Note that the grading of this extremely strong muscle is different from grading other muscles using MRC scale.

FOOT DORSIFLEXION AND INVERSION

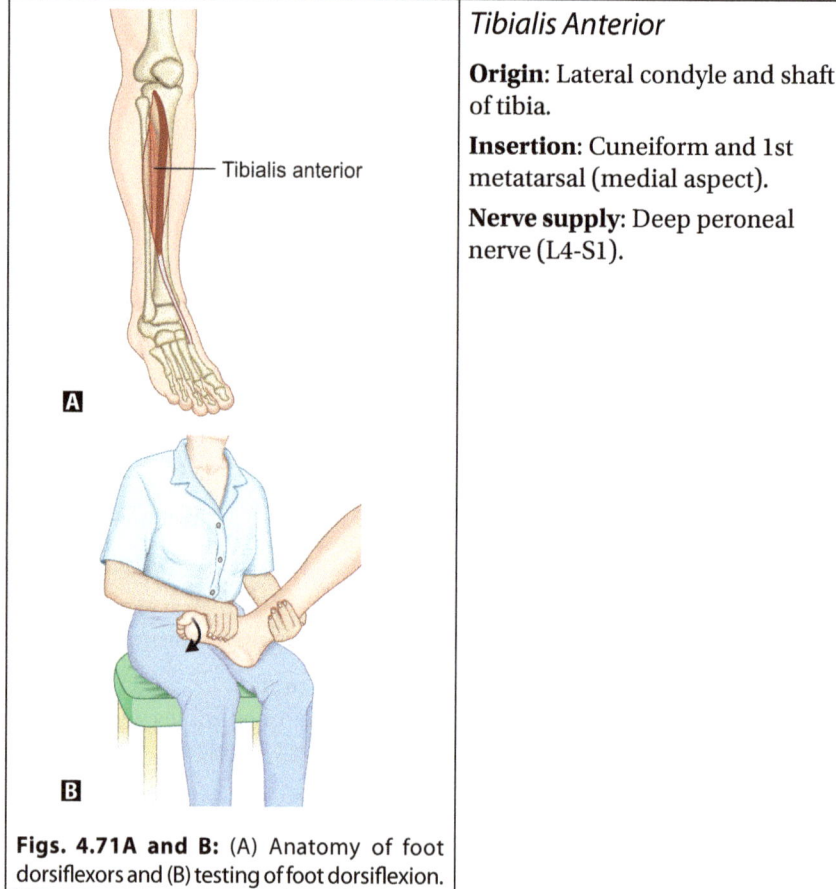

Tibialis Anterior

Origin: Lateral condyle and shaft of tibia.

Insertion: Cuneiform and 1st metatarsal (medial aspect).

Nerve supply: Deep peroneal nerve (L4-S1).

Figs. 4.71A and B: (A) Anatomy of foot dorsiflexors and (B) testing of foot dorsiflexion.

Methodology

Patient: Sitting, knee flexed and leg hanging freely over the edge of the cot.

Examiner: One hand supports the leg by holding it just above the ankle on its posterior aspect. The other hand is place over the dorsum of the foot and on its medial aspect near metatarsal heads. Resistance is applied in a downward and outward direction (as if everting the foot).

Test: Patient dorsiflexes ankle against examiner's resistance.

Caveats

- If the knee is not flexed, the stretch on gastrocnemius will prevent full range of dorsiflexion. Hence, knee must be flexed during the test
- Extensor hallucis longus and extensor digitorum longus can substitute for ankle dorsiflexion. This is identified by the fact that toes also dorsiflex during the movement. This can be avoided by keeping the toes relaxed.

FOOT INVERSION

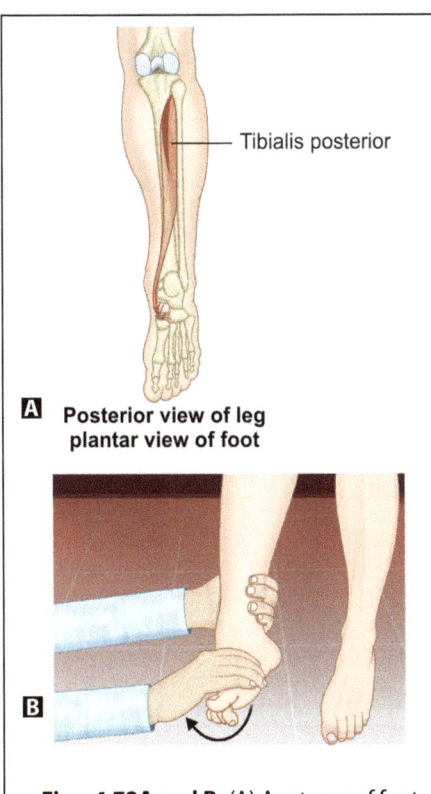

Tibialis Posterior

Origin: Inner posterior borders of tibia and fibula and the interosseous membrane.

Insertion: Tuberosity of navicular, medial cuneiform, bases of 2nd, 3rd and 4th metatarsals.

Nerve supply: Tibial nerve (L4, 5).

Figs. 4.72A and B: (A) Anatomy of foot invertors and (B) testing of foot invertors.

Methodology

Patient: Sitting, knee flexed, leg hanging freely at the edge of the cot, ankle slightly plantar flexed.

Examiner: Sitting in front of the patient, stabilizes the leg by holding it just above the ankle on its posterior aspect. The other hand is placed over the dorsum and medial aspect of the foot near metatarsal heads. Resistance is applied in an outward direction towards eversion.

Test: Patient is asked to turn the foot downward and inwards (as in trying to inspect the inner margin of the sole).

Caveats

Flexor digitorum longus and flexor hallucis longus can produce foot inversion. This is recognized by associated toe flexion and prevented by keeping the toes relaxed.

FOOT EVERSION

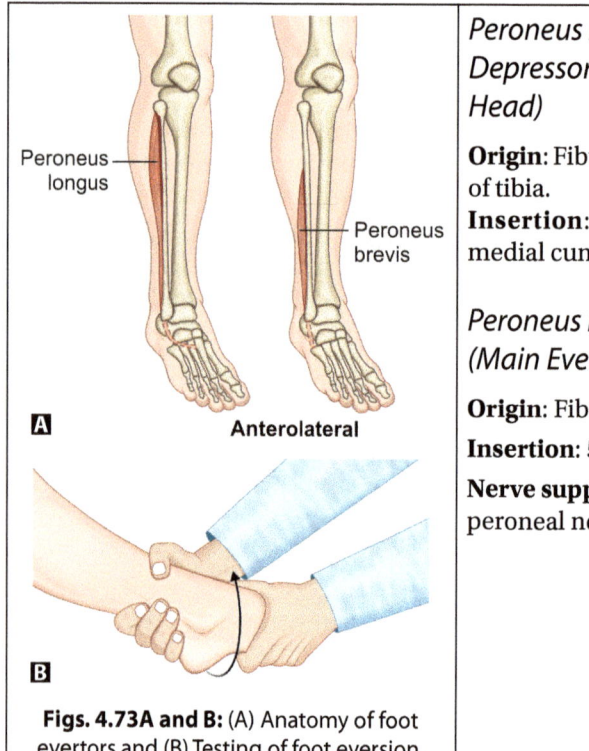

Peroneus Longus (Mainly Depressor at 1st Metatarsal Head)

Origin: Fibula and lateral condyle of tibia.

Insertion: 1st metatarsal and medial cuneiform.

Peroneus Brevis (Main Evertor)

Origin: Fibula

Insertion: 5th metatarsal

Nerve supply: Superficial peroneal nerve (L5, S1).

Figs. 4.73A and B: (A) Anatomy of foot evertors and (B) Testing of foot eversion.

Methodology

Patient: Sitting, with foot in neutral position.

Examiner: Sitting in front of the patient, grasps the leg above the ankle for stabilization. With the other hand, holds the foot over its dorsolateral aspect and applies downward and inward force.

Test: Patient presses the foot downward and outward (as if to inspect the lateral margin of the sole).

Modifications:
- The test can be done in supine position with examiner standing at the foot end
- Peroneus longus can be isolated by applying resistance under the 1st metatarsal head towards inversion and dorsiflexion patient depresses the foot.

Caveats

The toe extensors cause dorsiflexion and eversion. Hence, to test the peroneal muscles, the foot has to be plantar flexed and everted.

TOE METATARSOPHALANGEAL FLEXION

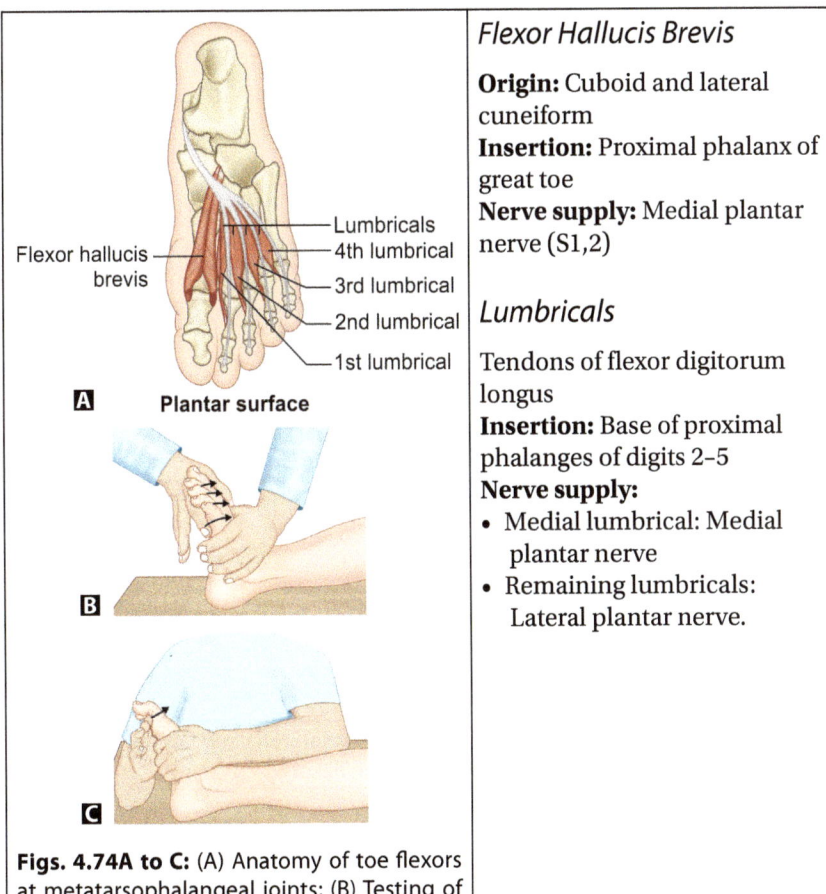

Flexor Hallucis Brevis

Origin: Cuboid and lateral cuneiform
Insertion: Proximal phalanx of great toe
Nerve supply: Medial plantar nerve (S1,2)

Lumbricals

Tendons of flexor digitorum longus
Insertion: Base of proximal phalanges of digits 2–5
Nerve supply:
- Medial lumbrical: Medial plantar nerve
- Remaining lumbricals: Lateral plantar nerve.

Figs. 4.74A to C: (A) Anatomy of toe flexors at metatarsophalangeal joints; (B) Testing of lumbricals and (C) flexor hallucis brevis.

Methodology

Patient: Sitting, leg relaxed and foot in neutral position.

Examiner: Holds the foot just below the ankle to stabilize it. To test FHB, Index finger of the other hand is placed beneath the proximal phalanx of the great toe and an upward force is applied. For lumbricals, resistance is applied under the proximal phalanges of 2nd to 5th toes

Test: Patient plantar flexes the toes at metacarpophalangeal joint against resistance.

Caveats

Flexor hallucis longus also causes flexion at metacarpophalangeal joint. This can be avoided by consciously giving resistance at the base of proximal instead of distal phalanx.

If flexor hallucis brevis is weak and FHL is strong, the DIP joint flexes and PIP joint extends (Hammer toe).

TOES PLANTAR AND DISTAL INTERPHALANGES FLEXION

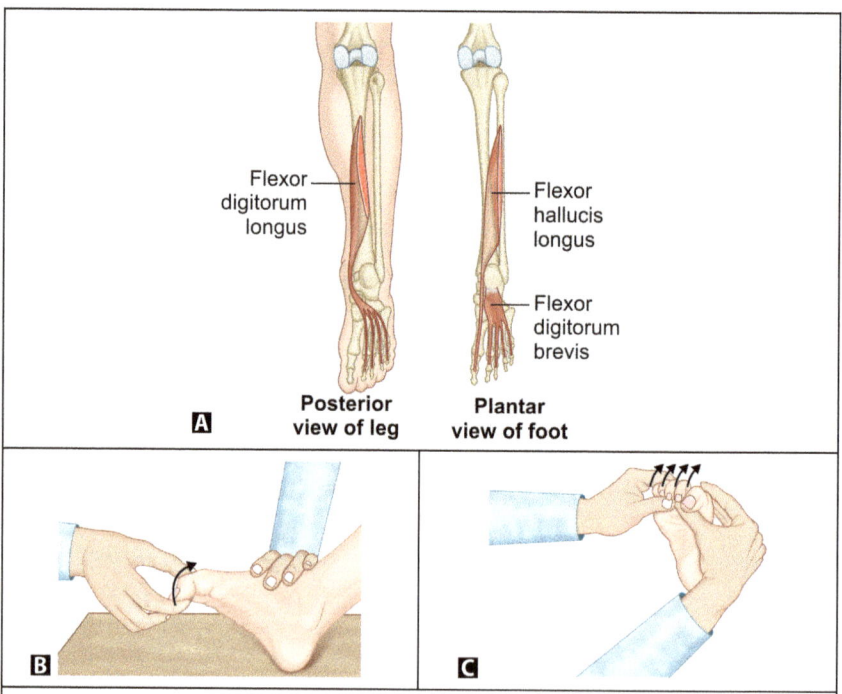

Figs. 4.75A to C: (A) Anatomy of toe flexors at interphalangeal joints and (B and C) testing of toe flexors.

Flexor hallucis longus: Tibial nerve (L5-S2)

Flexor digitorum longus: Tibial nerve (L5-S2)

Flexor digitorum brevis: Medial plantar nerve (S1, 2).

Methodology

Patient: Patient sitting, foot in neutral position.

Examiner: In front of the patient, one hand supporting the foot with four fingers on the dorsum and thumb on the sole of the foot. The other hand applies resistance under the middle phalanx for PIP flexion (Fig. 4.75B) and under the distal phalanx for DIP flexion assessment (Fig. 4.75C).

Test: Patient tries to curl the toes in against resistance.

Caveats

- Many patients cannot separate PIP from DIP flexion.
- Many patients cannot separate great toe from other toe flexion.

TOE DORSIFLEXION

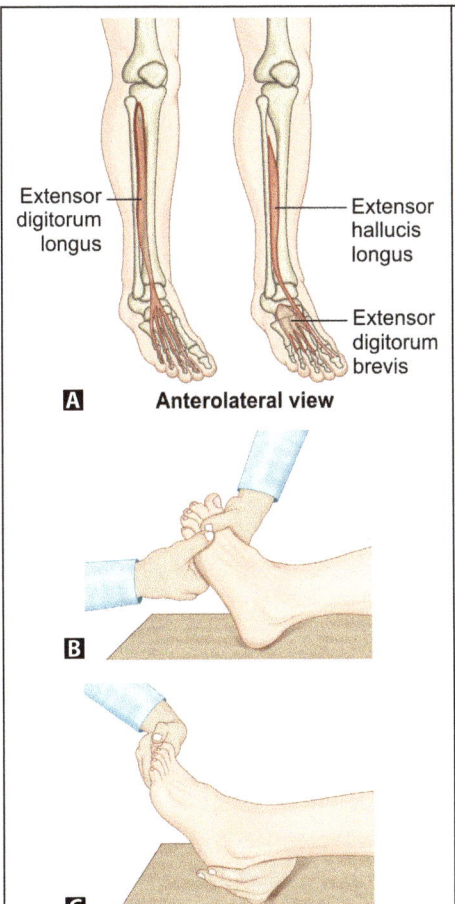

Extensor Digitorum Longus

Origin: Lateral tuberosity of tibia, shaft of fibula.
Insertion: Toes 2-5, middle and distal phalanx.

Extensor Digitorum Brevis

Origin: Calcaneus, talocalcaneal ligament.

Extensor Hallucis Longus

Origin: Shaft of fibula.
Insertion: Hallux, distal phalanx
Insertion: Toes 1-4.
Nerve supply: Deep peroneal nerve (L5, S1).

Figs. 4.76A to C: (A) Anatomy of toe dorsiflexors; (B and C) Testing of toe dorsiflexion.

Methodology

Patient: Supine with ankle in neutral position.

Examiner: Near the foot end of the bed. For lateral toe examination, one hand stabilizes the foot with four fingers on the sole and thumb on the dorsum. Thumb of the other hand applies resistance over the dorsum of proximal phalanges of the toes (Fig. 4.76B). For examination of great toe, one hand supports the heel and the thumb of the other hand applies resistance over the great toe at MP or IP joint (Fig. 4.76C).

Test: Patient tries to straighten the toes against resistance.

Caveats

Many patients cannot isolate dorsiflexion of great toe and other toes. Grading of these muscles is not reliable due to individual variability. Side to side comparison is better.

CHAPTER **5**

Examination of the Sensory System

GRK Sarma

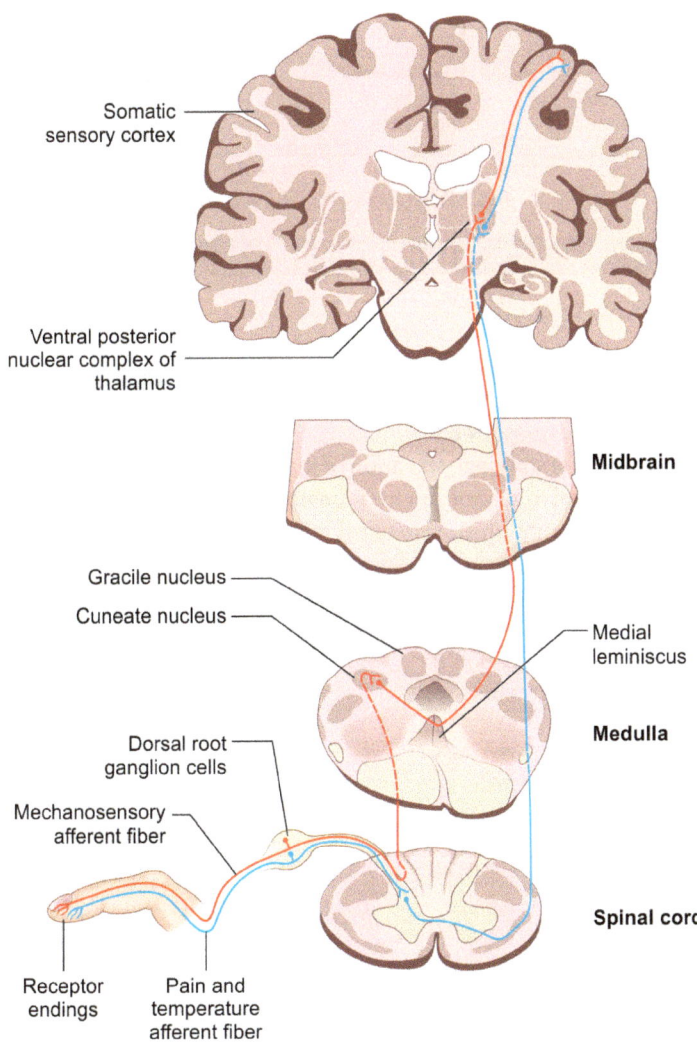

Fig. 5.1A: Proprioceptive pathways.

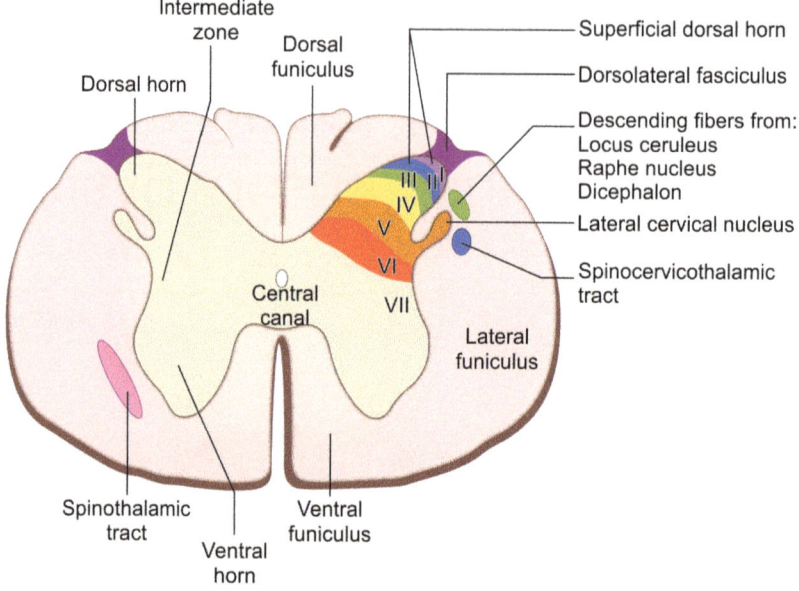

Fig. 5.1B: Dorsolateral funiculus.

PROPRIOCEPTION

PHYSIOLOGIC BASIS

- Proprioception consists of the sense of position and movement of the limbs and body in the absence of vision
- It includes two components:
  1. The sense of stationary position of the limbs (**limb position sense**) and
  2. The sense of limb movement (**kinesthesia**).
- The main receptors of muscles and joints and their afferent nerve fiber types are:

Receptor	Fiber type	Fiber diameter	Conduction velocity	Function
Muscle spindle primary afferents	Group Ia, myelinated	12–20 µ	70–120 m/s	Limb position kinesthesia
Golgi tendon organ	Group Ib, myelinated	12–20 µ	70–120 m/s	Limb position and kinesthesia
Muscle spindle secondary afferents	Group II, myelinated	6–12 µ	36–72 m/s	Only limb position
Joint capsule	Group III, thin myelinated	1–6 µ	4–36 m/s	Nociception at extreme joint position
Joint capsule	Group IV, unmyelinated	0.2–1.5 µ	0.4–2.0 m/s	Nociception at extreme joint position

Two principles help us to construct the entire details of the nerve fiber diameters and conduction velocities, just with the help of the '12–20 µ' value
 a. The diameter of one type of nerve fiber is roughly half of the preceding one
 b. The velocity can then be calculated by multiplying the diameter of nerve fiber with 6 [velocity (m/s) = diameter (µm) × 6)]

- Fibers carrying the proprioception pass through the dorsal roots, enter the dorsal horns of the spinal cord
- From here, there are **two pathways** for proprioceptive afferents:
    1. **Dorsolateral funiculus**; the major pathway for proprioception
    2. **Dorsal columns**; the minor pathway for proprioception
- Many of the 1st order proprioceptive afferents fibers synapse with 2nd order neurons in the dorsal horn, but some do not
- The 2nd order neuron fibers enter the ipsilateral **dorsolateral funiculus**, which is distinct from the **dorsal columns**, anatomically and functionally (Fig. 5.1A)
- These neurons synapse with 3rd order neuron in the lateral cervical nucleus (Fig. 5.1B), located just anterior to the dorsal horn in the C1 and 2 segments of the cord
- The 3rd order neurons cross the midline in the cord and ascend to reach the medial lemniscus in the medulla
- Some 1st order neurons that do not synapse in the dorsal horns enter the dorsal columns and synapse in the nuclei of the dorsal columns; the gracile nuclei (for lumbosacral segments) and the cuneiform nuclei (for cervicothoracic segments)
- Fibers in the dorsal columns are topographically arranged with the distal segments represented medially and the proximal segments laterally
- Axons of neurons in the gracile and cuneate nuclei form the medial lemniscus that crosses the midline and ascends in the medulla to reach the ventral posterolateral (VPL) nucleus of the thalamus
- Proprioceptive afferents from face area synapse in the main sensory nucleus of trigeminal nerve. Its post-synaptic neurons form the trigeminal lemniscus, which ascends parallel to the medial lemniscus to reach the ventral posteromedial (VPM) nucleus of thalamus
- Thalamocortical projections from VPL and VPM nuclei travel through the posterior limb of internal capsule to terminate in the post central gyrus, synapsing with neurons that encode position and movement
- The somatotopic organization is preserved at all levels
- In addition to the above tracts, unconscious proprioceptive sensations are carried by the spinocerebellar tracts.

METHODOLOGY

- Historical clues to abnormal proprioception are:
    - Incoordination of the upper limbs
    - Clumsiness in walking
    - Frequent stumbling
    - Difficulty standing upright with the eyes closed (wash basin symptom)
    - Involuntary movements (pseudoathetosis)
- The three most important principles to remember while examining joint position sensation are:
    1. *Sensitivity of the test is inversely related to the speed of joint movement.* This implies that if the joint is moved quickly up or down,

even a patient with mild or moderate proprioceptive defect may perceive the movement correctly. If the joint is moved **slowly over 1-2 seconds**, it may bring out the defect more reliably.
  2. ***Sensitivity of the test is inversely proportional to the amplitude of the movement.*** This implies that the test movements have to be in small range, as low as **1°** in fingers and **3°** in toes.
  3. ***Examiner's force must be applied in parallel to the plane of movement to avoid stimulating the pressure receptors.*** This implies that the examiner must hold the joint on either side (medially and laterally) while moving it in up and down direction. Conversely, while moving the joint in horizontal plane, the examiner's fingers must be placed above and below the joint
- Test the distal joints first and if these are abnormal, move proximally. In grossly impaired cases, even hip joint movement may not be perceived and it is important to document the extent of the deficit to better monitor the course of illness
- First demonstrate the test to the patient with eyes open and ensure that both of you understand what he means by "up" and "down"
- Patient has to understand that the movements will be random and not sequentially up and down
- Patient has to understand that he should respond only if the examiner asks (after completing the joint movement)
- Ask the patient to close his eyes
- Stabilize the proximal component of the joint (e.g. proximal phalanx) with one hand
- Hold the joint on its either side with your thumb and forefinger gently
- Move the joint over few degrees very slowly over 1-2 seconds in random direction
- In fingers 1° movement, and in toes, 3° movement can be appreciated normally
- After completing the movement, ask the patient to report the new position.
- If the patient cannot indicate the correct direction of movement, assess if he at least perceives the joint movement
- Stand close to the patient and ask him to stand with eyes open and then closed for 1 minute. If patient loses balance and sways excessively or even falls with eye closed (positive Romberg test), it indicates grossly impaired proprioception.

OTHER TESTS

- Parietal copy test: Ask patient to close his eyes. Place one hand or foot in a particular position and ask him to imitate that position with the other hand or foot
- Arm drift: Ask patient to out stretch his both hands with eye closed and observe for a drift
- Pseudoathetosis: Ask patient to out stretch his hands with eyes closed and observe for irregular slow movements (piano playing movements) of fingers. This occurs with severe proprioceptive loss.

INTERPRETATION

- Inability to perceive the joint position and movement indicates a lesion along the proprioceptive pathway
- Further localization is possible with the help of other neurological signs
- If the deep tendon reflexes are impaired, it indicates peripheral nerve or root level lesion. If they are brisk, it indicates spinal cord lesion
- Impaired proprioception in one upper and lower limbs with preserved proprioception over the face suggests contralateral high cervical cord lesion
- If facial proprioception is also impaired, it indicates a contralateral brainstem (mid pons or above) or thalamic level lesion
- A positive Romberg test is seen if joint position sense is impaired at knee or above level. It will be negative if the proprioceptive defect is limited to toes or ankle
- There are certain clinical clues to differentiate ataxia from proprioceptive defect (sensory ataxia) from cerebellar ataxia (Table 5.1).

Table 5.1: Clinical differentiation between sensory ataxia and cerebellar ataxia.

	Sensory ataxia	Cerebellar ataxia
Joint position sensation	Impaired	Preserved
Romberg's test	Positive	Negative (except in severe cases)
Pseudoathetosis	Present	Absent
Tendon reflexes	Absent/ present	Present (pendular)
Speech	Normal	Dysarthria
Nystagmus	Usually absent	Usually present
Effect of eye closure on limb ataxia	Markedly worse	No major effect

Caveats

- If the joint is moved too rapidly, a falsely normal joint position sense will be recorded
- If the joint is moved in large amplitudes, a similar error could occur
- If the examiner applies pressure perpendicular to the plane of movement, the patient can gather information on joint position from pressure receptors, even if JPS is impaired
- If the examiner moves the joint sequentially instead of randomly, patient may score well in the test
- While testing large joints like hip and knee, tactile stimulation of pressure receptors cannot be avoided. This must be taken into account while interpreting the results.

VIBRATION

PHYSIOLOGIC BASIS

- Vibration sensation results from the rhythmic simultaneous activation of multiple receptors, leading to synchronous discharge among many afferent fibers

- The receptors responsible for vibration sense include:
  - Merkel disk receptors and Meissner's corpuscles in the superficial layers of the skin
  - Pacinian corpuscles in deeper layers of skin, between layers of muscle, and in periosteum
- A particular range of frequencies stimulates each of these specific receptors as follows:
  - Low frequency (5-15 Hz): Merkel disc receptors
  - Mid frequency (20-50 Hz): Meissner's corpuscles
  - High frequencies (60-400 Hz): Pacinian corpuscles
- The total number of sensory nerve fibers activated by a vibrating stimulus determines the intensity of vibration
- The frequency of receptor firing determines the vibration frequency perceived
- The receptor afferents are myelinated and include both large diameter (group Ia, diameter 12-20 micrometers, conduction velocities 72 to 120 m/s) and medium diameter (group Ib, diameter 6-12 μm, conduction velocities 36 to 72 m/s) fibers
- The afferents pass through the dorsal root and enter the dorsal horn of the spinal cord
- Similar to the proprioceptive fibers, some of these afferents enter the dorsal columns and some enter the dorsolateral funiculus. Their further course parallels the proprioceptive pathway up to the post central gyrus, except that they terminate on different groups of thalamic and cortical neurons
- Though the pathways are similar, the proprioceptive and vibratory sensations may be differentially involved in certain diseases.

METHODOLOGY

- Explain the test to the patient
- Ensure that he understood the test and can differentiate between vibration and no vibration of the tuning fork over an expectedly normal region of the body
- Avoid testing the head area as control, as vibration here is "heard", in addition to being "felt"
- Ask the patient to close his eyes
- Set the 128 Hz tuning fork into motion by striking against a firm body (e.g. rubber head of a reflex hammer).
- Immediately place the base of the tuning fork against the body part. Start with the great toe and move up the malleoli of ankle, shin, anterior superior iliac spine, spinous processes, digits, wrist, olecranon of elbow, clavicle, sternum and the cervical spinous processes
- Ask the patient to report if he feels the vibration or not
- To check the reliability, strike the tuning fork into vibration, touch the tines with your hands and stop the vibration, and place the non-vibrating base

of the fork on the body part. Patient must accurately identify vibrating and non-vibrating stimuli without errors
- To check the vibration threshold, strike the fork with decreasing intensity to determine the least strength of vibration that can be perceived. Compare this threshold with yours on identical body part. A more accurate quantitative method to change the intensity of vibration is to use the Rydel Seiffer tuning fork
- Another way to quantify the vibration sensation is to time the duration of perception after the fork is set into vibration
- Normally, the duration of perception is ≥10 seconds in lower limbs and ≥20 seconds in upper limbs.

INTERPRETATION

- Selective involvement of JPS and vibration in a patient with peripheral neuropathy points to a demyelinating neuropathy (e.g. AIDP)
- Radiculopathies and plexopathies, in contrast, involve all modalities including touch and pain sensations
- Spinal cord lesions (compressions, demyelination, vascular lesions) usually produce a clear demarcation of sensory level and motor level
- Lesions involving only the dorsal column do not impair the JPS and vibration
- Lesions involving the dorsolateral cord impair the JPS and vibration
- Involvement of JPS and vibration on one side and pain and temperature on the other side is typically seen in Brown Sequard (hemicord) syndrome. This dissociation occurs as pain fibers in the cord are crossed, while proprioceptive fibers are not
- Similarly, bilateral selective loss of pain and temperature below a level indicates anterior spinal artery occlusion (anterior cord syndrome)
- In contrast, occlusion of dorsolateral funicular arteries produces selective loss of JPS and vibration ipsilaterally below that level
- Brainstem lesions also can produce selectivity in sensory loss that includes face. Lateral lesions impair pain and temperature, medial lesions impair proprioception
- Large thalamic lesions produce pan-sensory loss contralaterally; smaller lesions can produce selective loss of different modalities
- Cortical lesions usually produce discriminatory sensory loss, preserving the primary sensations
- "Splitting" of sternum/forehead: If a patient can feel the vibration near the midline over sternum or forehead, but cannot feel it just across the midline a few milimeters away, it indicates psychogenic sensory symptom. This is because, the tuning fork placed on periosteum stimulates the Pacinian corpuscles across a wide area, and does not respect the midline
- Dissociation between joint position and vibration sensations can occur. In B12 deficiency, vibration is more severely affected, while in tabes dorsalis, joint position is more severely affected.

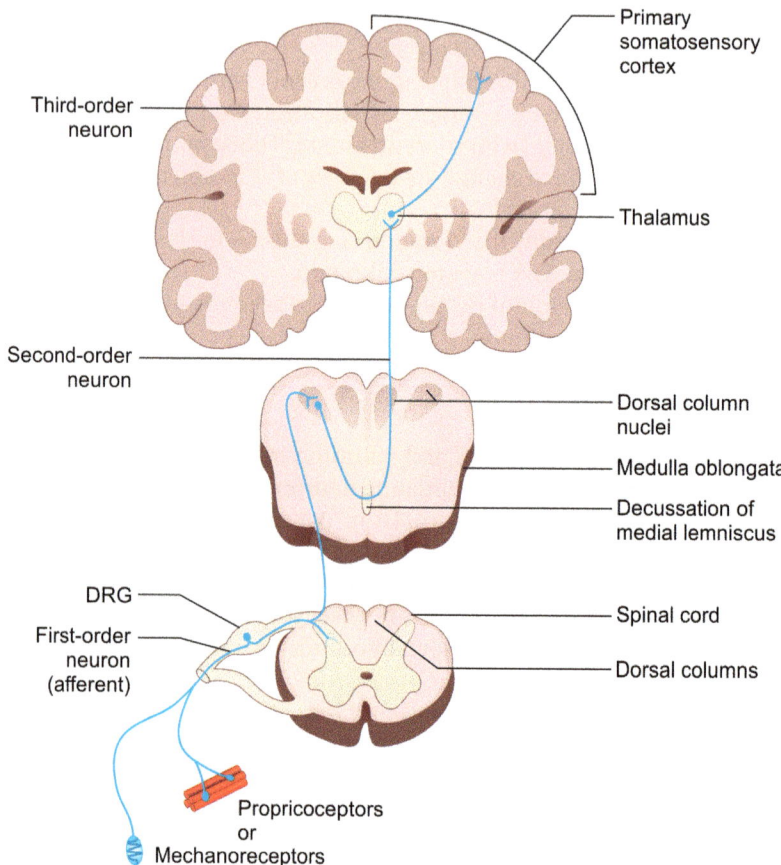

Fig. 5.2: Ascending pathways of tactile sensation.

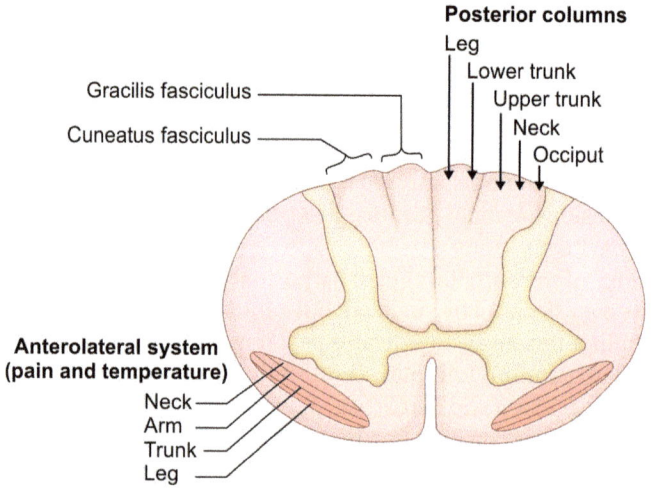

Fig. 5.3: Somatotopic organization tactile and nociceptive pathways.

TACTILE SENSATION

- Four mechanoreceptors exist in two layers of skin
  - Superficial layers (Meissner's corpuscles and Merkel discs)
  - Subcutaneous tissue (Ruffini endings and Pacinian corpuscles)
- In addition, in hairy skin, hair follicle receptors are present and detect hair displacement
- Meissner's corpuscles respond during the onset of skin stroking stimulation, and adapt rapidly
- Merkel disc receptors respond to pressure and adapt slowly
- Pacinian corpuscles respond to vibration and adapt rapidly
- Ruffini endings adapt slowly and respond to stretch
- The afferent fibers of all of these receptors afferents are myelinated and include both large diameter (group Aa, diameter 12-20 mm, conduction velocities 72 to 120 m/s) and medium diameter (group Ab, diameter 6-12 mm, conduction velocities 36 to 72 m/s) fibers
- Many pathways carry tactile sensation, explaining why diseases of spinal cord frequently spare it
- The afferents carrying tactile sensations are carried to higher centers by three different pathways:
  1. Some fibers enter the ipsilateral posterior columns without synapsing and ascend to reach gracile (below D8) or cuneate (above D8) nuclei. These fibers carry discriminatory sensations and tactile localization
  2. Some fibers cross to the opposite side and ascend in the anterolateral system, close to the spinothalamic tracts. These carry non-discriminatory light touch ("crude touch"), which does not help in tactile localization
  3. Some fibers enter the dorsolateral funiculus and synapse in the lateral cervical nucleus. Axons of the third order neurons reach the medial lemniscus and terminate in the VPL nucleus of thalamus.

METHODOLOGY

- A fine wisp of cotton, or feather or tissue paper is used as stimulus
- Ask patient to close his eyes or block his vision
- Select a nonhairy skin area for stimulation
- Gently touch the skin without exerting any pressure
- Stroke once across an area **not to exceed 1 cm** of skin
- Ask patient to report if he feels the touch
- Compare the response with homologous area on the other side
- Some patients are able to grade the sensation on 1-10 scale (the ten test). This is useful in delineating the length dependent impairment in peripheral neuropathies
- One can also score the response as per the international spinal injury standards as follows:
  0 = Absent

1 = Altered (impaired or partial appreciation, including hyperesthesia)
2 = Normal or intact (similar as on the cheek)
NT = Not testable
- Von Frey's hairs and Semmelweis monofilaments are designed to quantify the sensory impairment especially in diabetic neuropathies.

Interpretation

As tactile sensations are carried in multiple pathways, complete loss of touch sensation occurs with severe and complete cord lesions.

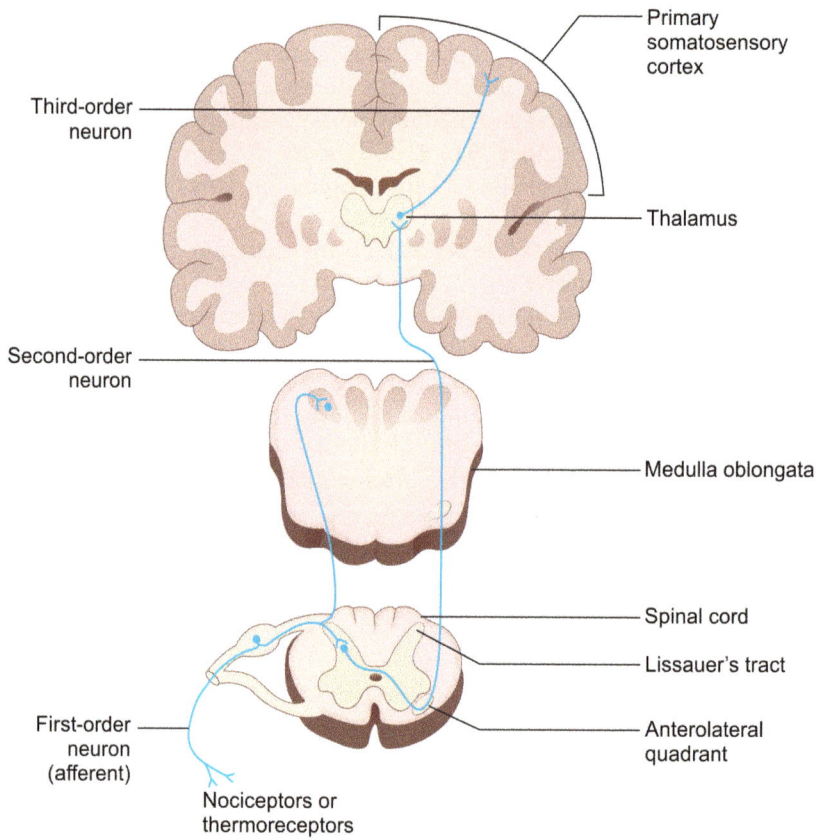

Fig. 5.4: Pain and temperature pathways.

PAIN AND TEMPERATURE (FIG. 5.4)

Physiologic Basis

- Receptors for pain and temperature are free nerve endings in the skin and mucosa. Some of them are unimodal while others are polymodal
- The afferent fibers are A δ and unmyelinated C fibers.

- First order neurons are located in the dorsal root ganglia at corresponding segmental levels
- Their axons enter the dorsolateral funiculus (Lissauer tract) and traverse one to two segments vertically before entering the dorsal horn
- 2nd order neurons are located in lamina I,II and V
- Most axons arising from these 2nd order neurons cross to the other side in anterior white commissure to form the spinothalamic tract [now known as the anterolateral system (ALS)].
- This tract is somatotopically organized, such that the more distal skin segments are represented more superficially, while the more proximal segments are represented more medially
- Few axons of 2nd order neurons enter the ipsilateral dorsolateral tract
- The spinothalamic tract enters the thalamus just medial to the inferior colliculus to terminate in the ventral posterolateral nucleus
- Fibers from the facial region travel through the trigeminal ganglion, enter the pons to reach the spinal nucleus of trigeminal nerve via the spinal tract of trigeminal nerve. The second order neurons pass through the trigeminothalamic tract, which runs close to the spinothalamic tract to terminate in the ventral posteromedial nucleus of the thalamus
- Thalamic radiations from the thalamus terminate in the post central gyrus. Those mediating pain also terminate on the limbic cortex
- Descending influences from the parietal cortex, thalamus, periventricular gray matter, brainstem reticular formation, nucleus raphe magnus, and periaqueductal gray matter can modulate the pain by regulating the activity of the dorsal horn cells.

Methodology—Pain Assessment

- Assessment of pain is inherently subjective, with many limitations. But reasonable information can be gathered by careful examination
- Stimuli used for testing pain are: Safety pins/ball pins/commercially available plastic sticks with one sharp and the other blunt tips. Avoid hypodermic needles as they are designed to pierce the skin in a relatively painless fashion.
- Whichever tool is used, must be discarded safely and not used to test another patient. This means that the pin wheel that comes in built with some reflex hammers is not ideal to test pain sensation in different patients.
- Patient has to close his eyes and report if he can feel the sharp and blunt stimuli, given in random fashion with the sharp and blunt ends of the instruments
- If patient can feel the pain sensation correctly, further refinement can be done by asking him to compare the test region with normal region on a scale of 1 to 10 or as percentage
- If in doubt, 8 out of 10 correct answers are suggested as a standard for accuracy; as this reduces the probability of correct guessing to less than 5%.

Methodology—Temperature Assessment

- Both hot and cold sensations are tested using water in test tubes
- Test tubes are filled with water at 10°C for cold and 40°C for hot sensation.
- These are brought into contact with the skin in random fashion, with patient's eyes closed
- Patient is asked to report the stimulus as hot or cold
- For research purposes, quantitative sensory testing methods are available.

Interpretation

- Selective involvement of pain and temperature (dissociated sensory loss) can occur in certain situations
- In small fiber neuropathies, pain and temperature are impaired with preserved tactile sensations
- In the spinal cord, central cord lesions like tumors or syringomyelia preferentially involve the decussating pain and temperature fibers to cause dissociated sensory loss
- In the spinal cord, anterior cord syndrome due to anterior spinal artery occlusion, involves the spinothalamic tracts, sparing the posterior columns to cause dissociated sensory loss below the level of lesion
- In the spinal cord and the brainstem, selectively placed lesions like demyelinating plaques, can involve spinothalamic tracts, causing dissociated sensory loss
- In extrinsic cervical compressive myelopathies, the outermost sacral fibers of the spinothalamic tracts are involved earlier, causing sacral sensory loss with other segments being intact. In intrinsic compressive lesions, sacral sparing occurs, while more proximal regions are involved. Thus, all patients with cord lesions must be examined for pain sensation in the sacral region.

Caveats

- If the stimuli are delivered in a regular fashion, the patients predict the response and report positively, even in the presence of sensory loss
- The examiner may be misled by such false positive responses. This can be avoided by randomly missing the stimulus and asking the patient if can feel the stimulus. Some patients continue to report "yes", showing the unreliability of their responses
- If the stimulus is delivered too rapidly, spatial summation can occur and produce erroneous results.

SEGMENTAL LOCALIZATION OF SENSORY LOSS

The following **key landmarks** have been recommended in the International Standards for the Classification of Spinal Cord Injury to localize the segment involved. These may be useful in rapid and accurate assessment of sensory level in patients with spinal cord disease. In patients with radiculopathies or peripheral neuropathies, more detailed mapping of area of abnormal sensations and a knowledge of the dermatomal patterns is required (figures)

C2: At least one cm lateral to the occipital protuberance at the base of the skull. Alternately, it can be located 3 cm behind the ear.

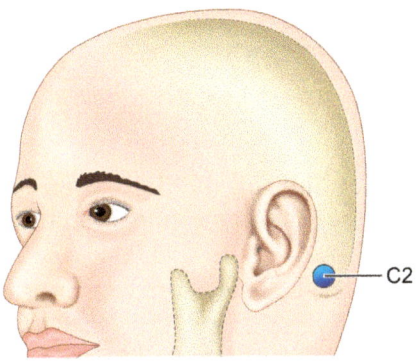

C3: In the supraclavicular fossa, at the midclavicular line.

C4: Over the acromioclavicular joint.

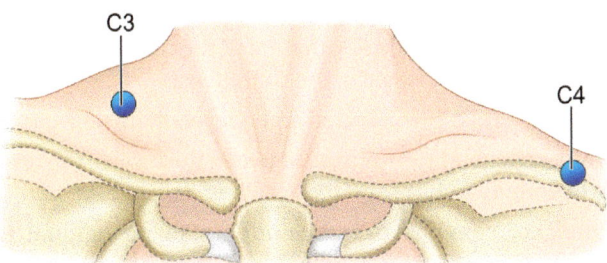

C5: On the lateral (radial) side of the antecubital fossa just proximal to the elbow

C6: On the dorsal surface of the proximal phalanx of the thumb.

C7: On the dorsal surface of the proximal phalanx of the middle finger.

C8: On the dorsal surface of the proximal phalanx of the little finger.

T1: On the medial (ulnar) side of the antecubital fossa, just proximal to the medial epicondyle of the humerus.

T2: At the apex of the axilla.

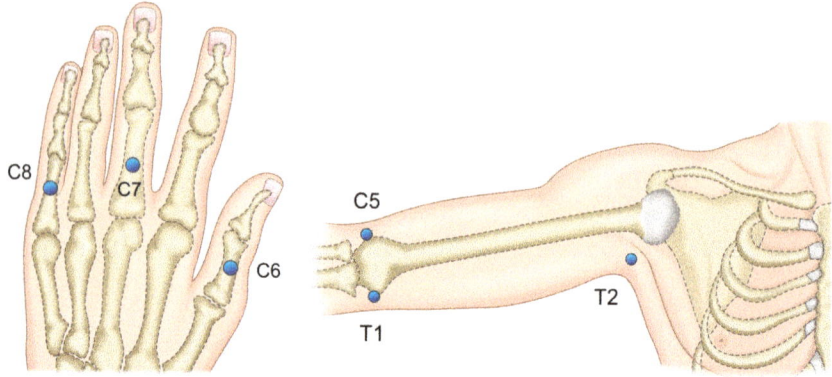

T3: At the midclavicular line and the third intercostal space, found by palpating the anterior chest to locate the third rib and the corresponding third intercostal space below it.

T4: At the midclavicular line and the fourth intercostal space, located at the level of the nipples.

T5: At the midclavicular line and the fifth intercostal space, located midway between the level of the nipples and the level of the xiphisternum.

T6: At the midclavicular line, located at the level of the xiphisternum.

T7: At the midclavicular line, one quarter the distance between the level of the xiphisternum and the level of the umbilicus.

T8: At the midclavicular line, one half the distance between the level of the xiphisternum and the level of the umbilicus.

T9: At the midclavicular line, three quarters of the distance between the level of the xiphisternum and the level of the umbilicus.

T10: At the midclavicular line, located at the level of the umbilicus.

T11: At the midclavicular line, midway between the level of the umbilicus and the inguinal ligament.

T12: At the midclavicular line, over the midpoint of the inguinal ligament.

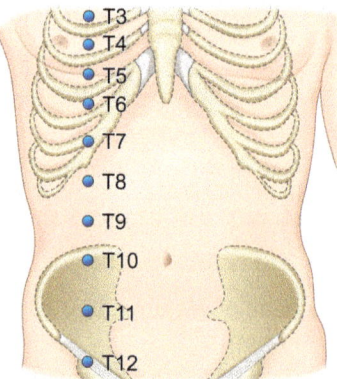

L1: Midway between the key sensory points for T12 and L2.

L2: On the anterior-medial thigh, at the midpoint drawn on an imaginary line connecting the midpoint of the inguinal ligament and the medial femoral condyle.

L3: At the medial femoral condyle above the knee.

L4: Over the medial malleolus

L5: On the dorsum of the foot at the third metatarsal phalangeal joint.

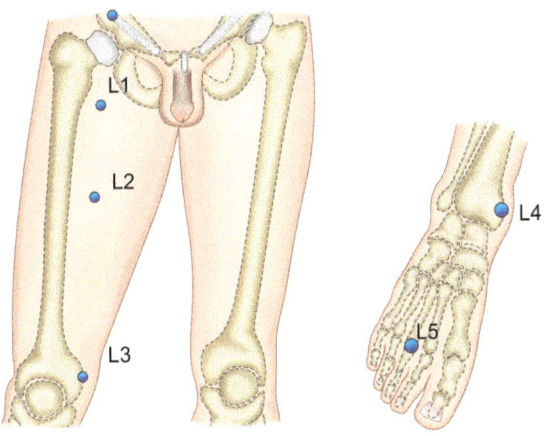

S1: On the lateral aspect of the calcaneus.

S2: At the midpoint of the popliteal fossa.

S3: Over the ischial tuberosity or infragluteal fold (depending on the patient their skin can move up, down or laterally over the ischii).

S4/5: In the perianal area, less than one cm. Lateral to the mucocutaneous junction.

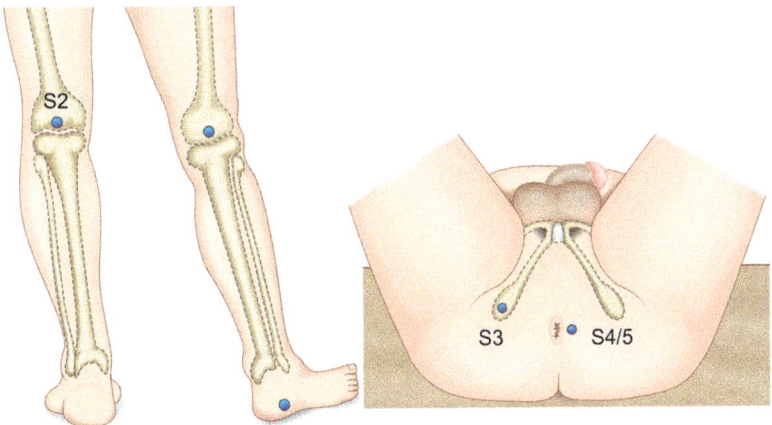

BIBLIOGRAPHY

1. Chhetri SK, Gow D, Shaunak S, et al. Clinical assessment of the sensory ataxias; diagnostic algorithm with illustrative cases. Pract Neurol. 2014;14:242-51.
2. Dyck PJ, et al. Assessing decreased sensation and increased sensory phenomena in diabetic polyneuropathies. Diabetes. 2013;62:3677-86.
3. Gardner EP, Martin JH, Jessell TM. The bodily senses. In: Kandel ER, Schwartz JH, Jessell TM, (Eds). Principles of neural science. New York: McGraw-Hill, 2000:430-50.
4. Gilman S. Joint position sense and vibration sense: anatomical organisation and assessment. J Neurol Neurosurg Psychiatry. 2002;73:473-7.
5. Kirshblum SC, et al. International standards for neurological classification of spinal cord injury (Revised 2011). The Journal of Spinal Cord Medicine. 2011;34(6):535-46.

CHAPTER 6

Reflexes

GRK Sarma

DEEP TENDON REFLEXES

Physiologic Basis
- These are monosynaptic reflexes, comprising of muscle spindle afferents and alpha motor neuron efferents. Both these components, therefore, influence the reflex excitability
- The sensitivity of the muscle spindle can be altered by the gamma motor neuron activity, which is in turn influenced by segmental and supraspinal inputs (discussed in detail in the previous section on muscle tone)
- The reflex excitability also depends on the force and speed with which the spindle is stretched. Hence, a heavy hammer produces a brisker reflex than a light hammer.

Method: General Principles
- Choose a good hammer and persist with the same type. In general, a heavy hammer with quality rubber head is a good choice. Smaller, lighter hammers are easy to carry, but often fail the real test bedside
- Develop the correct technique of patient and examiner positions, limb position, site, direction and force of the tendon tap. These are described for each reflex separately
- Because of wide range of normality, start with an assumption that 'the change in the reflex is **not** pathological'. The objective of the examination then is to disprove this hypothesis by adjusting the patient variables and examiner variables
- If both these variables are addressed, then the alteration of the reflexes is more likely to be due to a disease state
- Patient variables include age, body posture, position of the limb, state of mind, apprehension, level of alertness, body constitution, sedative drugs, room temperature.

Different types of reflex hammers in clinical use (Figs. 6.1 to 6.6).

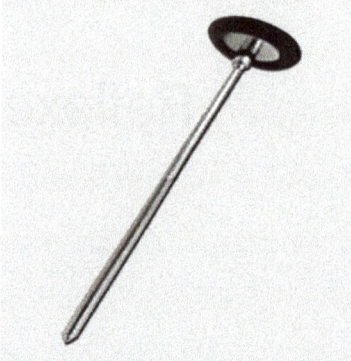

Fig. 6.1: Babinski hammer; looks like Queen square hammer, but has a detachable handle.

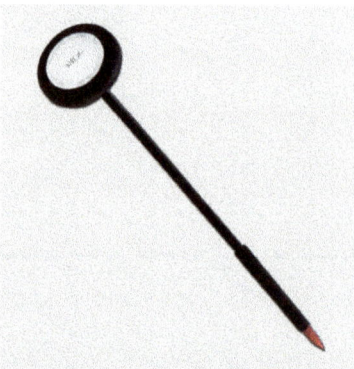

Fig. 6.2: Queen square hammer has a heavy, plastic mold and a long handle, with a pointed tip for plantar or abdominal reflex.

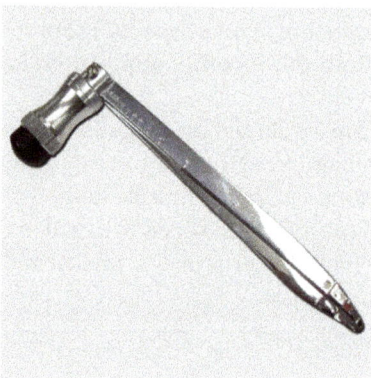

Fig. 6.3: McGill reflex hammer with 2 point discriminator.

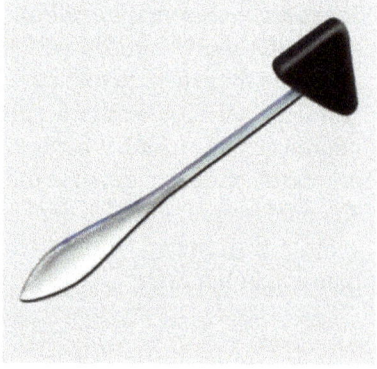

Fig. 6.4: Taylor hammer (Tomahawk hammer): Lighter than European ones, popular in the USA.

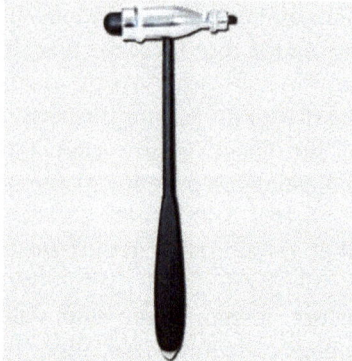

Fig. 6.5: Troemner hammer; a heavy hammer; the smaller head is for percussion myotonia, the larger for DTR.

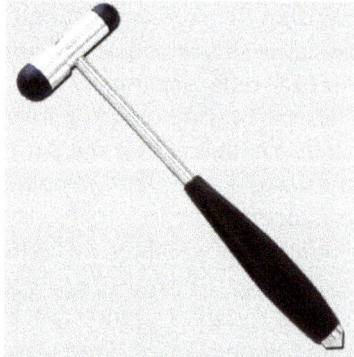

Fig. 6.6: Babinski Buck reflex hammer: There is a brush at the handle tip for cutaneous testing.

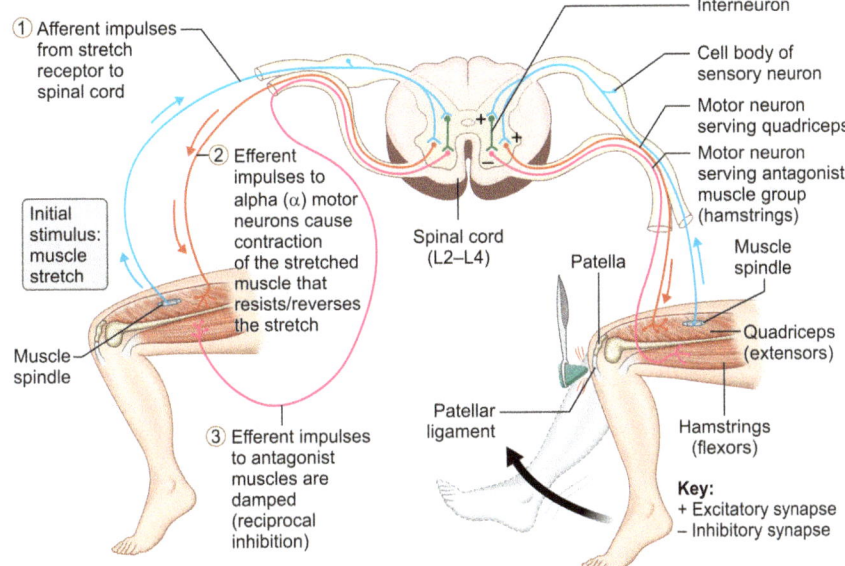

Fig. 6.7: Pathways in patellar reflex generation and reciprocal inhibition of knee flexors.

- Examiner variables include the type of hammer used, the site, direction, force and the speed of the stimulus and the examiner's perception of what is normal
- Patient must be relaxed. If needed, engage the patient in conversation to distract his attention
- Some patients, especially children, are apprehensive at the sight of the hammer. A sample, mild percussion demonstrates that the examination would not be a painful experience
- If a reflex is not obtained in a particular posture, try another (for example, sitting/ kneeling on the stool, etc.)
- If a reflex is not elicited, try Jendrassik maneuver (locking the fingers of one hand with those of another and pulling them apart as hard as possible) or clenching the jaws or fist. This maneuver must coincide with the tendon tap, as the effect is short lasting (less than 5–6 seconds)
- Consistently use one particular type of hammer to develop the subjective feel of "normal" for a given force
- Feel and tap the tendon, not the muscle. Directly tapping any muscle produces a local contraction (idiomuscular contraction)
- If possible, examiner's free hand may be placed over the muscle to feel the contraction and differentiate the true reflex from transmitted movements and also to identify minimal contraction that is inadequate to produce visible movement
- The direction of the tap has to be adjusted so as to produce the muscle stretch
- Use increasing force of the tap, but avoid pain

- If using a rigid hammer (Taylor/McGill hammer), the fulcrum of the movement must be at the wrist, not the shoulder or elbow. The latter generate excessive force and are likely to be painful
- This is achieved by consciously stabilizing your elbow and shoulder
- If using a flexible hammer (Queen square hammer), this problem is minimized, but the accuracy of the impact of the stimulus needs to ensured by practice
- When eliciting a reflex, elicit it on both sides, look for asymmetry and then move on to the next reflex
- The tendon reflexes may be examined in the following sequence to avoid errors of omission:
  - Jaw jerk
  - Trapezius reflex
  - Pectoralis reflex
  - Biceps reflex
  - Supinator reflex
  - Triceps reflex
  - Finger flexion reflex
  - Knee jerk
  - Hamstring reflex
  - Adductor reflex of the thigh
  - Ankle jerk.

Methodology of Individual Reflexes

A. Jaw jerk (trigeminal nerve):
  - Ask the patient to open the jaw to 1/3
  - Place your finger on the chin
  - Tap your finger with reflex hammer in an oblique direction that pulls open the jaw further (mandible pulled down)
  - Normally, this jerk is just elicitable.

B. Trapezius reflex (C3,4):
  - Place a finger on trapezius muscle, parallel to the spine
  - Strike the finger with a reflex hammer
  - Normally, slight elevation of shoulder is seen
  - Exaggerated reflex is seen in pyramidal tract lesions above C3 segment

C. Pectoralis reflex (C5-T1; medial and lateral pectoral nerves):
  - Patient's arm mildly abducted, place your fingers on the tendon of pectoralis major (not the muscle bulk) near its insertion on the humerus
  - Tap your fingers to stretch the muscle
  - Normal response is adduction and internal rotation at the shoulder
  - It may be difficult to elicit in some healthy individuals. Asymmetry is more relevant
  - Brisk reflex indicates a corticospinal tract lesion above C5 level.

D. Biceps reflex (C5, 6, musculocutaneous nerve):
- Flex the patient's elbow to 90°, support the semipronated forearm on his thigh or your forearm
- Place your thumb on the biceps tendon, slightly stretch the tendon and tap it with reflex hammer to produce a sudden stretch
- The biceps contracts and flexes the elbow
- In reflex overflow, there may be wrist flexion, finger flexion and thumb adduction
- Sometimes, the biceps reflex may be absent, but reflex overflow is present (inverted biceps reflex). It indicates C5, 6 cord segment lesion with involvement of pyramidal tracts (radiculomyelopathy).

E. Supinator reflex (brachioradialis reflex) (C5, 6; radial nerve):
- Patient's elbow is supported by examiner's hand with his thumb over the biceps tendon
- Patient's elbow is semiflexed, forearm mid-pronated (as if in a sling)
- Identify the tendon at its insertion over the base of styloid process, just lateral to the radial artery
- Tap the tendon just above the insertion
- Observe for 3 components:
  1. Contraction of brachioradialis causing supination of forearm and elbow flexion is normal
  2. Contraction of biceps suggests reflex overflow
  3. Finger flexion also suggests reflex overflow
- In inverted supinator reflex, the reflex itself is absent, but there is finger flexion.

F. Triceps reflex (C7, 8; radial nerve):
- Flex the patient's elbow to 90°, support the semipronated forearm on your forearm or patient's lap
- If patient is in supine position, the forearm is rested over his abdomen with elbow semi-flexed
- Identify the triceps tendon at its insertion over the olecranon process and tap it just above
- The triceps contracts and produces elbow extension
- If the triceps reflex is absent, but the biceps contracts, it is called inverted triceps reflex.

G. Finger flexion reflex (C8, T1, median and ulnar nerves):
- Patient's hand in supine position, resting on the table, fingers curled up and minimally grasping the examiner's fingers
- Tap your fingers in a direction that extends the patient's fingers
- Normal response is flexion of fingers including the thumb
- It may be absent in normal individuals. Therefore, asymmetry is more significant
- Brisk flexion of fingers and adduction of thumb are pathological and suggest corticospinal tract lesion.

H. Knee reflex (Patellar reflex) (L2-4; femoral nerve):
   - Patient sitting at the edge of the cot with legs hanging freely. Examiner's hand may be placed on the quadriceps muscle to feel the muscle contraction
   - Patient may also be examined in supine position, knees slightly passively flexed by placing examiner's forearm under it
   - Tap the tendon briskly with the hammer
   - Quadriceps contracts briskly to produce knee extension
   - Observe for contraction of ipsilateral adductors contralateral quadriceps and adductors which indicate reflex overflow.
I. Adductor reflex (L 2-4, obturator nerve):
   - Patient in supine or seated position
   - Tap over the medial epicondyle of femur near the adductor tubercle
   - Ipsilateral adductor muscles contract to produce adduction of thigh
   - Unilateral absent reflex suggests either L2-4 root lesion or obturator nerve entrapment. If the knee jerk (also L2-4) is preserved, the latter is likely
   - Marked contralateral thigh adduction is suggestive of corticospinal tract disease.
J. Medial hamstring reflex (L5, tibial component of sciatic nerve):
   - Patient in supine position, thigh abducted, externally rotated, knee semiflexed
   - Place your fingers on the medial hamstring tendon and tap with the hammer
   - Knee flexion is the normal response.
K. Lateral hamstring reflex (S1, tibial component of the sciatic nerve):
   - Patient in lateral recumbent position
   - Place your fingers on the lateral hamstring tendon and tap with the hammer
   - Knee flexion is the normal response
   - Absent reflex indicates S1 radiculopathy.
L. Ankle reflex (S1, tibial nerve):
   - Patient supine, with the thigh externally rotated, abducted, knee semiflexed (frog-like postion)
   - It may be useful to have the leg being examined partly crossed over the other
   - Patient may also be standing with knee semiflexed and supported on a chair, so that the foot projects beyond the edge of the chair
   - Slightly dorsiflex the foot with one hand and tap the tendon just above its insertion on the calcaneus with the hammer. It may be needed to tap the tendon at different angles of stretch before declaring the reflex absent
   - Gastrosoleus muscle contracts and plantar flexes the ankle
   - Absent ankle jerk suggests either peripheral neuropathy or radiculopathy. If lateral hamstring reflex (also S1) is preserved, the former is likely.

Observation: General Principles

- Observe the following:
  - Symmetry
  - Force needed to elicit the reflex
  - The force of contraction
  - The speed of contraction
  - Duration of contraction
  - Duration of relaxation
  - Overflow of the reflex to other muscles.
- Deep tendon reflexes are graded as follows by convention:
  - 0: Absent reflex inspite of reinforcement (unequivocally abnormal)
  - 1+: A slight but definitely present response. This level of response may be considered normal for some reflexes (e.g. ankle jerk), but abnormal for other, more lively reflexes (e.g. knee reflex)
  - 2+: Brisk response (normal)
  - 3+: Very brisk response, but still not unequivocally abnormal, not associated with Babinski sign, abnormal superficial reflexes, spasticity and clonus
  - 4+: Markedly hyperactive reflexes, often with reflex overflow, spasticity, clonus and Babinski sign (unequivocally abnormal)
- Reflex overflow (reflex spread): When a particular tendon is percussed, adjacent or even contralateral muscles may contract due to increase in reflexogenic zone. Normally, minimal finger flexion while eliciting brachioradialis reflex is acceptable. Marked finger flexion and thumb adduction is pathological. With knee jerk, contraction of ipsilateral adductors, contralateral quadriceps or adductors is pathological.

Interpretation

- There is a wide range of normality of tendon reflexes from hyporeflexia to hyperreflexia and even clonus. Therefore, tendon reflexes must not be interpreted in isolation
- Hyporeflexia (diminished or absent reflex) indicates either a lesion in the reflex arc itself (sensory neuropathy/radiculopathy/ganglionopathy/anterior horn cell/motor root/plexus/peripheral nerve), or an acute lesion in the supraspinal pathways (as in acute stroke, spinal trauma or myelitis)
- Hyper reflexia (brisk reflexes) indicates a lesion in the descending pathways above that particular level. For example, if the finger flexion reflex is brisk and the biceps reflex is normal, the lesion is above C8, T1 but below C5, 6.
- An absent reflex suggests a lesion in the reflex arc of that segment as shown in the Table 6.1. Further localization to sensory or motor components can be made by associated segmental sensory loss or segmental weakness, wasting and fasciculations.

Table 6.1: Segmental innervations of tendon reflexes.

Reflex	Root
Jaw jerk	Trigeminal nerve
Trapezius	C3, 4
Pectoralis	C5, 6
Biceps	C5, 6
Supinator	C5, 6
Triceps	C7
Finger flexion	C8, T1
Knee	L3, 4
Hamstring	L4, 5
Adductor	L2, 3
Ankle	S1

- Tendon reflexes are preserved in primary muscle disease until an advanced stage
- They are also preserved in myasthenia gravis, but reduced in Lambert Eaton syndrome.

Caveats

- Apparent reflex asymmetry can be produced by asymmetric positioning of the limbs
- Apparent reflex asymmetry can be produced by head turning to one side. Therefore, patient must keep the head straight during examination.

BIBLIOGRAPHY

1. Campbell WW. DeJong's the neurologic examination, 7th edition. Wolters Kluwer/Lippincott Williams & Wilkins. 2013.
2. Dick JP. The deep tendon and the abdominal reflexes. J Neurol Neurosurg Psychiatry. 1976;39:905-8.
3. Dick JPR. The deep tendon and the abdominal reflexes. J Neurol Neurosurg Psychiatry. 2003;74:150-3.
4. Fuller G. Neurological examination made easy. 4th edition. New York: McGraw-Hill, 2000.
5. Gregory JE, Wood SA, Proske U. An investigation in to the mechanism of reflex reinforcement by the Jendrassik' Manoeuvre. Exp Brain Res. 2001;138:366-74.
6. Lanska DJ. The Babinski reflex hammer. Neurology. 1999;53:655.
7. Perloff MD, Leroy AM, Ensrud ER. Teaching video neuroimages: the elusive L5 reflex. Neurology. 2010;75:e50.
8. Watson JC, Broaddus WC, Smith MM, et al. Hyperactive pectoralis reflex as an indicator of upper cervical spinal cord compression. Report of 15 cases. J Neurosurg. 1997;86:159-61.

SUPERFICIAL REFLEXES

In this section 4 reflexes are discussed:
1. Superficial abdominal reflex
2. Cremasteric reflex
3. Superficial anal reflex
4. Bulbocavernosus reflex.

SUPERFICIAL ABDOMINAL REFLEX

Physiological Basis

- This is a polysynaptic reflex
- It is equivalent to the late response seen in the blink reflex
- It appears after 6 months of age, as myelination of pyramidal tracts progresses
- The afferents and efferents of the abdominal reflex are:
    - Epigastric: T7–T9 intercostal nerves
    - Upper abdominal reflex: T9–T11 intercostal nerves
    - Lower abdominal reflex: T11–L1 intercostal, iliohypogastric and ilioinguinal nerve.

Method

- Patient in supine position
- Encourage patient to relax and explain that you will stroke his abdomen
- If abdomen is not relaxed, ask patient to flex at hips and breathe slowly
- Stimulate each quadrant at a time by lightly stroking with blunt object (key/pencil)
- Stimulus to be applied from lateral to medial, both in non-segmental and segmental distribution
- The exact segment can be mapped by extending a particular intercostal space from thoracic cage anteriorly over the abdomen.

Observation

- Watch for contraction of the muscles in the stimulated quadrant
- Watch the direction of movement of umbilicus
- Note if the reflex fatigues after few repetitions.

Interpretation

- Normally, the umbilicus moves towards the side of stimulation. This does not fatigue with repetition of stimulus
- If the reflex fatigues after few stimuli, it may indicate an early pyramidal tract lesion

- If the umbilicus does not move towards the side of stimulation, it suggests an abnormality in the afferent or efferent arc of the reflex at that level
- If the umbilicus moves towards the opposite side of the stimulus (inverted reflex), it is even more definitive of an abnormal abdominal reflex
- **Segmental** loss of abdominal reflex indicates a lesion in the afferent or efferent pathway at that segmental level (e.g. surgical injury to the intercostal nerve)
- Loss of all abdominal reflexes **below** a particular segment indicates a spinal lesion above that level
- Loss of all abdominal reflexes on **one side** indicates a cerebral lesion or a spinal lesion above T7 level
- The reflex is exaggerated in anxiety state and in extrapyramidal disease
- In patients with scoliosis, absence of abdominal reflex on one side may suggest underlying syringomyelia
- Dissociation of reflexes, that is loss of abdominal reflex with exaggerated deep tendon reflexes suggests pyramidal tract disease. In contrast, exaggeration of both deep tendon reflex and abdominal reflex suggests anxiety state.

Caveats

- Abdominal reflex may be absent in normal persons with obese abdomen, multiparous women or previous abdominal surgeries
- Heavy stimulation may elicit the deep abdominal reflex, which is exaggerated in pyramidal tract lesions.

SUPERFICIAL ANAL REFLEX

Physiological Basis

The reflex is mediated by inferior hemorrhoidal nerve (S2-S5).

Method

Stroke the perianal skin gently with a blunt object.

Observation

Look for puckering or contraction of external anal sphincter.

Interpretation

Absence of anal reflex indicates a lesion in S2-S5 segments (cauda equina/conus lesions).

BULBOCAVERNOSUS REFLEX

Method

- Explain the test to the patient

- Insert your gloved finger in the patient's rectum
- Pinch the glans penis (or clitoris).

Observation

Feel for the tightening of anal sphincter around the gloved finger.

Interpretation

Absence of bulbocavernosus reflex indicates a lesion in the S2-S5 segments (cauda equina/conus medullaris lesions).

Caveats

This reflex is not reliably elicited in females and is difficult to interpret.

CREMASTERIC REFLEX

Physiological Basis

The innervation is through ilioinguinal and genitofemoral nerves (L1-L2).

Method

- Patient in supine or standing position
- Stroke the inner and upper aspect of thigh
- Stimulus has to be from above downwards and medially.

Observation

Watch for the movement of testicle and scrotum on the side of the stimulus.

Interpretation

- Normally the scrotum and testicle on the side of stimulation are pulled up by the cremasteric contraction
- Absent response indicates pyramidal tract lesion above L1, or any breach in the reflex arc
- Exaggerated reflex has no significance.

Caveats

The reflex may be absent in the elderly men, in those with hydroceles or previous scrotal surgery.

PLANTAR REFLEX AND THE BABINSKI SIGN

Physiologic Basis

- When the sole of a foot is stimulated by a **non-noxious** stimulus, four possible results may be seen:
    1. No response

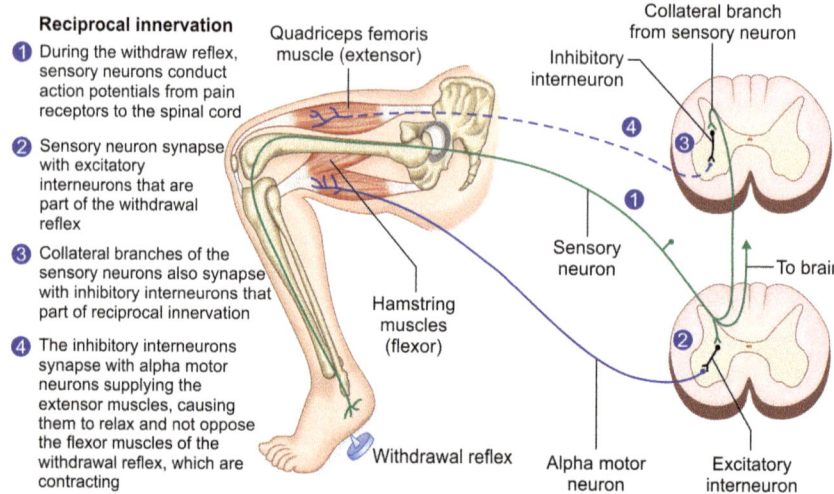

Fig. 6.8: Physiological basis of plantar reflex and the Babinski sign.

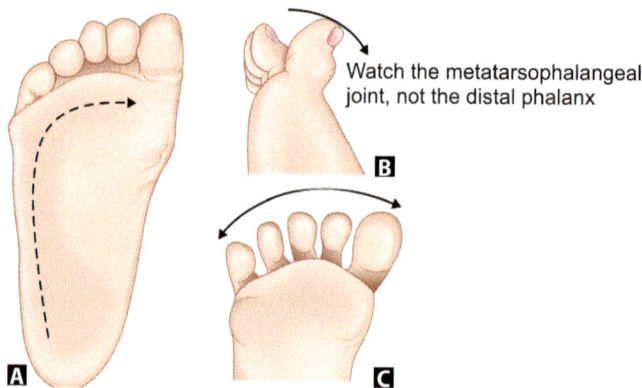

Figs. 6.9A to C: The stimulus and the responses of the Babinski reflex. (A) The stimulus stops short of the ball of the great toe; (B) Dorsiflexion of great toe; (C) Fanning of the toes.

    2. Normal superficial flexion reflex
    3. Voluntary withdrawal response, which is a normal response to tickle
    4. Spinal flexion withdrawal response which is an abnormal response to non-noxious stimulus, but is a normal response to noxious stimulus.
Sometimes, "equivocal response" is reported when one is not certain of the response.
- Normal plantar reflex is a superficial/cutaneous reflex, much like an abdominal reflex, and consists of plantar flexion of all the toes in response to stimulation of sole of the foot. Its afferents arise from S1 dermatome, and traverse through the tibial nerve, integrate in spinal segments S1. The efferents arise from S1 segment, traverse the tibial nerve to the toe flexor muscles

- In contrast, the pathological Babinski sign is a spinal defense flexion reflex. The afferents are similar to the normal reflex, but the integration occurs at L4, 5 S1, 2 segments and the efferents are carried through the peroneal nerve to the toe dorsiflexors. Supraspinal influences are from the basal ganglia, primary motor area, premotor area. The reflex is abolished by lesions of basal ganglia. Primary motor area may influence toe dorsiflexion and the premotor area may influence toe fanning
- During maturation of pyramidal system, toe dorsiflexion is eliminated from the flexion withdrawal response. In pyramidal tract dysfunction, the toe dorsiflexion re-emerges on plantar stimulation, along with knee flexion, tensor fasciae latae contraction
- This spinal flexion withdrawal reflex is different from voluntary withdrawal response seen in sensitive/anxious individuals (see "caveats" section).

Method

- Patient supine, hip and knee extended, heel resting on the bed
- All the thigh and leg muscles must be clearly visible. It is not enough to just focus on the toes
- Explain to the patient that his foot will be scratched and that he should let his legs "sleep"
- Avoid flexing the knee which can abolish the reflex
- Usual objects for stimulation include the tip of a key, match stick, or a wooden applicator
- Stimulus must be threshold one, i.e. as light as is sufficient to elicit the response
- Avoid painful stimuli and tickling
- Reinforce by head turning to opposite side
- If no response is obtained, increasingly firmer stimulation is needed
- The stimulus is started from the plantar aspect of the heel and drawn slowly anteriorly over 5-6 seconds, along the lateral margin of the sole up to the metatarsophalangeal joint level and then curved medially, stopping short of the ball of the big toe
- If the foot is hypersensitive, hold the foot at the ankle and elicit the reflex.

Observation

- Observe the metatarsophalangeal joint of the big toe (not the distal phalanx)
- Note the direction of movement of toes, presence of fanning (separation) of toes
- Watch and feel for contraction of tensor fasciae latae and hamstrings
- Watch if the response occurs as soon as the stimulus is applied (the voluntary withdrawal response) or is elicited as the summation of stimulus occurs over several seconds.

Interpretation

As mentioned above, one of the four responses need to be noted and interpreted.
- If no response is elicited, it may be due to interruption of the reflex arc at any level (afferent fibers, spinal segments or efferent fibers). An absent response with intact reflex arc is abnormal and carries the same significance as the Babinski sign
- Plantar flexion of all toes, more prominent in small toes, is the normal response
- Slow, tonic or clonic dorsiflexion of great toe and small toes with fanning of toes is the Babinski sign. Sometimes, there may be extension followed by flexion or vice versa
- Sometimes, there may be no toe movement, but only hip and knee flexion and contraction of tensor fasciae latae. This is also an abnormal response
- Presence of Babinski sign indicates that there is a dysfunction or lesion of the pyramidal fibers destined to the foot muscles
- Absence of Babinski sign suggests that the pyramidal tract fibers destined to the foot muscles are intact. It does not exclude lesion involving the rest of the pyramidal tract fibers
- Early and rapid rather than slow flexion of ankle, knee and hip suggest voluntary withdrawal reflex. This indicates that either the patient is too sensitive or the stimulus is tickling.

Caveats

- In patients with foot deformities like pes cavus, use alternate stimulation sites and look for contraction of tensor fasciae latae and hamstrings
- Pseudo-Babinski sign is the response that mimics Babinski sign in the absence of corticospinal tract disease. This can occur in exaggerated voluntary withdrawal reflex, with over-zealous stimulation, in chorea or athetosis. This is differentiated from true Babinski sign by the absence of hamstring contraction. Moreover, the pseudo-Babinski sign is eliminated by pressure over the ball of great toe, unlike the true Babinski sign
- In patients with thick soles, no response may be seen on stimulation of the sole. Hence, alternative methods of stimulation must be attempted
- If the short flexors of the toes are paralyzed, there may be an extensor response even in the absence of pyramidal tract disease
- In acute spinal shock, even if the pyramidal fibers to the foot are involved, no response may be elicited in the acute stage
- If the stimulus is over the medial aspect of the foot, there is a greater chance of eliciting the toe flexion rather than extension, even in pyramidal tract disease
- Sometimes, an impression of toe dorsiflexion is obtained when the whole foot dorsiflexes as part of voluntary withdrawal response. Therefore, contraction of extensor hallucis longus muscle must be observed to ensure that there is true dorsiflexion of the toe

- If dorsiflexion of the toe occurs in the absence of tensor fasciae latae contraction, it could be an erroneous method of stimulation. Therefore, watching and feeling for tensor fasciae latae contraction is important during stimulation
- Voluntary withdrawal reflex can closely mimic the Babinski sign. It is differentiated by the fact that Babinski sign does not fatigue easily. The voluntary reflex may precede or outlast the stimulus and does not involve contraction of tensor fasciae latae.

Alternate Methods

A number of variations in eliciting this reflex have been described. Their main use is in patients with over-sensitive soles, in severe foot deformities, in foot amputees.
- Oppenheim reflex: Firmly stroke the shin of tibia from above downwards with thumb and index finger.
- Gordon reflex: Squeeze the calf muscle hard
- Chaddock reflex: Apply a light stroke below the external malleolus.

BIBLIOGRAPHY

1. Bassetti C. Babinski and Babinski sign. Spine. 1995;20:2591-4.
2. Boes CJ. The history of examination of reflexes. J Neurol. 2014;261(12):2264-74.
3. Brazis PW, Masdeu JC, Biller J. Localization in clinical neurology, 6th edition, Philadelphia: Wolters Kluwer/Lippincott Williams & Wilkins; 2011.
4. Campbell WW. DeJong's The Neurologic examination, 7th edition. Wolters Kluwer/ Lippincott Williams & Wilkins; 2013.
5. Canning DA. Cremasteric reflex and retraction of a testis. J Urol. 2003;169(4):1604.
6. Dick JP. The deep tendon and the abdominal reflexes. J Neurol Neurosurg Psychiatry. 1976;39:905-8.
7. Dick JPR. The deep tendon and the abdominal reflexes. J Neurol Neurosurg Psychiatry. 2003;74:150-3.
8. Fujimori T, Iwasaki M, Nagamoto Y, et al. The utility of superficial abdominal reflex in the initial diagnosis of scoliosis: a retrospective review of clinical characteristics of scoliosis with syringomyelia. Scoliosis. 2010;5:17.
9. Kumar SP, Ramasubramanian D. The Babinski sign - a reappraisal. Neurol India. 2000;48:314-8.
10. PG HM Raijmakers, M Castro Cabezas, JA Smal, et al. Teaching the plantar reflex. Clin Neurol Neurosurg. 1991;93 (3):201-4.
11. Van Gijn J. Equivocal plantar response: a clinical and electromyographic study. J Neurol Neurosurg Psychiatry. 1976;39:275-82.
12. Van Gijn J. The Babinski reflex. Postgrad MedJ3. 1995;71:645-8.
13. Van Gijn J. The Babinski sign and pyramidal syndrome. J Neurol Neurosurg Psychiatry. 1978;41:865-73.
14. Yngve D. Abdominal reflexes. J Pediatr Orthop. 1997;17(1):105-8.

PATHOLOGIC OR PRIMITIVE REFLEXES

PICTORIAL PRETEST

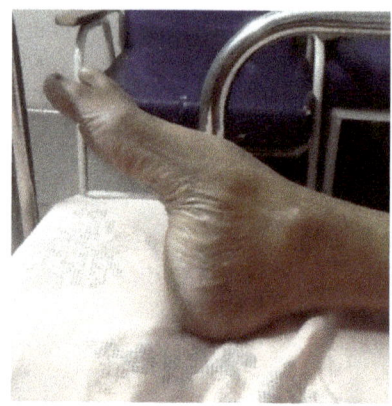
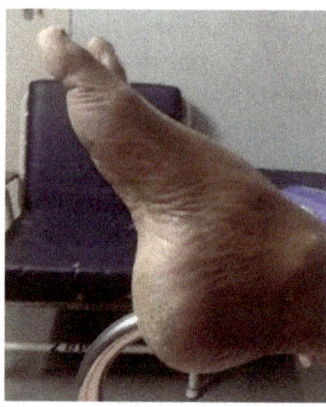

Fig. 6.10A   **Fig. 6.10B**

A. This 60-year-old man was admitted with **left hemiplegia** due to stroke. After 4 weeks, he was noted to have severe stiffness of his right sided limbs. A repeat MRI did not show any left hemispheric lesion.

Questions

1. Comment on his foot position when it was lifted off the bed (Fig. 6.10A) and when it was placed on the bed (Fig. 6.10B).
2. Can you explain the physiological basis of this finding especially, without an MRI evidence of left hemispheric lesion?

B. In the same patient, the examiner placed his fingers (Fig. 6.10C) in the palm without any specific instructions.

Questions

1. What is this patient's response and its physiological basis?
2. How can the examiner make the patient release his fingers?

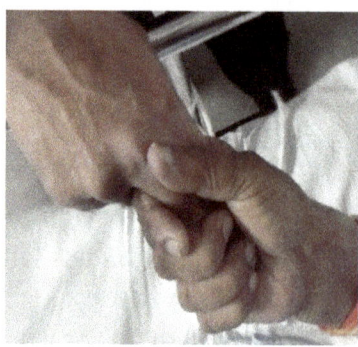

Fig. 6.10C

PRIMITIVE REFLEXES

Physiological Basis

- The primitive reflexes are a group of behavioral motor responses which are found in normal early development, are subsequently inhibited, but may be released from inhibition by cerebral, usually frontal, damage
- These involve more complex motor responses than simple stretch reflexes that are also "disinhibited" in disease states
- Anencephalic infants demonstrate a positive grasp reflex in both the hands and feet, indicating that the cerebral hemispheres are apparently not necessary for the reflexes. These reflexes could be segmental reflexes, inhibited by higher brain centers
- Most of these reflexes can be elicited in the neonate and the infant, but these decrease or disappear with age. They may re-appear in old age and in disease states
- The anatomical basis of these reflexes is not established, but frontal lobe disease is a consistent association.

Interpretation

- Primitive reflexes are not of great localizing value or lateralizing value, but they assist in establishing an organic basis of patient's condition
- In early infancy, if the primitive reflexes are not elicitable (especially unilaterally), a lower motor neuron lesion like plexus/root/peripheral nerve) involvement is suggested
- Some apparently healthy adults may exhibit these reflexes, but utilization behavior, oral reflexes, and asymmetric primitive reflexes are more likely to be pathological
- Multiple primitive reflexes in combination may be most predictive of organic (usually frontal lobe) disease
- Presence of primitive reflexes in an apathetic patient with normal brain imaging may be helpful in suggesting the presence of an organic neurodegenerative process, particularly affecting the frontal lobes, rather than a primary psychiatric disorder
- Habituation to the stimulus, that is, the reflex ceases after the stimulus is applied several times, is said to occur more often in normal individuals than in patients with neurologic disease.

GRASP REFLEX

Physiologic Basis

- In 1891, Robinson tested more than 60 infants under 1 month old and found that they were able to hang on to a horizontal rod by their hands unsupported for at least 10 seconds. Such reflex was even stronger in infant monkeys, suggesting a phylogenetic basis for human grasp reflex, which became redundant.

- Early descriptions suggested that unilateral grasp responses were due to lesions of the contralateral frontal lobe, possibly as a result of failure of the frontal lobe to inhibit parietal lobe function
- More recently lesions in the supplementary motor cortex (located just anterior to the foot area on the medial surface of the frontal lobe) and cingulate gyrus have been implicated in the etiology of these responses, although there is no consensus
- Contradictory to these observations, lesions of the frontal lobes may sometimes abolish these reflexes, and grasping is often bilateral, even with a unilateral lesion
- Eliciting the grasp reflex requires dual stimuli
- The first is a distally moving deep pressure over a specific area of the palmar surface of the hand, which elicits a brief muscular contraction (the "catching phase")
- This then develops into a strong "holding" phase only if traction is made on the tendons of the flexor or adductor muscles now in contraction, the response being maintained by continued traction
- Opposition of the thumb may also be noted, possibly dependent on the size and nature of the object that is grasped.

Methodology and Observation

- The examiner's hand is gently inserted into the palm of the patient's hand
- A distraction such as conversation with the patient is useful
- The palmar surface is stroked or simply touched especially between the thumb and the forefinger
- The flexor surfaces of the fingers are stimulated also by the examiner's fingers
- The stimulus should be in a distal direction
- With a positive response, the patient grasps the examiner's hand with variable strength and continues to grasp as the examiner's hand is moved
- Ability to release the grip voluntarily depends on the activity of the reflex; some patients can do so easily, while others can even be lifted off the bed
- A foot grasp reflex can be elicited by stroking gently the plantar surface medially especially over the metatarsophalangeal joints, with a blunt object such as the handle of a reflex hammer
- The lateral surfaces of the foot bend as if to make a cup out of the plantar surface. The toes adduct causing hollowing of the sole with some wrinkling.

Interpretation

- Grasp relfex is normal up to 1 year of age. The palmar grasp usually disappears by 6 months and the foot grasp by 12 months
- Presence of a grasp reflex in adults indicates frontal lobe disease, especially, contralateral supplementary area
- Sometimes, it may indicate ipsilateral or bilateral frontal lobe disease. This ipsilateral grasp reflex is more often seen with right frontal lesions.

Caveats

The grasp reflex may diminish if the dorsum of the hand is stroked, and thus the reflex may not be present if the patient's hand (palm uppermost) is rested in the examiner's palm.

PRIMITIVE ORAL REFLEXES

Physiologic Basis

- The primitive oral reflexes include the sucking, rooting, and snout reflexes, which all may be considered as appropriate feeding responses in infants
- They are seen in disorders that affect the frontal lobes, such as dementias, metabolic encephalopathies, closed head trauma, and hydrocephalus
- A significant number of normal individuals (up to 10%) can have suck and snout reflexes.

Methodology and Observation

Suck Reflex

- The suck reflex is elicited by lightly touching or tapping on the lips with an object such as a tongue blade, reflex hammer, or the examiner's finger
- At times the reflex is obtained merely by approaching the lips with an object
- The suck reflex consists of sucking movements by the lips.

Snout Reflex

- The snout reflex is brought about by gentle pressure on the upper lip near the philtrum lightly
- The contraction of the muscles causes puckering or protrusion of lips to resemble a snout.

Rooting Reflex

- Gently stroke the cheek (tactile rooting) and observe if the mouth turns towards the site of stimulus
- Bring an object like a reflex hammer into the visual field and observe the patient's mouth turning towards it (visual rooting).

Caveats

- These oral primitive reflexes must not be mistaken for orolingual **dyskinesias**
- Snout reflex must not be confused with "**pouting reflex**". This is a muscle stretch reflex elicited by tapping (instead of pressure) over the upper lip. It is a normal response that becomes exaggerated in pyramidal tract disease.

- Some authors use the terms pout and snout reflex inter changeably, but the basic difference between them must be understood irrespective of the term used.

PALMOMENTAL REFLEX

Physiologic Basis

- Stimulation of the thenar eminence can cause an involuntary contraction of the mentalis muscle of the chin. This reflex is known as the palmomental or palm-chin reflex
- The reflex may be present in healthy people of all ages
- The common afferent pathway consists of the cutaneous and muscular receptors of the thenar eminence and the median nerve
- The common efferent pathway involves the motor nuclei of the facial nerve. Longer latencies may involve the thalamus and motor cortex and shorter latencies may result from brainstem integration of the reflex
- Cortical inhibition of reflex and decussating brainstem pathways is lost with aging and disease states.

Methodology and Observation

- Stroke the thenar eminence at the wrist in a proximal to distal direction up to the base of the thumb using a sharp object such as the pointed end of a reflex hammer, key, paper clip, or fingernail
- The stimulus should cause discomfort but not pain
- Contraction of the ipsilateral, contralateral, or both mentalis muscles may be observed
- In pathological states, the reflex may be elicitable by stimulation of the hypothenar eminence, palmar aspect of the thumb, forearm, chest, abdomen, or even the sole
- If positive, repeat the stimulus at least 5 to 6 times to look for persistence of the reflex.

Interpretation

- In healthy people the trigger or release area is confined to the palm and the response is weaker, short lived, and easily fatigable by 5th stimulus
- A strong, sustained, and easily repeatable contraction of the mentalis muscle, which can be elicited by stimulation of areas other than the palm, is more likely to indicate cerebral damage
- The reflex is not of value in identifying the site of cerebral pathology. A unilateral palmomental reflex may be due to a contralateral/ ipsilateral/ bilateral lesions
- In a patient with facial palsy, prominent palmomental reflex provides an evidence for upper motor neuron lesion
- Palmomental reflex is more commonly observed in patients with psychoses, advanced Parkinson's disease and in dementias.

ANSWERS TO THE PRETEST

A. When the foot is placed in contact with the bed, the forefoot developed flexion posture, with toe adduction. This contraction relaxed after the foot was lifted off the bed passively. This is suggestive of foot grasp reflex, triggered by contact with the bed. A grasp reflex usually suggests contralateral supplementary motor area lesion, but ipsilateral and bilateral grasp reflex can occur with unilateral frontal lesion. This ipsilateral grasp reflex is more common with right frontal lesions, as in this patient.
B. The patient exhibited a prominent palmar grasp reflex, which has the same significance and physiologic basis as the foot grasp reflex. The grasp can be released by stroking the dorsal aspect of the hand.

BIBLIOGRAPHY

1. deNoordhout AM, Delwaide PJ. The palmomental reflex in Parkinson's disease. Arch Neurol. 1988;45:425-7.
2. Fujimori T, Iwasaki M, Nagamoto Y, et al. The utility of superficial abdominal reflex in the initial diagnosis of scoliosis: a retrospective review of clinical characteristics of scoliosis with syringomyelia. Scoliosis. 2010;5:17.
3. Futagi Y, Toribe Y, Suzuki Y. The Grasp Reflex and Moro Reflex in Infants: Hierarchy of Primitive Reflex Responses. International Journal of Pediatrics. 2012;2012:191562.
4. Isakov E, Sazbon L, Costeff H, Luz Y, Najenson T. The diagnostic value of three common primitive reflexes. Eur Neurol. 1984;23:17-21.
5. Mori E, Yamadori A. Unilateral hemispheric injury and ipsilateral instinctive grasp reaction. Arch Neurol. 1985;42:485-8.
6. Owen G, Mulley GP. The palmomental reflex: a useful clinical sign. J Neurol Neurosurg Psychiatry. 2002;73:113-5.
7. Robinson L. Darwinism in the nursery. Nineteenth Century. 1891;30:831-2.
8. Schott JM, Rossor MN. The grasp and other primitive reflexes. J Neurol Neurosurg Psychiatry. 2003;74:558-60.
9. Whittle IR, Miller JD. The palmomental reflex (letter). Surg Neurol. 1986;26:520-1.

CHAPTER 7

Examination of Coordination

GRK Sarma

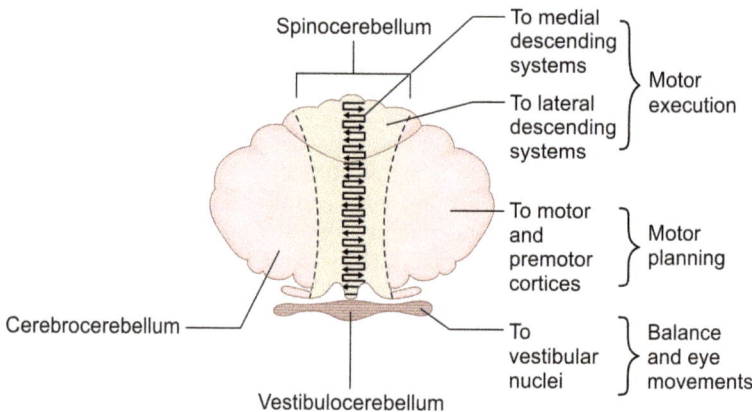

Fig. 7.1: Physiological systems of cerebellum.

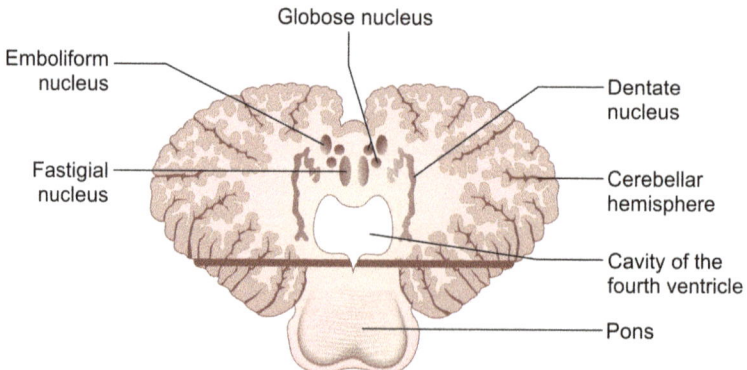

Fig. 7.2: Nuclei of cerebellum.

BASIC PRINCIPLES

- Coordination is defined as the normal use of motor, sensory and synergizing functions in the smooth performance of a movement. The various muscle groups that must be synergized during an action include agonists, antagonists, synergists and fixators. The cerebellum is considered the center of coordination of movement.
- A defect in any one of the pyramidal, extrapyramidal, somatosensory, cerebellar or vestibular systems can impair coordination. However, the term incoordination or ataxia is used if smooth action is impaired in the absence of significant abnormality of power, tone, sensations and involuntary movements.
- The cerebellum is functionally divided into 3 systems: The vestibulocerebellum (archicerebellum), the spinocerebellum (the paleocerebellum) and the cerebrocerebellum (the neocerebellum).

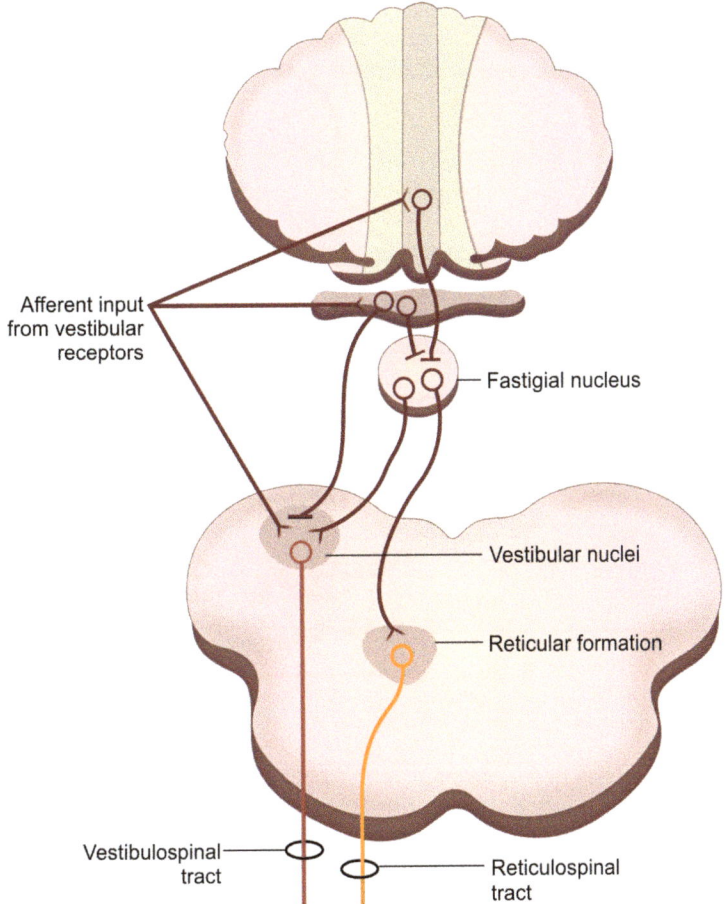

Fig. 7.3: Vestibulocerebellum and its connections.

- Cerebellar disease can manifest with either disturbance in stance and gait due to midline/vermian disease or incoordination of limbs due to ipsilateral hemispheric disease. Pancerebellar disease presents with the combination of the above two syndromes.
- The classical signs of cerebellar disease include:
    - Hypotonia
    - Dysequilibrium
    - Dyssynergia which can manifest in the form of dysarthria, ataxia, dysmetria, decomposition of movement, intention tremors, dysdiadochokinesis, rebound phenomenon
- Nonorganic illness must be considered when neurological findings are inconsistent.

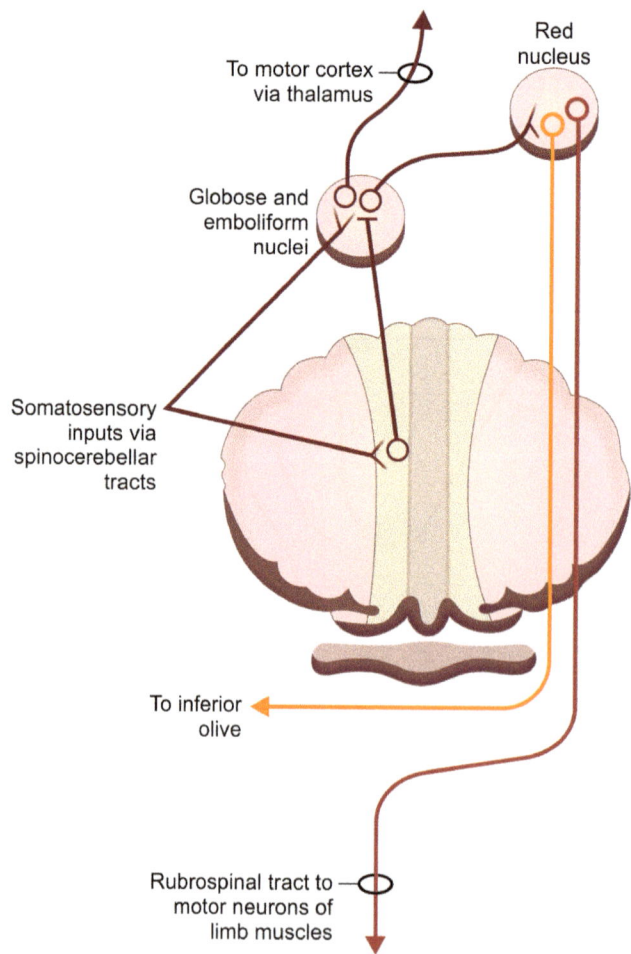

Fig. 7.4: Spinocerebellum and its connections.

TESTING OF STATION/STANCE

Physiological Basis

- Control of postural equilibrium is a function of vestibulocerebellum, spinocerebellum and their connections.
- The vestibulocerebellum (flocculonodular lobe and adjacent vermian cortex) receives inputs about the orientation of head and body in space from vestibular receptors of the kinetic and static labyrinths through the vestibular nuclei. It projects its efferents back to vestibular nuclei which give rise to medial and lateral vestibulospinal tracts that synapse with anterior horn cells innervating axial and proximal limb muscles respectively. The vestibular nuclei also project via the medial longitudinal fasciculus to the ocular motor nuclei of cranial nerves III, IV and VI to coordinate the eye movements.
- The spinocerebellum (vermis and intermediate zones) receives inputs from lower limbs (through ventral and dorsal spinocerebellar tracts) and upper limbs (through cuneocerebellar tract). Its efferents arising from the fastigial nucleus synapse with vestibular nuclei and midbrain reticular formation which control axial muscles. Its efferents from globose and emboliform nuclei reach contralateral precentral region (through superior cerebellar peduncle) and red nucleus. The precentral region gives rise to the anterior corticospinal tract and the red nucleus gives rise to the rubrospinal tract, which control the tone of the axial and proximal limb muscles.

Method

- Observe in supine, seated and standing position
- Observe with the patient standing with feet together, with eyes open and then closed
- Then observe the patient standing with one foot directly in front of the other
- Note his balance after giving a little push to one side and then the other
- Then observe him standing on one foot and then on the other.

Observation

- Swaying to one or both sides
- Tilting of the body or head to one side
- Oscillations of the body, and head
- Note if the swaying is markedly worse with eyes closed
- Difficulty in standing on one foot but not the other.

Interpretation

- Above abnormalities on one side indicate ipsilateral vestibulocerebellar/spinocerebellar system or their connections

- Marked worsening with eye closure suggests sensory ataxia (somatosensory or vestibular)
- Abnormalities on above tests without side to side preference indicate vermian lesion
- If a patient is able to stand on one foot, but not the other, he is likely to have lesion involving the ipsilateral cerebellum or its connections
- If he is unable to maintain his balance when pushed to one side, but not the other, this again suggests an ipsilateral cerebellar lesion.

Caveats

- In psychiatric conditions or malingering, Romberg sign may appear to be positive. However, the swaying is mostly at the hips in contrast to true Romberg sign, in which, the swaying is at the ankles
- Mild swaying when eyes are closed can occur in some normal individuals
- Even in cerebellar disease, the unsteadiness worsens with eyes closed. Only a disproportionate worsening indicates sensory ataxia.

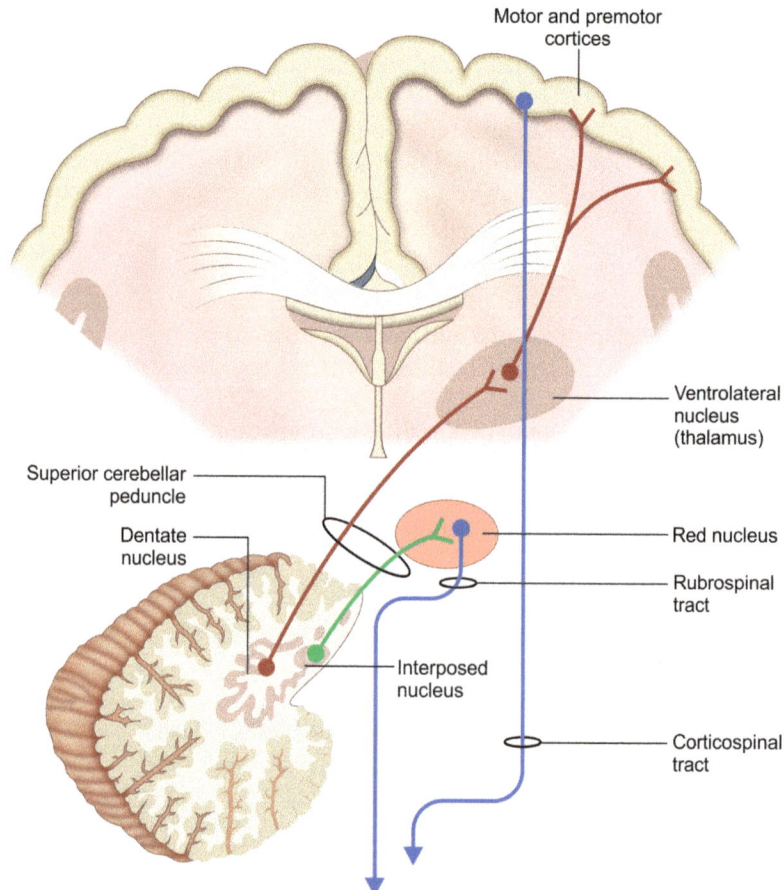

Fig. 7.5: Neocerebellum and its connections.

- In patients who are grossly unsteady with eyes open, it is neither possible, nor necessary to test with eyes closed
- Vestibular disease can impair performance in above tests and can be differentiated only with the help of other tests.

PAST POINTING

Physiological Basis

- The pontocerebellum (neocerebellum) is important in planning and execution of fine coordinated movements of the limbs
- It comprises of lateral cerebellar cortex which receives inputs from contralateral cerebral cortex through pontine nuclei and from inferior olivary nucleus
- It projects via Purkinje cell axons to the dentate nucleus which projects via superior cerebellar peduncle to contralateral red nucleus and thalamic lateral nucleus. The latter in turn projects to the premotor (area 6) and motor cortex (area 4). These cortical areas give rise to the corticospinal tracts that control the planning and execution of the coordinated movements of the limbs
- The double decussation explains ipsilateral signs in a hemispheric cerebellar lesion.

Method

- Patient sits or stands directly in front of the examiner at arms distance
- Examiner and patient stretch their arms forward so that their index fingers just touch each other
- The patient fully raises or lowers his arm and brings it back to original position to touch examiner's finger
- This is repeated several times on one side and then the other side. Both arms can also be tested simultaneously
- Test is done with eyes open and then with eyes closed.

Observation

- Watch for drifting of arm outward from the target (examiner's fingertip)
- Subtle drift is accentuated with eye closure
- The more number of times the test is repeated, the greater is the drift.

Interpretation

- If the ipsilateral arm drifts **outwards** (away from the midline) from the target, it suggests ipsilateral lesion in neocerebellar system or its connections
- In bilateral cerebellar disease, both arms drift outward from the target.

Caveats
- Vestibular disease can also cause arm drift
- However, in vestibular disease, **both** arms drift **towards** the side of the disease (in the direction of the slow phase of the nystagmus).

POSITION HOLDING

Physiological Basis
This is a test for the integrity of spinocerebellum and vestibulocerebellum and their connections.

Method
- The patient stands with both arms stretched forward at horizontal level
- Observe for some time for any drift
- If no drift is noted, ask patient to close his eyes, with arms still stretched
- Observe for any drift
- Finally tap the patient's wrists down and observe the arm's displacement.

Alternate Methods
- With patient supine, ask him to raise his legs in the air one at a time and hold for several seconds
- With the patient seated, ask him to extend his knee and hold it for several seconds
- Tap the extended limb to look for degree of displacement.

Observation
- Watch for drift of the limb
- Watch for oscillations, side to side or up and down
- Watch for the degree of arm displacement and if any swinging up and down on tapping the wrist.

Interpretation
- In unilateral cerebellar disease, the ipsilateral arm drifts outwards and either up or down, especially with eyes closed
- The ipsilateral limb has a typical posturing with wrist flexion, and excess pronation
- Marked arm displacement and swinging up and down few times on tapping the wrist are seen in ipsilateral cerebellar disease.

Caveats
- Pyramidal tract disease can also cause arm drift on stretching the arm horizontally. This can be differentiated from cerebellar disease only by

associated signs like hypertonia rather than hypotonia, and dysmetria, dyssynergia
- Sydenham's chorea can also cause identical arm drift.

FINGER-TO-NOSE TEST

Physiological Basis

This is a test of integrity of neocerebellum or its connections involved in the upper limb movements.

Method

- The patient may stand or sit or lie down
- The arm is abducted and extended to 90°
- The patient has to move the arm and touch the tip of his nose with the tip of his index finger and bring it back to its original position
- The test is done slowly and then rapidly
- The test is done with eyes open and then eyes closed.

Variations of Finger Nose Test

- **Nose-to-finger test**: Patient touches the tip of his nose and the examiner's fingertip, which is first held stationary and then moved to different positions
- **Finger-to-finger test**: Patient holds both arms abducted and extended in horizontal position. Patient brings both hands together with index fingers touching each other in midline. Repeat the test with eyes closed.

Observation

- Watch for the accuracy and smoothness or lack of it (dyssynergy, i.e. the movement is broken down into individual components)
- Watch if the patient stops before reaching the target (hypometria) or overshoots it (hypermetria)
- Watch if patient has marked incoordination only with eyes closed
- Watch for intention tremor as the finger approaches the target
- In the finger to finger test, watch if one hand crosses the midline to touch the other.

Interpretation

- Unilateral hypometria, hypermetria and dyssynergia are seen with ipsilateral lesion involving the neocerebellum or its connections
- Marked worsening of incoordination with eyes closed suggests sensory ataxia
- During the finger-to-finger test, with unilateral cerebellar disease, the ipsilateral hand fails to reach the midline and often sags down. The normal hand crosses the midline to reach the other.

Caveats

- A common cause of poor performance in this test is the patient's inability to understand what exactly needs to be done. Repeated explanation and demonstration may be needed to make the patient understand
- Finger to nose incoordination may be confused with intention tremor. In the latter, there is a side to side oscillatory movement which develops as the finger approaches the target or shortly afterwards
- Patients with nonorganic illness can trick the examiner into believing that they have incoordination in this test. Observing the patient's spontaneous actions like holding a cup, buttoning his shirt and reaching for objects is important. A dissociation between spontaneous actions and formal testing like finger nose test is a clue to the nonorganic basis.

HEEL-KNEE-TOE TEST

Physiological Basis

This test the integrity of ipsilateral neocerebellum or its connections involved in the lower limb movements.

Method

- Patient in supine or sitting position
- Patient has to place one heel on his opposite knee
- Then, he has to run his heel down along the shin to stop at the great toe
- He has to lift the heel again and place it back on the knee and repeat the movement
- Test is repeated several times and then again with eyes closed
- Test is repeated on the opposite side.

Observation

- Watch for accuracy of placement of heel on the knee
- Watch for smoothness or lack of it as the heel runs down along the shin
- Watch for side to side wavering of the heel while moving downwards.

Interpretation

In cerebellar disease, the ipsilateral heel cannot be placed accurately on the knee. As the heel runs down the shin, there is side to side wavering.

Caveats

- Heel-to-knee incoordination may be confused with intention tremor. In the latter, there is a side to side oscillatory movement which develops as the heel approaches the target or shortly afterwards

- Sensory ataxia may cause heel knee incoordination, which markedly worsens with eye closure.

DYSDIADOCHOKINESIS

Physiological Basis

This is an inability to efficiently perform rapid alternating movements that require stopping one action and follow it immediately by its diametric opposite action. This is a function of neocerebellum and its connections that coordinate smooth switching on and off of agonists and antagonists.

Method

- Patient sits with elbows flexed or extended and forearms completely supinated with palms facing upwards
- Ask him to repeatedly pronate and supinate the forearms as rapidly as possible
- Repeat the test with clenched fist.

Alternate Methods

- Opening and closing the fist
- Flexing and extending individual fingers
- Touching the tip of the thumb with the tip of each finger in sequence
- Tapping the table top with the palm or individual finger tips
- Tapping the palm of one hand alternating with palm and dorsum of the other hand
- Dorsiflexion and plantar flexion of ankle or the toes
- Tapping the floor with the sole of one foot
- Protruding and retracting the tongue or side to side movement of the tongue.

Observation

- Watch for rate, rhythm, accuracy and smoothness of the movements
- Watch for superimposition of wrist flexion-extension instead of forearm supination-pronation.

Interpretation

- Decomposition of the movement into coarse, irregular and slow components is indicative of a lesion in the ipsilateral neocerebellum or its connections
- Superimposition of wrist flexion-extension or even finger extension while attempting forearm supination-pronation is typical of ipsilateral cerebellar disease.

Caveats

- Pyramidal or extrapyramidal diseases can also impair performance on this test. However, the movement is simply slowed and labored but not irregular and decomposed as in cerebellar disease
- Even in normal individuals, dominant hand performance is better than the nondominant hand and should not be mistaken for true dysdiadochokinesis
- In mild cerebellar dysfunction, the initial movements may appear normal, but after several attempts, the movement decompensates. If the patient is not tested for sufficient time, this fatigability may be missed.

REBOUND TEST

Physiological Basis

This tests the ability to contract the antagonist muscles immediately after relaxation of the agonists, which is a function of ipsilateral neocerebellum and its connections.

Method

- Patient sits with shoulder adducted, forearm flexed and supinated, fist clenched tightly
- Elbow may or may not be supported on the table
- Pull the wrist tightly against patient's resistance
- Keep your free arm over the face of the patient to protect it from the rebound flexion
- Suddenly release the wrist.

Observation

Observe if the patient's elbow flexion is adequately and instantaneously checked as soon as you release his wrist.

Interpretation

If the patient cannot stop the contraction of elbow flexion and switch to elbow extension, this indicates a lesion in the ipsilateral neocerebellum or its connections.

Caveats

- Rebound may be absent in cerebellar disease
- It may be elicited in some normal individuals
- It may be elicited in a spastic limb
- Therefore, rebound elicited unilaterally in the absence of significant weakness or spasticity is more significant.

BIBLIOGRAPHY

1. Campbell WW. In: DeJong's the neurological examination, 7th edition. Wolters Kluwer/ Lippincott Williams & Wilkins; 2013.
2. Diener HC, Dichgans J. Pathophysiology of cerebellar ataxia. Mov Disord. 1992;7: 95-109.
3. Inhoff AW, Diener HC, et al. The role of cerebellar structures in the execution of serial movements. Brain. 1989;112:565.
4. Oberdick J, Sillitoe RV. Cerebellar zones. History, development and functions. Cerebellum. 2011;10(3):301-306.
5. SH. Narabayashi H. analysis of intention tremor. Clin Neurol Neurosurg. 1992;94(Suppl):S130-S132.
6. Subramony SH. Approach to ataxic disorders. Handbook Clin Neurol. 2011;103: 389-98.

CHAPTER 8

Examination of Gait

GRK Sarma

GAIT ASSESSMENT

Physiologic Basis

- Gait is a complex **motor** and **mental** skill that requires integration of mechanisms of locomotion with those of balance, motor control, cognition and musculoskeletal function
- Locomotion is achieved by a continuous flow of integrated signals performing the alternate **advancing, loading** and **unloading** of lower limbs
- Mesencephalic tegmentum and lateral-dorsal portion of ponto-mesencephalic junction and posterior subthalamic nucleus are the important lower centers that generate the gait cycle
- The activity of this "**locomotor center** (especially the **pedunculopontine** nucleus in the pontomesencephalic junction)" is integrated with polymodal sensory inputs (vision, proprioception, vestibular) and cerebral, brainstem and cerebellar processing and musculoskeletal execution of the movement.

Gait Cycle (Figs. 8.1A and B)

- Gait is systematically analyzed by breaking it into a series of "gait cycles". Each cycle starts with one foot taking off from the ground and ends with that foot ready for the next take off
- One gait cycle thus consists of a stance phase and a swing phase for each leg alternating with the other.

Definitions of Common Terms Used in Gait Assessment

- **Stance phase:** During this, the leg remains in contact with the ground, while the other leg moves forward
- **Swing phase:** During this, the leg moves forward while the body is supported by the other leg
- **Single support phase:** When the body is supported by only one leg, it is the single support phase

Examination of Gait

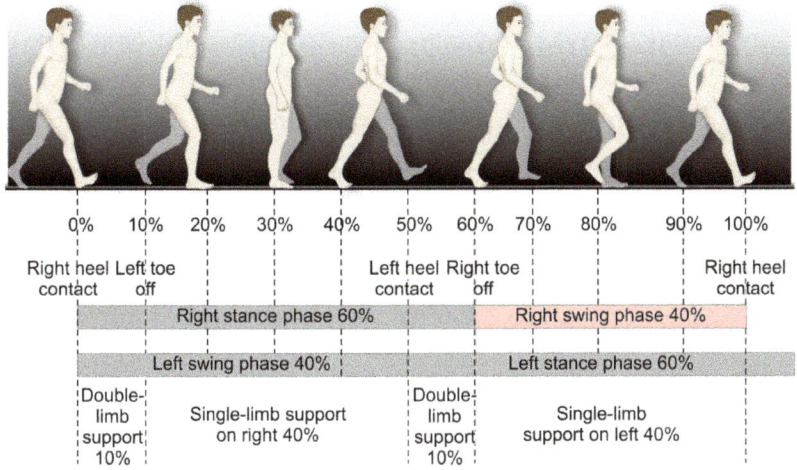

Fig. 8.1A: The gait cycle.

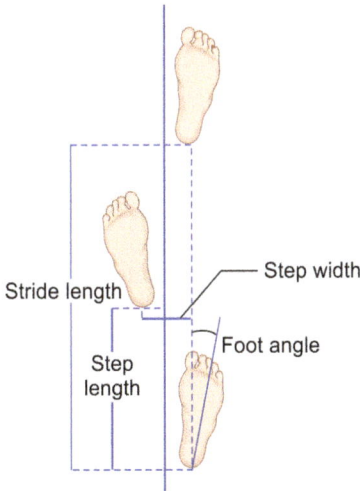

Fig. 8.1B: Several distance measures help to describe a typical gait cycle.

- **Double support phase:** When the body is supported by both legs, it is the double support phase
- **Step length:** The distance between ground contact of one foot and the next ground contact of the opposite foot
- **Stride length:** The distance between ground contact of one foot and the next ground contact of the same foot
- **Step width:** The perpendicular distance between similar points on both feet during two consecutive steps
- **Foot angle:** The angle between the long axis of the foot and the line of progression
- **Cadence:** Number of steps in one minute (normally 100–130/min)

- Thus, the gait cycle can be summarized sequentially as follows: Double support (10%) → right single support (or left swing) (40%) → double support (10%) → left single support (or right swing) (40%).

The approximate normal values of various parameters of gait cycle are given below:

Parameter	Normal value (approximate)
Right single support	40%
Left single support	40%
Right swing	40%
Left swing	40%
Double support	20%
Cadence	100–130/min
Stride length	1.3 m
Step length	0.7 m
Step width	0.6 m
Foot angle	5°

Methodology

Assess the following aspects:
- **Rising ability from sitting**: Ask patient to stand from a chair with his arms crossed. This tests the strength of hip extensors, knee extensors and general postural control as well as initiative.
- **Standing capacity**: Ask patient to stand at his comfortable position and then with feet together, then on one leg at a time for 5 sec, then tandem stand (one foot in front of another) for 30 seconds and finally test Romberg's sign, and pull test.
- **Walking ability**: Assess normal walking in an open space.
    - Patient should be walking at his most comfortable speed for 7-10 meters, preferably with a turn at mid distance (3-5 meters forward, turnaround, 3-5 m backward)
    - Assess turning around, look for freezing/imbalance
    - The timed up and go test (TUaG) test: Ask patient to get up from chair and walk 3 meters, turn 180° and return to the chair. Normal persons take less than 10 seconds to complete the task. If a patient takes longer than 14 seconds, it is abnormal and indicates increased risk of fall. Taking longer than 30 seconds indicates severe gait disorder.

Assess the following (accurate estimation of these parameters requires analysis in a gait laboratory. Clinical assessment is at best an approximation):
- Stride length
- Cadence
- Step width
- Stance phase and swing phase

- Single support phase
- Double support phase.

INTERPRETATION

- Common neurological conditions causing gait disturbance are described below in terms of the gait cycle described earlier
- Such systematic description allows more complete characterization of the gait abnormality and identification of unusual features in an otherwise "typical gait".

Parkinson's disease	
Parameter	Observation
Rising up	Hesitant
Posture	Generalized flexion (trunk, upper and lower limbs), bent spine (Camptocormia) lateral flexion (Pisa sign), mild neck flexion
Equilibrium	Impaired postural reflex occurs late in illness; tends to fall en-bloc especially forward, reduced associated movements
Step initiation	Delayed, hesitant
Stride length	↓ (marche a petits pas)
Stride linearity	Linear
Stride cadence	↓, freezing (especially at obstacles, narrow passages or multitasking) may show festination (chases own center of gravity). Rest tremor may appear during walking
Step width	↓
Swing phase	Markedly ↓, reduced arm swing
180° turning	Slow, may freeze

Atypical parkinsonism	
Parameter	Observation
Rising up	Slow
Posture*	Excess neck flexion (MSA) or extension (PSP), trunk extension (PSP)
Equilibrium*	Impaired **early with frequent falls** especially backward, ataxia may be added (MSA)
Step initiation	Hesitation
Stride length	↓
Stride linearity	Linear/irregular (MSA)
Stride cadence*	↓, **festination rare**
Step width*	↑ in MSA due to ataxia component
180° turning	Impaired

*Parameters which differentiate this condition from idiopathic Parkinson's disease (also highlighted in bold)

Normal pressure hydrocephalus/Binswanger's disease

Parameter	Observation
Rising up	Slow
Posture*	Upright, normal facial expression
Equilibrium	Impaired
Step initiation	Hesitant
Stride length	↓
Stride linearity*	Linear, sometimes irregular (ataxia component)
Stride cadence*	↓, **exaggerated arm swing (military gait)**
Step width	↓

* Parameters which differentiate this condition from idiopathic Parkinson's disease (also highlighted in bold)

Spastic gait

Parameter	Observation
Rising up	Slow
Posture*	Wernicke-Mann attitude (upper limb flexed at all joints, lower limb extended)
Equilibrium	Preserved in mild cases. Impaired with severe spasticity
Step initiation*	Preserved, but labored
Stride length	↓, (range of hip, knee and ankle movements reduced)
Stride linearity*	Scissoring/circumduction, with contralateral trunk flexion
Stride cadence*	↓, no freezing
Step width*	May be slightly widened for balance. If bilateral, scissoring results (adductor spasticity)
Swing phase%	↓ (but absolute time in increased due to slowness). Foot take off is incomplete, drags on the ground, often with plantar flexed, inverted foot
180° turning	Labored

* Parameters which differentiate this condition from idiopathic Parkinson's disease (also highlighted in bold)

Cerebellar gait

Parameter	Observation
Rising up	Unsteady
Posture	Wide based, hips slightly flexed to lower the center of gravity. Unsteady in severe cases. 3 Hz anteroposterior trunk tremor in anterior lobe lesions
Equilibrium	Impaired in vermian lesion. Sways to lesion side in lateral cerebellar lesions
Step initiation	Normal
Stride length	Irregular
Stride linearity	Irregularly variable
Stride cadence	↓
Step width	↑
Swing phase%	↓
180° turning	Sways

Some Descriptive Terms for Gait Disorders

- Duck gait (waddling gait): Proximal weakness
- Cock gait: Manganese toxicity (feet dystonia)
- Dromedary gait (camel gait): Chorea
- Stamping gait: Sensory ataxia
- High stepping gait (equines gait): Peroneal weakness
- Flail gait: Peroneal and tibial weakness (Fig. 8.2)
- Military gait: NPH (exaggerated arm swing)
- Bouncing gait: Spastic ataxic gait (MS, ACM, hydrocephalus), cerebellar truncal tremors, action myoclonus of the legs.

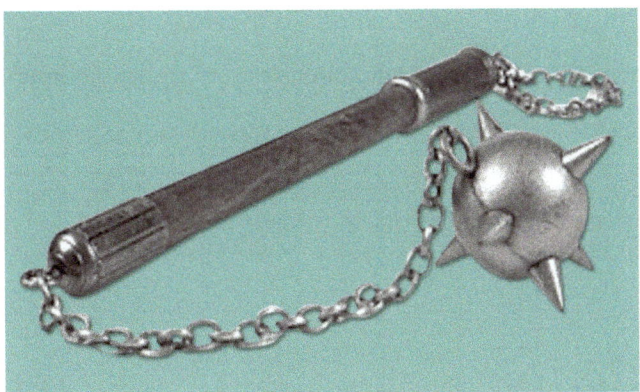

Fig. 8.2: A flail.

Conditions Causing Tilt of the Trunk to One Side

Neurological causes (variable with posture, reduce in supine/sleep)
- Truncal dystonia
- Parkinsonism (Pisa sign)
- Acute vestibular lesion (ipsilateral tilt)
- Thalamic stroke (tilt away from lesion side)
- Basal ganglia stroke (tilt away from lesion side)

Spinal deformities

Causes of Involuntary Leg Movements on Standing

- Orthostatic tremor
- Essential tremor
- Cerebellar truncal tremor
- Action myoclonus of legs
- Ankle clonus

CAVEATS

- Senile gait: Some elderly individuals exhibit a slow gait with minimal forward flexion to compensate for age-related mild disequilibrium. They do not have other signs of parkinsonism, which should not be over diagnosed
- Depressed individuals also exhibit a slow gait that may appear like early parkinsonism
- Dopa-responsive dystonia (DRD) may be mistaken for spasticity because of stiffness, brisk reflexes, and toe dystonia mimicking Babinski sign
- Psychogenic gait disorder may be bizarre, of sudden onset, inconsistent, distractible and resolve dramatically.

BIBLIOGRAPHY

1. Chambers G, Sutherland D. A practical guide to gait analysis. Am Acad Ortho Surg. 2002;10:222-31.
2. Dickson M, Farley CT, Full RJ, et al. How animals move: an integrative view. Science. 2000;288:100-6.
3. Oatis CA. Kinesiology: The mechanics and pathomechanics of human movement, 2nd edition. Wolters Kluvers/Lippincott Williams; 2004.

CHAPTER 9

Examination of Movement Disorders

GRK Sarma

GENERAL APPROACH TO MOVEMENT DISORDERS

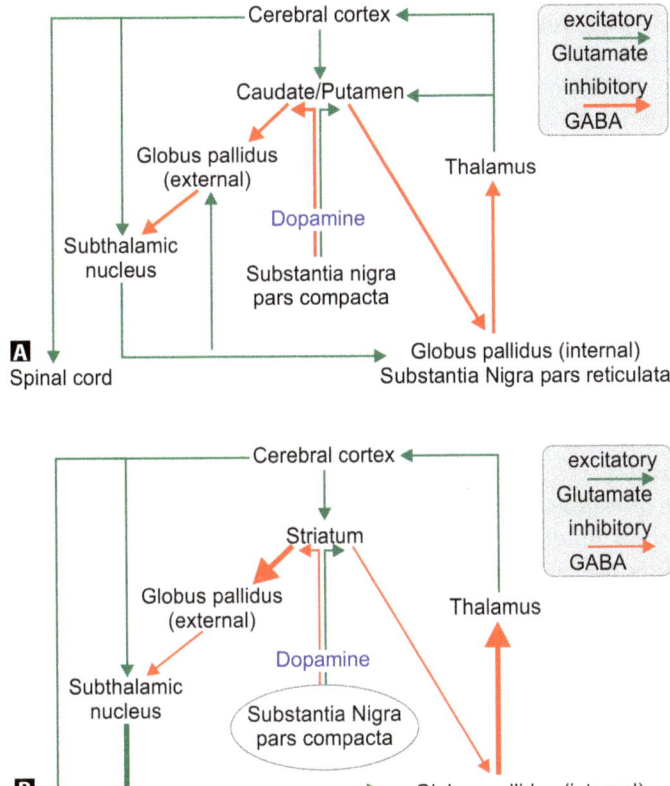

Figs. 9.1A and B

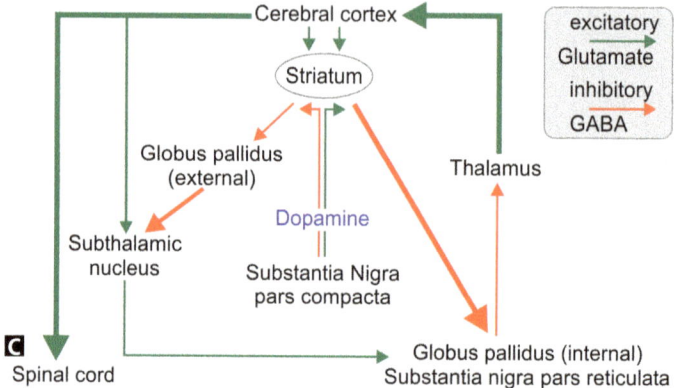

Fig. 9.1C

Figs. 9.1A to C: Schematic representation of basal ganglia circuits in health (A), and in hypokinetic (B) and hyperkinetic (C) movement disorders.

- This chapter provides a basic framework of clinical evaluation of movement disorders
- The most important step in the evaluation of patients with movement disorders is to correctly identify the phenomenology. This is easier said than done because many patients have mixed disorders (e.g. tremor plus dystonia). In an unusual movement disorder, psychogenic cause is always a possibility but is difficult to prove
- A detailed history with special attention to drug history and family history is important
- A meticulous examination, supplemented by the clinic/home video recording if necessary, completes the clinical assessment
- While assessing an abnormal movement, the following questions need to be answered. Synthesizing these responses usually leads to correct recognition of the movement disorder(s) and the possible differential diagnoses
- These questions are more or less applicable to most movement disorders with some modification in the individual case. Using this simple scheme, it is possible to describe the various movement disorders in a systematic manner
- These questions about the involuntary movement under consideration are:
    - Where is it?
    - How is it?
    - When is it seen?
    - What increases it?
    - What decreases it?
    - Whether it can be suppressed?
    - What else is there?
    - Finally, What is it?

- How these questions are relevant is discussed with examples below:
    - Where is it?
        - Parkinson's disease is typically asymmetric in onset, while atypical Parkinsonism is usually symmetric
        - Chorea involving the lower face is seen in tardive dyskinesia, while chorea involving upper face is seen in Huntington's disease
        - Dystonia of feet is primary in children and secondary in adults
    - How is it?
        - Describe the movement as is seen
        - Slow/fast: The movement disorders are classified into hypokinetic and hyperkinetic types based on the speed of the movement (Box 9.1 and Flowchart 9.1)
        - Rhythmic or not: For example, tremor is rhythmic, while polyminimyoclonus is arrhythmic
    - When is it seen?
        - Rest: For example, rest tremor of Parkinson's disease
        - Posture: For example, orthostatic tremor occurs only on standing, disappears while walking
        - Action: For example, task specific dystonias
        - Sleep: Palatal myoclonus, spinal myoclonus, periodic movements of sleep, tics can persist in sleep
    - What makes it more? (here, it may be better to ask open ended questions and then ask for specific triggers):
        - High carbohydrate meal worsens paroxysmal non-kinesogenic dystonia
        - Loud noise triggers brainstem myoclonus
    - What makes it less?
        - Alcohol reduces essential tremor and myoclonic dystonia
        - Walking backwards may relieve dystonia of feet
    - Can it be suppressed?:
        - Tics can be voluntarily suppressed
        - Dystonia can be suppressed by sensory tricks
    - What else is there?
        - Associated sensory symptoms: PLMT, RLS and phantom dyskinesias; tics may be associated with a vague discomfort or unusual sensation in the prodrome before the movement.
        - Associated neurological signs like pyramidal signs, cerebellar signs, eye movement abnormalities, cognitive impairment, etc. provide clue to the diagnosis
        - Associated systemic signs (For example, KF ring in Wilson's disease, short stature in mitochondrial disease)
- What is it? This is the final question to be answered after taking all the above information into account. The movement disorder(s) has or have to be clearly defined so as to permit further clinical diagnosis
- Movement disorders are generally classified as hypokinetic and hyperkinetic disorders (Flowchart 9.1)

> **Box 9.1:** Broad classification of movement disorders.
>
> A. Hypokinetic disorders: Parkinsonism
> B. Hyperkinetic disorders:
>   - Jerky movements:
>   - Myoclonus
>   - Chorea
>   - Tics
>   - Non-jerky movements:
>   - Dystonia
>   - Tremors

- The defining features of hypokinetic disorders are:
  - Slowness of movement
  - **Fatiguing (decrement)** of repetitive alternating movements (finger or foot tapping)
  - Poverty of associated movements (blink, arm swing)
- Fatiguing of repetitive movements differentiates true hypokinetic disorders from slowness of movement seen in pyramidal and cerebellar disorders
- Hyperkinetic movement disorders may be distinguished by their salient and defining clinical features as shown in the Flowchart 9.1.

Flowchart 9.1: Hyperkinetic movement disorders.

```
                    Hyperkinetic
                      movement
                      disorders
    ┌──────────┬──────────┬─────────┬──────────┬──────────┐
  Flowing   Shock-like  Rhythmic  Sustained  Sterotyped
                                  postures
   ┌───┴───┐                                  ┌─────┴─────┐
 Small   Large                           Distractible  Suppressible
amplitude amplitude
   │       │         │         │          │          │        │
 Chorea Ballism  Myoclonus   Tremor    Dystonia  Stereotypies Tics
```

- Often, patients have more than one movement disorder and such combination provides a hint to the underlying disease (Table 9.1)

Table 9.1: Combination of movement disorders and its usual etiology.

Combinations of movement disorders	Usual etiology
Parkinsonism + myoclonus	Multiple system atrophy (MSA)
Parkinsonism + myoclonus + asymmetric severe rigidity	Corticobasal degeneration
Chorea + dystonia + parkinsonism	Huntington's disease
Dystonia + tremor	Primary dystonia
Tremor + dystonia + parkinsonism	Wilson's disease
Myoclonus + ataxia	Mitochondrial disease, Unverricht-Lundborg disease, celiac disease

- Finally, certain conditions are confused with movement disorders. Such pitfalls must be avoided (Box 9.2).

Box 9.2: Mimics of some movement disorders.
- Facial dystonia:
  - Ptosis
  - Apraxia of eyelid opening
  - Trismus
  - Focal seizure
- Limb dystonia
  - Contracture
  - Spasticity
  - Myotonia
  - Neuromyotonia
  - Pseudoathetosis
  - Tonic spasms
  - Focal seizures
- Cervical dystonia
  - Congenital torticollis
  - Sandifer syndrome
  - Dropped head syndrome (neuromuscular weakness)
  - Retropharyngeal abscess
  - Atlantoaxial subluxation
- Parkinsonism
  - Slowness of normal ageing
  - Depression
  - Hypothyroidism
  - Catatonia
  - Spasticity

BIBLIOGRAPHY

1. Abdo WF, et al. The clinical approach to movement disorders. Nat Rev Neurol. 2010; 6:29-37.
2. Burn DJ. Approach to the patient with a movement disorder. Acnr; 27-8.
3. Deuschl G[1], Bain P, Brin M. Consensus statement of the Movement Disorder Society on Tremor. Ad Hoc Scientific Committee. Mov Disord. 1998;13 (Suppl) 3:2-23.
4. Kishore A, Calne DB. Approach to the patient with a movement disorder and overview of movement disorders. In: Watts RL, Koller WC (Eds). Movement disorders: neurologic principles and practice. McGraw Hill (New York). 1997; PP. 3-14.

TREMOR

Physiologic Basis

- Definition: Tremor is a rhythmic oscillatory movement of a body region about a fixed point due to synchronous or alternating contraction of antagonistic muscles.
- Four different mechanisms have been considered important in the pathogenesis:
    1. Mechanical oscillations of the extremity: Present in any outstretched limb due to the mass-spring effect (mechanical effect of weight of the limb on the ligaments and muscles)
    2. Reflexes that elicit and maintain the tremor. The mechanical oscillations of the limb elicit a stretch reflex by activating the muscle spindles. In sympathetic activated states, the muscle spindles are sensitized, increasing this tremor
    3. Central oscillators: Inferior olive and its connections can switch to an oscillatory mode in disease states due to hypersynchronization.
    4. Impaired feed forward or feed backward loops in the central systems: Deep cerebellar nuclei are important in stopping a movement when it needs to, by feed forward and feedback mechanisms. In disease states, this mechanism fails causing to and fro overshoots manifesting as intention tremor.
- Tremors are classified based on the activation condition as shown in Flowchart 9.2. This has a bearing on the phenomenology and localization of the tremor.

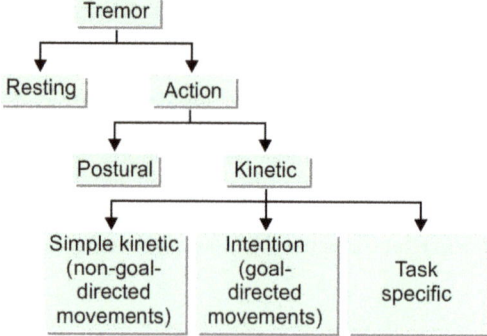

Flowchart 9.2: Classification of tremors.

- **Resting tremor** occurs in a body part that is not voluntarily activated and is completely supported against gravity. It increases by mental or physical activation of other body regions like contralateral hand or gait. It decreases or disappears during the onset of voluntary action of the involved limb.
- **Re-emergent tremor** is the resting tremor that reappears when the voluntary activity is sustained. For example, a resting tremor disappears on raising the arm and stretching out the hand only to reappear after a latency. If there is no latency, it is a feature of essential tremor.

- **Action tremor**: Tremor that appears during voluntary muscle contraction. This includes postural and various kinetic tremors
- **Postural tremor**: It is present when actively maintaining a position against gravity. In some patients, there is a position specific tremor (occurs only a particular posture).
- **Kinetic tremor**: It occurs during a voluntary movement. As is clear from the names, kinetic tremors may be simple kinetic (during non-goal directed movements), intention (during goal directed movements) or task specific (primary writing tremors, musicians tremors, etc.).

Method

- Examine the patient with minimal clothing as possible, from head to toe, systematically observing each body region.
- Examine the patient during common activities of daily living, as described in The Essential Tremor Rating Scale (TETRAS) (speaking, carrying a plate, feeding with spoon, pouring water, drinking from a glass, dressing, writing, using keys)
- Describe the tremor by the following variables (which are similar to all movement disorder evaluations):
    - Is it tremor? (a regular rhythmic oscillatory movement)
    - Where is the tremor (Topography)
    - How fast or slow is it (Frequency)
    - What body part condition increases it? (Activation condition—rest, posture, movement)
    - What manipulations reduce it? (Relieving condition)
    - Are there signs of other system involvement (pyramidal, extrapyramidal, cerebellar)?

Topography (Head-to-Toe)

- Head: More often in ET than PD
- Face and Jaw: More often in PD than in ET
- Chin: More often in PD than ET
- Palate
- Voice: More common in ET than PD
- Trunk
- Upper limb
- Lower limb
- Bilateral/unilateral

Frequency (Tremorogram is Required to Measure the Exact Frequency)

- Low frequency: < 4 Hz
- Medium frequency: 4–7 Hz
- High frequency: >7 Hz

Regular/Irregular

True tremor is regular and has a relatively constant frequency and amplitude in a given position. If the amplitude and frequency vary with time it raises the possibility of cortical myoclonus than true tremor. Tapping the tips of fingers of the outstretched hand may elicit a cortical myoclonic jerk.

Activation Condition

Head: Observe in neutral position for at least 10 seconds. Use the tip of the nose as the landmark to assess the amplitude of the tremor.

Face and Jaw: Observe at rest and during facial muscle activation by closing the eyes, smiling, opening the mouth, pursing the lips.

Voice: Ask an open ended question to listen to the voice. If there is no obvious tremor, ask him to say extended "aaah" and "eeeh" for 5 seconds and listen for tremor. It may be graded using TETRAS scale as follows:
- 0 = Normal.
- 1 = Slight voice tremulousness, only when "nervous".
- 2 = Mild voice tremor. All words easily understood.
- 3 = Moderate voice tremor. Some words difficult to understand.
- 4 = Severe voice tremor. Most words difficult to understand.

Upper limb

Rest: Keep the limb supported completely against gravity, and get all voluntary activity eliminated. If this is not done, postural tremor might emerge. To confirm the resting tremor, give mental activity (counting backwards), contralateral hand movements and ask patient to walk. Resting tremor must increase during these activities.

Ask patient to rhythmically move his un-involved limb (tap the hand or foot/close and open the fist/supinate-pronate the forearm) at a frequency different from the patient's tremor. The tremor frequency changes to match that of the activated limb in psychogenic tremor (entrainment).

Passively move the limb with tremor to feel the increased muscle tone. During the examination, the tremor fluctuates along with the variable and inconsistent hypertonia (co-activation sign) in psychogenic tremor.

Posture:
i. **Forward outstretched postural tremor:** Subjects should bring their arms forward, slightly lateral to midline and parallel to the ground for 5 seconds. The wrist should also be straight and the fingers abducted so that they do not touch each other.
ii. **Lateral "wing beating" postural tremor (Fig. 9.2):** Subjects will abduct their arms parallel to the ground and flex the elbows so that the two hands do not quite touch each other and are at the level of the nose. The fingers are abducted so that they do not touch each other. The posture should be held for 20 seconds.

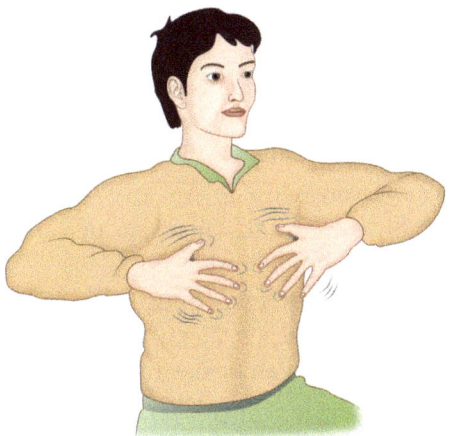

Fig. 9.2: Wing beating tremor

Kinetic tremor:
  i. **Finger nose test** patient makes a fist and then extends out the index finger. Ask him to touch a set object or the examiners finger located to the full extent of their reach, which is located at the same height (parallel to the ground) and slightly lateral to the midline. He then touches his own nose and repeats this back and forth three times. Only the position along the trajectory of greatest tremor amplitude is assessed.
  ii. **Archimedes spiral:** See next Topic
  iii. **Handwriting:** Paper is placed on a table in a position that suits patient's habitual style of writing. The writing hand should not be supported by the other hand. Using ballpoint pen, he is asked to write in cursive letters, few lines.
  iv. **Feeding with a spoon:** This can be assessed using a home video also (saves clinician's time) and graded as per TETRAS scale as follows:
   - 0 = Normal
   - 1 = Slightly abnormal. Tremor is present but does not interfere with feeding with a spoon
   - 2 = Mildly abnormal. Spills a little.
   - 3 = Moderately abnormal. Spills a lot or changes strategy to complete task such as using two hands or leaning over.
   - 4 = Severely abnormal. Cannot feed with a spoon.
  v. **Drinking from a glass**
   - 0 = Normal.
   - 1 = Slightly abnormal. Tremor is present but does not interfere with drinking from a glass.
   - 2 = Mildly abnormal. Spills a little.
   - 3 = Moderately abnormal. Spills a lot or changes strategy to complete task such as using two hands or leaning over.
   - 4 = Severely abnormal. Cannot drink from a glass or uses straw or sippy cup.

vi. **Pouring**
   - 0 = Normal.
   - 1 = Slightly abnormal. Tremor is present but does not interfere with pouring.
   - 2 = Mildly abnormal. Must be very careful to avoid spilling but may spill occasionally.
   - 3 = Moderately abnormal. Must use two hands or uses other strategies to avoid spilling.
   - 4 = Severely abnormal. Cannot pour.

vii. Similarly, effect of tremor on activities of daily living like carrying a plate, using a key, dressing, etc. can be easily examined bedside or using a home video.

Lower limb tremor
  i. Raise each lower limb horizontally parallel to the ground for 5 seconds. Then perform a standard heel to shin maneuver with each leg, three times.
 ii. Standing: Patient stands, unaided if possible. The knees are 4-5 inches apart and are flexed 10-20°. The arms are down at the patient's side. Tremor is assessed at any point on the legs or trunk.

Relieving Factors

- Alcohol (from history, or examine the home video of the tremor after patient consumes his habitual amount)
- If patient has head tremor, turn the head to various positions to see if it varies (this happens in dystonic tremor, but not in essential/cerebellar tremor)
- If the patient has head tremor, see if it is relieved by sensory tricks or arm elevation (happens in dystonic tremor)
- If patient has foot tremor, see if it disappears on ankle plantar flexion and increases on dorsiflexion. These features indicate that he has ankle clonus and not true tremor
- If the tremor disappears on movement of the involved limb, it suggests a resting tremor.

Other Signs

- Reflexes (hyporeflexia is seen in neuropathic tremor)
- Cerebellar signs
- Froment's sign, rigidity, bradykinesia, postural imbalance
- Signs of thyrotoxicosis
- Look for Keiser-Fleischer ring

Interpretation

Based on Activation Method

- **Rest tremor** requires a **central oscillator** (in the Guillain-Mollaret's triangle and its connections especially with substantia nigra). The usual causes are: Parkinson's disease, rubral tremor (Holme's tremor), palatal tremor. The Parkinson's disease tremor may have a classical pill rolling appearance due to the alternate contractions of agonist and antagonist muscle groups involved.
- **Postural tremor** is due to the interaction of **peripheral (neuromuscular) inputs and the central generator**. Therefore, the usual causes are exaggerated physiological tremor (8-12 Hz), essential tremor, postural orthostatic tremor (classified as a variant of essential tremor) neuropathic tremor, and dystonic tremor.
- Goal-directed action tremor (**intention tremor**) is due to impaired function of **cerebellum** or its connections (especially via the **dentato rubrothalamic** pathway). The usual causes are: cerebellar lesions, rubral tremor (Holme's tremor), and thalamic lesions.
- **Task specific** tremor for example, on writing, is due to **dystonic tremor (primary writing tremor)**.

Based on the Frequency

- Low frequency (less than 4 Hz): All rest tremors
- Mid frequency (4-7 Hz): Most postural tremors
- High frequency (>7 Hz): Severe forms of postural tremors (orthostatic tremor, exaggerated physiological tremor, essential tremor)
- Drugs can cause all frequencies of tremors depending on the mechanism. Sympathomimetics (antidepressants) exaggerate the physiological tremor (fast frequency), while lithium and flunarizine act on the central generator (low frequency).
- Similarly alcohol withdrawal can cause all frequency tremor. In withdrawal state, there is catecholamine excess with fast tremor, while in chronic toxicity, cerebellar degeneration causes slow tremor.

Caveats

- In all patients with complaints of "clicking tinnitus", examine the palate so as to not miss palatal tremor
- In all patients with complaints of "leg tremor", manipulate the foot to see its influence. Ankle clonus is sometimes mistaken for foot tremor, but can be exacerbated by dorsiflexion and reduced by plantar flexion of the foot. Wrist clonus also can be similarly modified by manipulation
- In all patients with irregular appearing finger tremors, consider cortical myoclonus. Examine for hypersensitivity to tapping the outstretched hand and fingers

- In patients with "head tremors", consider dystonic tremor vis a vis essential/cerebellar tremor. Dystonic tremor varies with head position and sensory tricks like touching various head regions and arm elevation
- Vocal tremor is to be differentiated from spasmodic dysphonia
- Psychogenic tremors can be confusing. These are suggested by some clues
    - Sudden onset
    - Inconsistency
    - Distractibility
    - Entrainment
    - Coactivation
- A common situation is to differentiate essential tremor from early parkinsonian tremor. The following points help in this differentiation (Table 9.2):

Table 9.2: Differences between essential tremor and parkinsonian tremor.

	Essential tremor	Parkinsonian tremor
Head tremor	++	–
Voice tremor	++	–
Chin tremor	–	++
Jaw tremor	–	++
Leg tremor	–	++
Laterality	Bilateral	Unilateral
Resting tremor	–	++
Responds to	Alcohol	l-dopa

BIBLIOGRAPHY

1. Berendse HW, Van Laar T. Tremor. In: Wolter EcH, van Laar, Berendse T (Eds). Parkinsonism and related disorders. VU University Press; 2007.
2. Deuschl G, Volkmann J, Raethjen J. Tremors: Differential diagnosis, Pathophysiology and therapy. In: Jankovic J, Tolosa E (Eds). Parkinson's disease and movement disorders, 5th edition. Wolters Kluver/Lippincott William & Wilkins; 2007.
3. Examination of a patient with tremor. In: Bhidayasiri R (Ed). Movement disorders: a video atlas. Humana Press; 2012.
4. Fahn S, Jankovic J (Eds). Principles and practice of movement disorders. 2007.

ARCHIMEDES SPIRAL DRAWING (SPIROGRAPHY)

Introduction
- The Archimedes spiral drawing demonstrates the frequency, amplitude and direction of a tremor, eliminating the stylistic differences of handwriting.
- In contrast to the normal handwriting which needs brief breaks between words, spirography demands one continuous pen movement. Thus abnormal movements of hypokinesia, tremor and dystonia are more easily appreciated during spirography.
- Archimedes spiral drawing test has a number of possible variations: free hand drawing or drawing over a predrawn spiral; tracing over the lines of the spiral or drawing between the lines; drawing clockwise or counterclockwise, drawing from inside out or from outside in.
- Here, a method published in a recent article in Movement Disorders by Haubenberger, et al. is elaborated further, as the authors reported good inter-rater reliability using this. However, there is no consensus on which is the best method to assess this test.

Objectives
The drawings can be used:
- To assess the tremor characteristics
- To assess the movement characteristics in patients with parkinsonism.

Methodology
- Patient should not have taken coffee or tea
- Copying over a predrawn spiral is preferred to free hand drawing.
- The spiral may contain about 5 loops, spaced at 1.5 cm gaps in a clockwise direction
- The width of the entire picture is therefore about 7.5 cm
- Patient traces the spiral from inside out
- Patient's arm must be unsupported
- He draws in the gap between the lines.

Interpretation
- The spiral of Parkinson's disease patient is smaller than normal with tighter turns. There are no action tremors. The oscillations become more widely spaced as the patient speeds up towards the outer sections of the spiral The abnormalities are asymmetric in idiopathic Parkinson's disease (PD)
- In essential tremor, the tremor is unidirectional along 8 O'clock- 2 O'clock axis in the right hand and along 10 O'clock-4 O'clock axis in the left hand. The amplitude of tremor is symmetric in both hands and is consistent with repeated tasks. The tremor axis remains the same if the patient is made to draw vertical, horizontal or oblique lines joining corners of a page
- In dystonic tremor, the tremor is seen in all segments of the spiral, is irregular and jerky and its axis is not constant. If patient is made to write a phrase repeatedly, the letters progressively become illegible

- Functional (psychogenic) tremor affects both hands but there is variation in amplitude and frequency between the right and left spirals. The tremor affects both hands but there is variation in amplitude and frequency between the right and left spirals. The amplitude changed from small to large within a single spiral. There is a consistent amplitude during straight line drawing; while the spirals were drawn quickly, there was freezing of drawing for straight lines.

Caveats

A PD patient may be unable to draw between the lines due to significant akinesia but manage to trace the spiral lines. Here, the lines provide the cues to initiate and maintain the movement. In such patients, tracing the lines may be accepted to assess tremor severity.

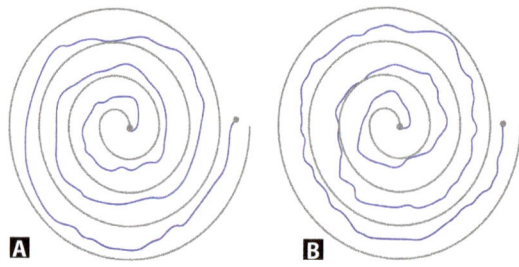

Figs. 9.3A and B: Archimedes spiral in mild tremor (A) and severe tremor (B).

BIBLIOGRAPHY

1. Deuschl G, Krack P, Lauk M, Timmer J. Clinical neurophysiology of tremor. J Clin Neurophysiol. 1996;13:110-21.
2. Deuschl G, Lohle E, Heinen F, Lucking C. Ear click in palatal tremor: its origin and treatment with botulinum toxin. Neurology. 1991;41:1677-9.
3. Deuschl G, Wilms H. Clinical spectrum and physiology of palatal tremor. Mov Disord. 2002;17 (Suppl 2):S63-6.
4. Elble R, et al. The Essential Tremor Rating Assessment Scale (TETRAS). Tremor Research Group (TRG). Mov Disord. 2008;23:S1-6.
5. Elble RJ. Diagnostic criteria for essential tremor and differential diagnosis. Neurology. 2000;54:S2-6.
6. Haubenberger D, Kalowitz D, Nahab FB. Validation of digital spiral analysis as outcome parameter for clinical trials in essential tremor. Mov Disord. 2011;26(11):2073-80.
7. Heilman KM, Orthostatic tremor. Arch Neurol. 1984;41:880-1.
8. Louis ED, Levy G, Cote LJ, Mejia H, Fahn S, Marder K. Clinical correlates of action tremor in Parkinson disease. Arch Neurol. 2001;58:1630-4.
9. Louis ED. Essential tremor: evolving clinicopathological concepts in an era of intensive post-mortem enquiry. Lancet Neurol. 2010;9:613-22.
10. Muthuraman M, Hossen A, Heute U, Deuschl G, Raethjen J. A new diagnostic test to distinguish tremulous Parkinson's disease from advanced essential tremor. Mov Disord. 2011;26:1548-52.
11. Raethjen J, Deuschl G. Tremor. Curr Optin Neurol. 2009;22:400-5.

DYSTONIA

Definition

- Dystonia is defined as a hyperkinetic movement disorder characterized by involuntary, **patterned, sustained** or repetitive muscle contractions of opposing muscles. This results in abnormal posturing or movement or both. The EMG activity of dystonia usually exceeds 100 ms.
- The specific features of dystonia that need to be looked for are:
    - "Patterned" contraction in contrast to random movements of some other hyperkinetic movement disorders. Patterned contraction implies that the same muscle groups are activated repeatedly or in a sustained fashion.
    - Sustained contraction which implies that at least at the peak of the movement, the contraction is prolonged. Thus, even if the movement is jerky like a myoclonus, at its peak, the contraction will be sustained.
    - The movement involves co-contraction of antagonistic muscle groups. This may be evident clinically or can be demonstrated by EMG recordings
    - Gestes antagonists: Performing some specific voluntary movements may alleviate the dystonia by inhibiting the dystonic motor program outflow. Example: keeping a pencil or pen in the mouth may inhibit the facial dystonia. The *gestes antagonistes* normally involve a body part that is different from (and often contiguous with) the one affected by the dystonia that is alleviated.
- Sensory tricks: A variety of sensory stimuli alleviate the dystonia. Example: touching the neck may suppress the cervical dystonia
- Overflow: Dystonia extends to a contiguous body region where it is not observed as an independent phenomenon. Example: Overflow to the upper limb in patients with cervical dystonia.

Physiologic Basis

Though dystonia is clinically a motor disorder, there is evidence to suggest that it is likely a disorder involving motor and sensory cortices as well as the sensorimotor integration. The proposed mechanisms of development of dystonia are:
- Decreased motor cortical surround inhibition that is required for precise isolation of muscle groups during an act. This results in overflow to contiguous muscle groups and co-contraction of antagonists
- Increased neuronal plasticity in the motor cortex. This may explain certain segmental dystonias that develop with repetitive occupational activities (writer's cramp)
- Abnormal activation of sensory cortex during activities like writing, causing abnormality of the motor cortex activity. This is supported by the abnormal sensory evoked potentials and thickened sensory cortex in some patients with dystonia.

Dystonia Classification

Dystonia can be classified as follows:

By Etiology

- Primary (or idiopathic): Dystonia is the only clinical sign and there is no identifiable exogenous cause or other inherited or degenerative disease. Example: DYT-1 dystonia.
- Dystonia-plus: Dystonia is a prominent sign, but is also associated with another movement disorder. There is no evidence of neurodegeneration. Example: Myoclonus-dystonia (DYT-11).
- Heredodegenerative: Dystonia is a prominent sign, among other neurological features, of a heredodegenerative disorder. Example: Wilson's disease.
- Secondary: Dystonia is a symptom of an identified neurological condition, such as a focal brain lesion or drug. Examples: dystonia due to an infarct
- Paroxysmal: Dystonia occurs in brief episodes with normalcy in between. These disorders are classified as idiopathic (often familial although sporadic cases also occur) and symptomatic due to a variety of causes. This group includes paroxysmal kinesigenic dyskinesia (PKD; DYT-9), paroxysmal exercise-induced dystonia (PED) and non-kinesigenic form (PNKD; DYT-8).

By Age at Onset

- Early onset (variably defined as 20–30 years): Usually starts in a leg or arm and frequently progresses to involve other limbs and the trunk
- Late onset: Usually starts in the neck (including the larynx), the cranial muscles or one arm. Tends to remain localized with restricted progression to adjacent muscles.

By Distribution

- Focal: Single body region (e.g. writer's cramp, blepharospasm)
- Segmental: Contiguous body regions (e.g. cranial and cervical, cervical and upper limb)
- Multifocal: Non-contiguous body regions (e.g. upper and lower limb)
- Generalized: Both legs and at least one other body region (usually one or both arms)
- Hemidystonia: Half of the body (usually secondary to a structural lesion in the contralateral basal ganglia).

Methodology

- Ensure that the movement disorder in question is a hyperkinetic disorder with patterned muscle contraction

- Examine the patient with minimal clothing as possible, from head to toe, systematically observing each body region (ocular, facial, laryngeal, cervical, brachial, crural, truncal).
- Summarize the dystonia using the following variables, each having a diagnostic significance. These variable apply in most other movement disorder evaluations:
  - Age of onset:
    - Infantile
    - Childhood
    - Adult onset
  - Rapidity of onset:
    - Acute
    - Insidious
  - Course:
    - Static
    - Progressive
    - Fluctuating
  - Topography:
    - Focal
    - Segmental
    - Multisegmental
    - Generalized
    - Specify the body part involved (cranial, laryngeal, cervical, upper limb, lower limb, trunk, respiratory muscle, etc.)
  - Mobile/fixed dystonia: Whether the dystonia varies with posture/task/action or is fixed throughout the assessment. A fixed dystonia is likely a secondary dystonia, while primary dystonias are typically mobile and can be modulated by sensory tricks and other maneuvers.
  - Relieving maneuvers: Try various methods like
    - Head position (in torticollis)
    - Sensory tricks
    - Walking backwards
    - Distraction
    - Suggestion
    - Exercise (paradoxical dystonia)
    - Voluntary suppression (dystonic tic)
  - Aggravating/precipitating factors: Try
    - Suggestion
    - Posture
    - Head position (in torticollis)
    - Specific task
    - Walking
    - Vibration by tuning fork
  - Associated movement disorder: Note if there is additional tremor, myoclonus, tics

- Other system involvement or sparing: Pyramidal, cerebellar, sensory and cognitive functions
- Family history.

Interpretation

Variable	• = Primary dystonia • = Secondary dystonia
Age at onset: • Infancy • Childhood • Adulthood	• • • • •
Rapidity of onset: • Acute • Chronic	• • •
Course: • Static • Progressive • Fluctuating	• • • • See table for fluctuating dystonias
Topography: • Focal onset • Generalized • Upper limb/cranial • Lower limb • Hemidystonia	Adults: •, children: • Adults: •, children • Adults: •, children: • Adults: •, children • •
Mobility: • Mobile • Fixed	• •
Dystonia at rest	•
Task specific/action dystonia	•
Other systems involved	•

- Neurological examination can differentiate primary and secondary forms of dystonia, but confirming the etiology requires investigations (neuroimaging, genetic studies, metabolic studies)
- Metabolic cause has to be certainly sought in the following situations:
    - Very early onset dystonia
    - Typical clinical signs (Kayser-Fleischer ring)
    - Typical MRI findings (e.g. bat wing appearance, tiger-eye appearance)
    - Hepatic disease
    - Anemia
    - Abnormal lipid profile
- DYT1 gene test is indicated
    - In primary dystonia with onset before 30 years
    - In primary dystonia with onset after 30 years, if there is a family history of early onset dystonia

- Tuning fork induced vibration can bring out or exacerbate dystonia (group IA afferent impulse processing is defective). This is not-specific to any particular etiology
- Dystonic attacks in sleep may be paroxysmal hypnogenic dystonia/ frontal lobe seizures
- Dystonia is usually brought out on walking or exercise. In paradoxical dystonia, exercise relieves dystonia. Patients then prefer moving about, mimicking akathisia
- Diurnal variation of dystonia is characteristic of dopa responsive dystonia (evening exacerbation)
- Fluctuating dystonia is also seen in drug-induced dystonia, paroxysmal kinesogenic dystonia, hypnogenic dystonia, neurometabolic disorders (aminoacidurias), psychogenic dystonia, multiple sclerosis, transient ischemic attack, Sandifer syndrome and thyrotoxicosis
- In torticollis, a useful maneuver to identify the abnormal muscles and compensatory contraction of their antagonists, is head positioning. The dystonia is minimized with head turned in the line of action of the abnormal muscle and is maximized in the opposite direction
- Cervical torticollis/retrocollis after food intake are a feature of Sandifer syndrome due to gastroesophageal reflux
- Dystonia that disappears on distraction: Likely psychogenic.

Caveats

Overlap with Other Movement Disorders (Myoclonus, Tremor, Tics, Athetosis)

- Sometimes, jerky movements may be noted in patients with dystonia. These could represent either myoclonic dystonia or myoclonus dystonia. In the former, the dystonia itself has a rapid jerky appearance mimicking myoclonus. The latter is a specific syndrome where in myoclonus occurs in addition to dystonia and also involves body areas not involved by dystonia. Alcohol often relieves myoclonus-dystonia
- Similarly, dystonia and tremor must be differentiated from dystonic tremor. If the tremor is slow (2–5 Hz), it is more likely a manifestation of dystonia (dystonic tremor), whereas a faster frequency tremor is likely to be an independent one like essential tremor
- Athetosis also causes slow muscular contraction causing abnormal movements. This however, lacks the stereotyped patterned contraction that is characteristic of dystonia
- Tics can sometimes be slow and involve stereotyped muscular groups, mimicking dystonia (Dystonic tics). However, tics are preceded by an urge that is relieved by the movement and are suppressible
- Blepharospasm can be confused with apraxia of eyelid opening. Overactivity of eyelid muscles is seen in the former, but not the latter. Frontalis over activity is seen in the latter, but not the former. In difficult cases, EMG may be needed.

Overlap with Non-neurological Conditions

- In patients with painful deformed hand, in addition to rheumatoid arthritis, consider striatal hand
- In patients with stiff jaw, in addition to TMJ disease, consider oromandibular dystonia
- A number of other conditions mimic dystonia and need to be differentiated. (atlanto-axial dislocation, Arnold-Chiari malformation, posterior fossa mass lesion, Sandifer syndrome, congenital postural torticollis, etc.).
- In spasmodic dysphonia, adductor type is usually organic. The abductor type is either organic or more often psychogenic.

BIBLIOGRAPHY

1. Albanese A, Barnes MP, Bhatia KP, et al. A systematic review on the diagnosis and treatment of primary (idiopathic) dystonia and dystonia plus syndromes: report of an EFNS/MDS-ES Task Force. Eur J Neurol. 2006;13:433-44.
2. Albanese A. Dystonia: clinical approach. Parkinsonism and related disorders. 2007;13;S356-61.
3. Hallett M. Pathophysiology of dystonia. J Neural Transm. 2006;[Suppl]. 70:485-8.
4. Jankovic J. Dystonic disorders. In: Jankovic J, Tolosa E, (Eds). Parkinson's disease and movement disorders, 5th edition. Philadelphia: Lippincott Williams and Wilkins; 2007, pp. 321-47.
5. Obeso JA, Rothwell JC, Lang AE, et al. Myoclonic dystonia. Neurology. 1983;33:825-30.
6. Schrag A, Trimble M, Quinn N. The syndrome of fixed dystonia: an evaluation of 103 patients. Brain. 2004;127:2360-72.

CHOREA

Definition

- **Chorea** is defined as a movement disorder characterized by the continuous flow of random purposeless muscle contractions
- It is associated with a hypoactivity of subthalamic nucleus and increased firing rate of globus pallidus (pars interna)
- The phenomenon of chorea is not much different in different diseases. Thus, the correct diagnosis depends more on associated findings than on the phenomenology
- Ballism: When severe chorea results in flinging and violent movements, it is called ballism. The physiologic basis, however, is similar to that of chorea
- The etiological categories of chorea can be broadly classified as in Flowchart 9.3.

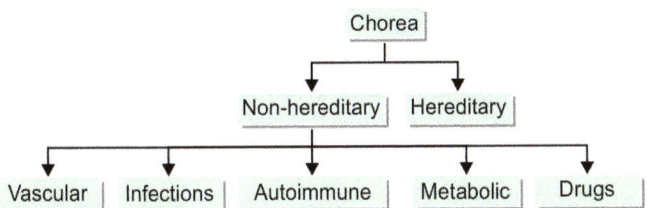

Flowchart 9.3: Etiology of chorea.

Methodology

The overall examination scheme is similar to other movement disorder assessment and attempts to answer the 5 basic questions:
1. Is it chorea?
2. Where is it? (topography)
3. What aggravates it?
4. What relieves it?
5. Which other systems involved?

Examination of Chorea

Confirm the diagnosis of chorea by observing the characteristics and excluding its mimics (see caveats section).

Topography

- Describe the topography from head to toe:
    - Facial movements: look for grimacing
    - Orolingual:
        - Observe at rest
        - Ask to protrude tongue and look for lacerations

- ♦ Ask him to keep the tongue protruded for 1-2 minutes and look for choreiform movements (Jack in the box phenomenon)
  - Vocal: Look for involuntary vocalizations (sounds, words) during examination
  - Truncal: Observe at rest and while walking
  - Limbs (proximal/distal):
    - ♦ Look for minimal snapping or fidgeting of fingers especially while walking
    - ♦ Ask patient to raise the upper limbs to a horizontally forward position
    - ♦ Watch for abnormal posturing of hands like arm drift, pronator drift, piano playing movements, spooning of hands (hyperextension of fingers, dorsiflexion of wrists)
    - ♦ Ask patient to grip the examiner's fingers and watch for involuntary grasping and releasing (milk maid's grip)
  - Unilateral/bilateral.

Aggravating Factors

- Note the movements after distraction (chorea increases, psychogenic movements decrease)
- Note if they increase while walking (chorea increases, psychogenic movements may decrease).

Relieving Factors

- Check from history if they disappear in sleep (chorea does)
- Ask patient to try suppressing the movements (tics are suppressible; chorea only partly suppressible).

Signs of Other System Involvement

- Cognitive assessment, especially frontal executive functions
- Look for hypotonia, pendular jerks
- Cerebellar signs (SCA)
- Peripheral neuropathy ⎫
- Amyotrophy ⎪
- Seizures ⎬ Neuroacanthocytosis
- Tongue mutilation ⎪
- Oromandibular dystonia ⎪
- Vocal tics ⎭
- Parkinsonism
- Dystonia
- Wing beating tremor: Wilson's disease
- Liver disease signs

- Renal failure signs
- SLE symptoms and signs
- Symptoms and signs of underlying cancer [small cell lung cancer (SCLC)]
- Arthritis
- Carditis: Sydenham's chorea.

Interpretation

There are few signs that are exclusive to a particular condition. These are:
- Chorea with mutilating orolingual dystonia: Acanthocytosis
- Chorea with motor impersistence: Huntington's disease.

There are other signs that are seen in few selected diseases and are listed in the subsequent Boxes 9.3 to 9.11:

Box 9.3: Chorea with parkinsonism or dystonia.
- Huntington's disease
- Wilson's disease
- Neurodegeneration with brain iron accumulation
- Mitochondrial disease

Box 9.4: Chorea with vocalizations.
- Huntington's disease
- Neuroacanthocytosis
- McLeod syndrome
- Wilson's disease

Box 9.5: Chorea with gaze abnormalities.
- Huntington's disease
- Ataxia telangiectasia
- Mitochondrial disease
- Spinocerebellar ataxia
- Wilson's disease

Box 9.6: Chorea with cerebellar ataxia.
- Spinocerebellar ataxia
- Dentatorubral-pallidoluysian atrophy (DRPLA)
- Friedreich's ataxia
- Ataxia telangiectasia
- Choreoacanthocytosis
- McLeod syndrome
- Mitochondrial disease
- Prion diseases

Box 9.7: Chorea with peripheral neuropathy.
- Choreoacanthocytosis
- Macleod's syndrome
- Friedreich's ataxia
- Mitochondrial disease
- Ataxia telangiectasia
- Spinocerebellar ataxias

Box 9.8: Common genetic conditions associated with chorea.
- Huntington's disease
- Benign hereditary chorea
- Dentatorubral-pallidoluysian atrophy
- SCA 17
- SCA 3
- Wilson's disease
- Neuroacanthocytosis
- Abetalipoproteinemia
- McLeod syndrome
- Ataxia telangiectasia
- Ferritin associated basal ganglia disease
- Gangliosidosis
- Lesch-Nyhan syndrome
- Niemann-Pick disease
- Aminoacidopathies

Box 9.9: Differential diagnosis of triad of 'movement disorder + dementia + behavioral change'.
- Huntington's disease
- Neuroacanthocytosis
- Wilson's disease
- Hallervorden-Spatz
- Ceroid lipofuscinosis
- Mitochondrial disease
- Vasculitis
- Human immunodeficiency virus

Box 9.10: Acquired metabolic causes of chorea.
- Thyrotoxicosis
- Hyperglycemia (non-ketotic)
- Hypoglycemia
- Non-Wilsonian hepatolenticular degeneration
- Renal failure
- Ketogenic diet

Box 9.11: Drugs that can cause chorea.
- Alcohol
- Anticholinergics
- Anti-epileptic drugs (phenytoin, valproate, lamotrigine)
- Calcium channel blockers (flunarizine, cinnarizine)
- Dopamine agonists
- Hormones (oral contraceptive pills)
- Levodopa
- Lithium
- Neuroleptics
- Stimulants (methylphenidate, amphetamine)
- Superselective serotonin reuptake inhibitors (fluoxetine, paroxetine)
- Tricyclic antidepressants

Caveats

- Tics may be confused with chorea, but are characterized by sensory urge and relief of tensions after the movement. They are also suppressible. In addition, tics reproduce normal human movements or vocalizations, whereas chorea produces non-purposive movements
- Chorea may be confused with myoclonus, but the latter lacks the continuous flow of movement that is typical of the former.

BIBLIOGRAPHY

1. Jankovic J, Tolosa E. Parkinson's disease and movement disorders. 5th edition. 2007: 236-45.
2. Wild EJ, Tabrizi SJ. The differential diagnosis of chorea. Pract Neurol. 2007;7:360-73.

MYOCLONUS (FLOWCHART 9.4)

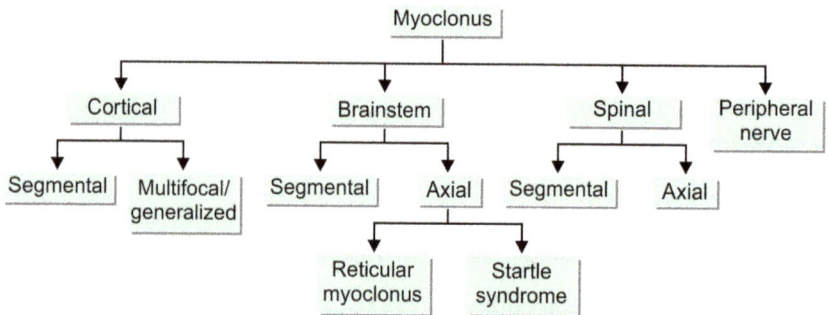

Flowchart 9.4: Myoclonus.

Physiologic Basis

- Definition: Myoclonus is a sudden brief shock-like jerk (usually ≤100 ms by EMG) caused either by active muscle contraction (positive myoclonus) or brief loss of muscle contraction in active postural muscle (negative myoclonus)
- The activity may involve the agonists and antagonists in a synchronous (e.g. post hypoxic) or asynchronous fashion (e.g. essential myoclonus), depending on the etiology
- Myoclonus may be caused by an abnormality anywhere from the cerebral cortex, brainstem, cerebellum, spinal cord to the peripheral nerves
- At each of these levels, it can be focal (or segmental) or multifocal (or multisegmental or axial)
- Cortical myoclonus:
  - Is due to hyperexcitability of sensorimotor cortex
  - It is mainly distal (distal muscles have larger representation in the cortex)
  - It can be multifocal
  - It appears or increases on activity
  - It is sensitive to touch/noise/light
  - It is modulated by sleep (decreases)
- Brainstem myoclonus:
  - In certain conditions, it can be due to a lesion involving the Mollaret's triangle. There are other types of brainstem myoclonus that are caused by other mechanisms
  - It is present at rest
  - It is not usually increased by physical activity
  - It is not decreased in sleep (e.g. palatal tremor)
  - A typical clinical feature is sound-sensitivity and sometimes light sensitivity

- Spinal myoclonus:
    - Is due to loss of inhibitory inter-neurons in the posterior horns
    - It can remain segmental or spread to adjacent segments causing axial myoclonus (propriospinal myoclonus)
    - It is present at rest
    - It is resistant to supraspinal influences like sleep or voluntary activity (unlike cortical myoclonus)
    - It is unresponsive to sound (unlike brainstem myoclonus)
    - It usually spares facial muscles (unlike brainstem myoclonus)
- Myoclonus can arise from peripheral nerves as in hemifacial spasms/in nerve tumors

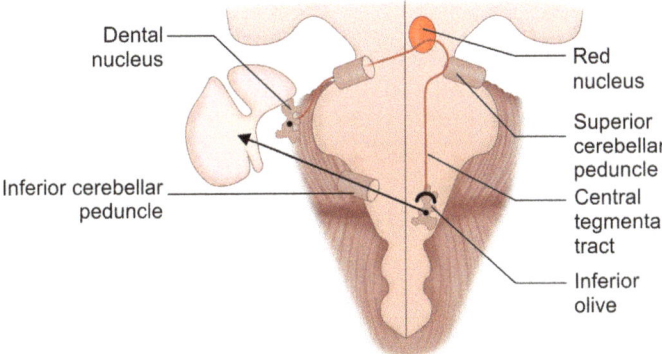

Fig. 9.4: Structures constituting the "Mollaretz's triangle" that is implicated in palatal myoclonus.

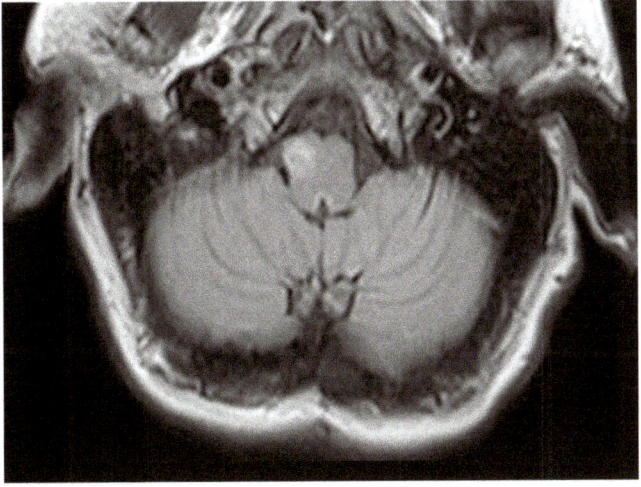

Fig. 9.5: Hypertrophied inferior olive in a patient with palatal myoclonus.

- Salient differences between the above categories of myoclonus are provided in the Table 9.3.

Table 9.3: Differences between cortical, brainstem and spinal myoclonus.

	Cortical	Brainstem	Spinal
Muscles	Distal	Cranial innervated +/- axial spread	Spinal innervated +/- axial spread
Action induced	Sensitive	May be sensitive	Not sensitive
Multifocal	Yes	No	No
Stimulus sensitive	Yes (touch/sound/light)	May be (sound/light)	No
Decrease in sleep	Yes	May be	No

Method

- A detailed history including the onset, progression, family history and drug intake is important
- The following steps are common to most movement disorders assessment and apply to myoclonus as well:
    - Is it myoclonus or not? (Ascertain the diagnosis of myoclonus).
    - Where is the myoclonus? (focal/segmental, axial, multifocal or generalized.)
    - What is the nature of myoclonus? (irregular/rhythmic)
    - What factors exacerbate it?
    - What factors inhibit/suppress it?
    - Is any other system involved? (cognitive, pyramidal, extrapyramidal, peripheral nerves)
- Differentiating myoclonus from other hyperkinetic disorders: See "caveats" section.

Topography

- From head to toe: Inspect the eyelids, facial muscles, palate, head and neck (sternomastoid jerks), diaphragm, trunk, limbs (proximal or distal)
- If multisegmental, describe the sequence of involvement of different regions.

Exacerbating Factors

- Examine the patient at rest
- Ask him to hold the limb against gravity and watch for positive or negative myoclonus
- Observe for myoclonus during various actions (drinking, eating, pouring, wearing clothes, standing, walking)
- Give a sudden unexpected loud noise (dropping a metal object/banging a door/clapping)
- Ask the patient to extend his forearm and wrist and give a brisk tap to the finger tips
- Tap the forehead of the patient with hand or gently with a reflex hammer.

Relieving Factors
- Check if myoclonus disappears on distraction
- Examine the patient in sleep if possible (the relatives may record a video when patient is asleep).

Other Systems
- Assess for short stature
- Look for cherry red spot, optic atrophy, retinitis pigmentosa in the fundus
- Assess higher mental functions (MMSE)
- Examine cerebellar signs, pyramidal signs, extrapyramidal signs
- Examine cranial nerves, including VIII nerve
- Examine peripheral nervous system for neuropathy.

Interpretation

Topographic Diagnosis

Focal (segmental) myoclonus: Can be from
- Cortical: Can be spontaneous/reflex/action triggered. It can be irregular or rhythmic. Examples are: Rasmussen's encephalitis/dysplasias/tumors etc. Neurophysiological investigations can establish the cortical origin in difficult cases.
- Brainstem: Involves brainstem innervated segments, like palate (palatal tremor/myoclonus), facial and ocular muscles. The usual frequency is 1.5–3 Hz. Palatal myoclonus can be essential or symptomatic (see Table 9.5 for differentiation)
- Spinal: Involves spinal segments at 0.5–3 Hz and persists during sleep. Thoracic or abdominal segments and diaphragm are common segments involved
- Peripheral nerve: as in peripheral nerve trauma/ tumor/ hemifacial spasm.

Axial myoclonus: Usually causes neck, trunk and hip flexion and arm abduction, i.e. involves axial and proximal appendicular muscles. This can arise from either the brainstem or the spinal cord. These can be differentiated by the spread of the muscle activity either by clinical examination or by multi-channel EMG recording of muscles at various levels. In spinal myoclonus, it starts from the involved spinal segment and spreads proximally and distally. In brainstem myoclonus, it starts from cranial innervated muscles (usually sternomastoid) and spreads down to the spinal segments.

Brainstem myoclonus (reticular or startle types):
- Causes an axial myoclonic jerk in the cranial innervated muscles and descends down to the spinal segments as well as ascends up along the other brainstem segments
- The two types (startle versus reticular) may further be differentiated (Table 9.4).

Table 9.4: Difference between startle and reticular myoclonus.

	Startle myoclonus	Reticular myoclonus
Spontaneous jerks	None	Common
Sensitive area	Mantle area (head, face, upper chest)	Limbs
Stimuli	Sound/light/touch	Touch
First response	Blink of the eyes, facial twitch	Sternomastoid contraction

Spinal cord (propriospinal):
- Spontaneous
- Starts in the thoracic/abdominal segments/diaphragm and ascends and descends from these levels.

Multifocal/generalized

Can be due to essential myoclonus/non-progressive idiopathic epilepsy syndromes/symptomatic epilepsies.

Other Clues to Diagnosis

- Myoclonus at rest suggests spinal or brainstem myoclonus, whereas action induced myoclonus suggests cortical origin
- Glass and colleagues, described a condition in which myoclonic jerks occurred predominantly or exclusively on assuming an upright posture (orthostatic myoclonus)
- Proximal weakness, short stature, deafness: Suggest mitochondrial disease [myoclonic epilepsy with ragged red fiber (MERRF) syndrome]
- Cerebellar signs: Suggest DRPLA, SCA, multiple system atrophy, MERRF
- Cherry red spot in fundus: Sialidosis
- Dementia: Creutzfeldt–Jakob disease (CJD), corticobasal ganglionic degeneration (CBGD), Alzheimer's disease, subacute sclerosing panencephalitis (SSPE), neuronal ceroid lipofuscinoses (NCL), sialidosis
- Myoclonus disappears on distraction: Psychogenic myoclonus
- Myoclonus that persists in sleep: Palatal tremor, spinal myoclonus
- Palatal myoclonus can be further categorized as Table 9.5.

Table 9.5: Comparison of essential palatal myoclonus and symptomatic palatal myoclonus.

	Essential palatal myoclonus (many "T"s in the list)	Symptomatic palatal myoclonus (many "L"s in the list)
Age	Teens	Late
Area of palate involved	Top of the palate	Lateral aspect
Muscle involved	Tensor veli palatini	Levator veli palatini
Cranial nerve involved	Trigeminal	Lower cranial nerves (IX, VII)
Click	Ticking noise	No (no tick)
Sleep	Turns off	Persists
Other cranial muscles	Not involved	Involved
Contralateral olivary hypertrophy on MR	No	Yes

- Ocular signs that help in diagnosis of myoclonus:
  - Cherry red spot: GM2 gangliosidosis, sialidosis
  - Optic atrophy: Neuronal ceroid lipofuscinosis, mitochondrial disease, Krabbe's disease
  - Retinitis pigmentosa; Neuronal ceroid lipofuscinosis
  - Opsoclonus: Opsoclonus-myoclonus syndrome
  - Vertical supranuclear gaze palsy: Progressive supranuclear palsy (PSP)
  - Horizontal gaze palsy: Gaucher's disease.
- Causes of cortical myoclonus:
  - Progressive myoclonic epilepsies
  - Juvenile myoclonic epilepsy
  - Post anoxic myoclonus
  - Creutzfeldt-Jakob disease
  - Metabolic encephalopathy
  - Corticobasal ganglionic degeneration
  - Alzheimer's disease
  - Multiple system atrophy
  - Juvenile Huntington's disease
  - SCA 6
  - DRPLA
  - Hashimoto's encephalopathy
  - Autoimmune encephalopathies
  - Celiac disease
  - Pellagra
  - Paraneoplastic encephalopathy
- Causes of brainstem axial myoclonus:
  - Brainstem lesions
  - Metabolic encephalopathies
  - CJD
  - SSPE
  - Opsoclonus myoclonus syndrome
  - Palatal myoclonus
  - Myoclonus dystonia
  - Hyperekplexia.

Caveats

- Physiological myoclonus (hypnic, normal startle response) must not be over diagnosed as pathological
- Tics may mimic myoclonus, but they are associated with an inner urge to move, relief of the tension by the movement, and are suppressible
- Chorea may mimic myoclonic jerks, but is characterized by flowing random movements rather than jerky movements
- Tremor may mimic myoclonus when both are distal. The former is by definition rhythmic and oscillatory. The latter is usually stimulus sensitive

when it is distal and semi-rhythmic or rhythmic (cortical myoclonus). In difficult cases, electrophysiology will help
- In a given patient, more than one form of myoclonus may occur. For instance, in posthypoxic myoclonus, cortical myoclonus may coexist with brainstem myoclonus
- Very small, hardly visible distal myoclonic jerks (mini polymyoclonus) are typical for MSA
- Psychogenic myoclonus can be difficult to prove. In such a situation, documenting the premovement (Bereitschaft's) potential indicates that the etiology is psychogenic.

BIBLIOGRAPHY

1. Fahn S, Frucht SJ, Hallett M, et al. Myoclonus and paroxysmal dyskinesias. Adv Neurol. 2002;89:361-76.
2. Gerschlager W, Brown P. Myoclonus. Curr Opin Neurol. 2009;22:414-18.
3. Glass GA, Ahlskog JE, Matsumoto JY. Orthostatic myoclonus: a contributor to gait decline in selected elderly. Neurology. 2007;68:1826-30.
4. Kojovic M, Cordivari C, Bhatia K. Myoclonic disorders: a practical approach for diagnosis and treatment. Ther Adv Neurol Disord. 2011;4(1):4762.
5. Lindahl A. Startles, jumps, falls and fits. Pract Neurol. 2005;5:292-7.
6. Lozsadi D. Myoclonus: a pragmatic approach. Practical Neurology. 2012;12:215-24.

TICS

Physiologic Basis

Definition

- Tics are relatively brief and intermittent involuntary movements (motor tics) or sounds (phonic tics). The latter are due to involvement of respiratory, pharyngeal, laryngeal, oral and nasal musculature.
- The characteristic features of tics that distinguish them from other movement disorders are as follows:
  - Repetitive stereotyped movements
  - Inner urge to produce the movement
  - Sense of discomfort preceding the movement
  - Relief of the sensory symptoms following the movement
  - Suppressibility of the movement associated with increasing discomfort
- The following summarizes the evidence regarding the pathogenesis of the prototype tic disorder—Tourette syndrome:
  - There is increased cortical excitability and decreased intracortical inhibition in these patients (transcranial magnetic stimulation studies)
  - There is increased activity of dopamine transporter causing increased dopamine concentration in the dopaminergic terminals in the striatum, limbic cortex and prefrontal cortex. There is also a stimulus dependent increase in dopaminergic transmission.
  - These changes result in the production of unwanted movements that manifest as tics as well as associated attention deficit hyperactivity, impulse control disorder and obsessive compulsive behavior in Tourette syndrome.

Classification of Tics

Motor Tics

A. Simple tics: Involve only one group of muscles and cause brief jerk like movement. They may be further divided into:
   - Clonic tics: Blinking, nose twitching and head jerking
   - Dystonic tics: Blepharospasm, bruxism and torticollis
   - Tonic tics: Tensing of abdominal muscles
B. Complex tics: Consist of coordinated, sequences movements resembling normal acts but are inappropriately timed and of inappropriate intensity. Examples: head shaking, touching, hitting, kicking, jumping, gesturing, burping, etc.

Phonic Tics

A. Simple tics: Sniffing, throat clearing, grunting, coughing, blowing, sucking, etc.

B. Complex tics: Meaningful verbalizations, profanities, echolalia, and palilalia.

Etiology of Tics

- Sporadic:
    - Transient tic disorder (< 1 year)
    - Chronic tic disorder (>1 year)
    - Tourette syndrome
    - Tic disorder not otherwise specified (Tourette criteria unfulfilled)
    - Primary dystonia and tics
- Inherited:
    - Tourette syndrome
    - Huntington's disease
    - Primary dystonia
    - Neuroacanthocytosis
    - NBIA
    - Wilson's disease
    - Lesch-Nyhan syndrome
    - Tuberous sclerosis
    - Duchenne muscular dystrophy
- Secondary:
    - Drugs (methylphenidate, pemoline, levodopa, dopamine receptor blockers, cocaine, carbamazepine, phenytoin, phenobarbitone, lamotrigine, antipsychotics)
    - Toxins (carbon monoxide)
    - Infections (encephalitis, CJD, neurosyphilis, rheumatic chorea)
    - Developmental disorders (static encephalopathies, autistic spectrum disorders)
    - Chromosomal disorders (Down's syndrome, Klinefelter syndrome and fragile X syndrome)
    - Others (head injury, stroke, schizophrenia, neurodegenerative disease).

Methodology and Observations

- Observe the pattern of movement according to the general scheme provided in the chapter on "Approach to movement disorders"
- Topography: Is it involving one or more body regions? Is it motor or phonic or both?
- When is it seen: Observe if it is seen more prominently at rest? Does it persist in sleep?
- Aggravating factors: This information has to be obtained both from history and during examination
- Relieving factors: Is the urge relieved by movement? Enquire the regions that have sensory discomfort preceding the movement (Figure 9.6).

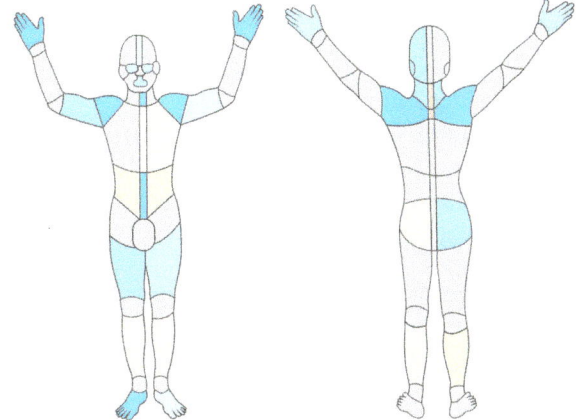

Fig. 9.6: Location of premonitory urges in Tourette's syndrome. Darker colors indicate more intense premonitory sensation.

- Check if it is suppressible: Ask the patient to control the movement for a specified time. Check if the patient develops increasing discomfort during this period.
- Look for associated phenomena (each of these may occur in 10–20% of Tourette's syndrome cases):
    - Coprolalia: Patient may utter profanities in a non-contextual manner
    - Copropraxia: Patient makes obscene gestures
    - Echolalia: Patient repeats examiner's words
    - Echopraxia: Patient repeats examiner's gestures
    - Palilalia: Patient repeats his own words, especially the last phoneme
    - Palipraxia: Patient rapidly repeats an action
- Also check for red flags which warrant further investigations:
    - Onset >18 years
    - Progressive (rather than waxing waning) course
    - Drug history
    - Dysmorphic features (chromosomal disorders)
    - Cognitive impairment
    - Impaired consciousness (seizures)
    - Features of attention deficit disorder
    - Myoclonus
    - Dystonia (e.g. NBIA, Wilson's disease)
    - Chorea (e.g. Acanthocytosis, Huntington's disease)
    - Neuropathy (Acanthocytosis)
    - Proximal muscle weakness (Duchenne muscular dystrophy)
    - Kayser-Fleischer ring (Wilson's disease)
    - Skin lesions (tuberous sclerosis)
    - Valvular heart disease (rheumatic heart disease)

Interpretation

- If the tics involve multiple body regions, including motor and vocal components, consider Tourette syndrome
- If the course is waxing and waning, it favors primary tic disorder. In contrast, relentless progression warrants search for secondary causes
- The Diagnostic and Statistical Manual of Mental Disorder-IV (DSM-IV) criteria for Tourette syndrome are as follows:
    - Onset<18 years
    - Duration >1 year
    - Multiple motor and at least one vocal tic
    - Unexplained by other conditions
- If the movements persist in sleep, it is a point in favor of tics. Few other movement disorders persist in sleep [palatal myoclonus, spinal myoclonus, restless legs syndrome (RLS) with moving toes].

Caveats

- Tics may be confused with a number of other movement disorders. The following differences may help in correct diagnosis (Table 9.6).

Table 9.6: Features of tics compared with other types of hyperkinetic motor disorders.

	Premonitory sensation	Suppressible	Unidirectional	Sudden	Rhythmic
Tics	+	+	+	+	–
Myoclonus	–	–	+	++	±
Dystonia	±	–	±	–	–
Chorea	–	–	+	+	–
Akathisia	+	+	±	–	±

- Coprolalia and echolalia may also be seen in some culturally determined startle syndrome (e.g. jumping Frenchmen of Maine). Complex vocal tics differ from these by their spontaneous occurrence in the absence of stimulus, while startle syndromes occur in response to sudden stimuli
- Myoclonus may mimic tics, but is faster, and is not preceded by the sensory symptoms
- Stereotypies are differentiated from tics by their bidirectionality and longer duration
- Compulsions, like tics, are also motor acts preceded by a sensory urge and relieved by performing the act. However, unlike tics, they are more complex and are more goal-directed.

BIBLIOGRAPHY

1. Chouinard S, Ford B. Adult onset tic disorders. J Neurol Neurosurg Psychiatry. 2000; 68:738-43.
2. Jankovic J. Phenomenology and classification of tics. Neurol Clin North Am. 1997;15:267-75.
3. Jankovic J. Tics and Tourette syndrome. In: Jankovic J, Tolosa E (Eds). Parkinson's disease and movement disorders. Wolter Kluwer/Lippincott Williams and Wilkins, 5th Edition. 2007.
4. Jankovic J. Tourette's syndrome. N Engl J Med. 2001;345:1184-92.
5. Kwak C, Dat Vuong K, Jankovic J. Premonitory sensory phenomenon in Tourette's syndrome. Mov Disord. 2003;18:1530-3.
6. Rickards H. Tourette's syndrome and other tic disorders. Pract Neurol. 2010;10:252-9.
7. Singer HS. Tourette syndrome: from behaviour to biology. Lancet Neurology. 2005; 4:149-59.
8. Stern E, Silbersweig DA, Chee K-Y, et al. A functional neuroanatomy of tics. Arch Gen Psychiatry. 2000;57:741-8.

CHAPTER **10**

Clinical Evaluation of Seizures and Epilepsies

SEIZURE SEMIOLOGY

Elisabeth Hartl, Soheyl Noachtar

PICTORIAL PRETEST

Case 1

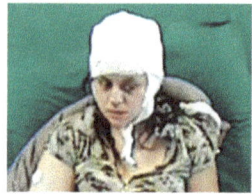
Seizure onset
+15 seconds
A

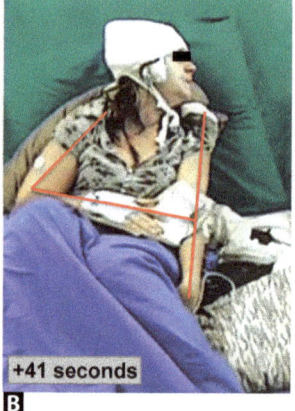
+41 seconds
B

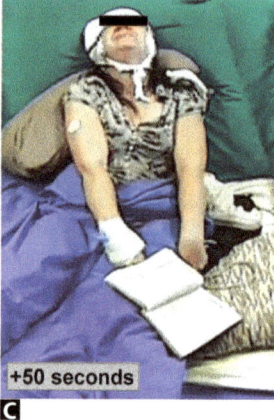
+50 seconds
C

Figs. 10.1A to C: Seizure semiology at different time points after onset; (A) Eye version to the left 15 seconds after seizure onset; (B) Sign of four, 41 seconds after seizure onset; (C) Bilateral tonic posturing 50 seconds after seizure onset.

This 31-year-old woman presented with recurrent episodes of sudden nausea, followed by smacking and repetitive opening and closing of the right hand as well as a dystonic posturing of the left hand since adolescence. Infrequently, her seizures also evolved into forced eye and head turning to the left (Fig. 10.1A) and tonic posturing of all limbs (Figs. 10.1B and C) with subsequent clonic jerks lasting for about one minute. During these episodes she could respond and follow commands until the generalized tonic posturing commenced. Afterwards she was confused and slowed for about 10 minutes.

Questions

1. How would you describe seizure semiology?
2. From which hemisphere do her seizures arise?
3. Which lobe is likely to generate this seizure semiology?

Case 2

A 22-year-old student was brought to hospital after his first generalized tonic-clonic seizure. He was on a party the night before and consumed alcohol. Regular alcohol abuse was denied. Upon presentation he had some bruises and a laceration of the left lateral tongue. The patient's reports revealed that since two years he sometimes has abrupt and very short lasting bilateral jerks of the proximal arms, especially in the morning. In addition, friends observed short episodes of few seconds with loss of consciousness, a staring face expression and reduced motor activity.

Questions

1. How would you classify his seizure semiology?
2. Which epilepsy syndrome does he most probably have?

Case 3

A 44-year-old man (Fig. 10.2) presented with recurrent seizures beginning with sickness and tiredness with subsequent loss of consciousness. His wife described an atony with drops from sitting position or his head falling to one side, followed by a tonic extension of the extremities and few body jerks. The episodes lasted for 15 seconds. Afterwards he was rapidly reoriented. MR scans were normal. Family history was negative for epilepsy.

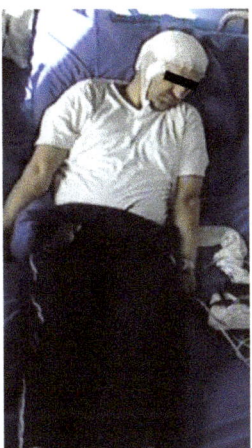

Fig. 10.2: Atonic head drop at seizure onset.

Question

1. Does he have epileptic or non-epileptic seizures?

(Answers and discussion are given at the end of the chapter).

INTRODUCTION

- An opportunity to analyze seizure semiology arises in the following situations:
    - A reliable history is obtained from an observant eye witness
    - A clear home video/smartphone recording of a seizure is available
    - Seizure occurring during the interview in the outpatient or inpatient setting
    - Seizure observed in the emergency department as in status epilepticus or clusters of seizures
    - Long-term video EEG recordings either as routine evaluations or as pre-surgical evaluations
- Whatever may be the situation, a systematic analysis of seizure semiology is invaluable in the proper diagnosis and management of these patients.

PHYSIOLOGICAL BASIS

Definitions

- Epilepsy is a disorder characterized by an enduring predisposition to generate epileptic seizures
- An epileptic seizure is a transient occurrence of symptoms due to abnormal excessive or synchronous neuronal activity in the brain
- Epilepsy diagnosis requires:
    - One unprovoked or reflex seizure and a probability of further seizures similar to the general recurrence risk (at least 60%) after two unprovoked seizures, occurring the next ten years
    - At least two unprovoked or reflex seizures occurring more than 24 hours apart
    - Diagnosis of an epilepsy syndrome
- The clinical signs (i.e. seizure semiology) are the clinical expression of the symptomatic brain region involved by the epileptic activity at that moment
- Epileptic activity has a tendency to spread over the brain which is reflected by the sequence of the seizure associated signs and symptoms. The initial seizure phenomena have a particular localizing signficance
- Semiology helps to classify the epilepsy syndrome (generalized vs. focal epilepsy) and thus to choose the adequate anticonvulsive medication
- Seizure semiology helps to localize the epileptogenic zone to identify patients who might be candidates for epilepsy surgery
- Semiology helps to differentiate between epileptic and non-epileptic seizures.

Seizure Semiology

Semiological seizure analysis encompasses four functional categories:
1. Perception
2. Consciousness

3. Motor activity
4. Autonomic system

During epileptic seizures all, several, or only one of these categories may be altered. Seizure symptoms can often only be assessed when specific clinical testing is performed during the seizure (see below). The above 4 categories are elaborated below:

Aura

Auras are epileptic seizures with exclusively subjective (perceptual) symptoms without concomitant objective symptoms.

Consciousness and motor activity are not altered during auras.

Somatosensory aura	• Paresthesia with clear somatotopic localization • Patients describe sensations like tingling, numbness, a "strange sensation" or in rare cases pain • Reflecting the somatotopic distribution, unilateral paresthesias tend to be restricted to the face and hand caused by epileptic activation of the contralateral somatosensory region (Brodmann area 1, 2, and 3)
Visual aura	• Simple visual hallucinations like white or colored phosphenes are typically caused by an epileptic activation of the primary visual cortex (Brodmann area 17 and/or 18) • Complex visual hallucinations like distortion of objects can be evoked by an epileptic activation of occipital or temporal association cortices
Olfactory aura	• Olfactory auras are difficult for patients to describe, usually they report a negative sensation • They occur most likely by an epileptic activation of the orbitofrontal part of the straight gyrus (gyrus rectus)
Auditory aura	• Simple acoustic hallucinations like sounds are due to an epileptic activation of the Heschl-Gyrus • Complex acoustic hallucinations like voices or melodies sometimes occur during epileptic activation of the temporal association cortex
Gustatory aura	Rare and difficult to describe, if at all they are perceived as a negative sensation
Psychic aura	• "Strange feeling" with altered perception of the inner and outer world • Patients describe déjà vu and jamais vu sensations, emotions like fear or illusions of altered distance to objects • Patients have the feeling that the sensations are unreal • They are most likely caused by an epileptic activation of the basal temporal lobe
Epigastric aura	• Vague, unpleasant feeling starting in the epigastrium with a tendency to rise upwards • Often it is accompanied by sickness • It is in all probability caused by an epileptic activation of the insula • It is especially common in patients with mesial temporal lobe epilepsy
Autonomic aura	• Autonomic alterations like tachycardia, sweating, changes of breathing • Caveat: Autonomic symptoms can also occur during seizures and can also follow other aura symptoms caused by the fear of seizure propagation • There is some evidence that isolated autonomic symptoms can be triggered by an epileptic activation of the basal frontal lobe and the anterior part of the cingulate cortex

Absence Seizure

- Absence seizures are characterized by a loss of consciousness accompanied by blank stare
- Motor activity is reduced, but discrete motor symptoms like blinking can be observed
- They usually have a short duration of few seconds with abrupt start and end
- Patients are amnestic for those episodes
- Traditionally, the term absence seizure is reserved for generalized epilepsies. However, recent research shows that this seizure type also occurs in focal epilepsies. To avoid terminological confusion when using the term absence in focal epilepsies, the term **dialeptic** seizure has been introduced for this seizure type
- If consciousness cannot be evaluated, like in babies or severely mentally incapacitated individuals, the term **hypomotor** seizure is used. They are characterized by reduced motor activity, but ongoing mild complex movements like sitting up or looking around or short tonic freezing.

Motor Seizure

These are seizures with motor signs as predominant ictal semiology.

Simple motor seizure

- Involuntary simple motor action differing from physiological movements by velocity, posturing or evolution
- Consciousness is usually not disturbed
- Simple partial seizures are caused by epileptic activation of primary (Brodman area 4, 6) and supplementary motor regions (mesial part of Brodman area 6)
- The term is only used if seizures are not further classifiable into one of the following categories:

Clonic seizure	• Repetitive, rhythmical, short contractions of different muscle groups, usually acromelic • Usually unilateral, caused by activation of Brodman area 4 and 6 • Bilateral clonic jerks are usually caused by an activation of the supplementary motor region
Tonic seizure	• Tonic contraction of one or more muscle groups, usually proximal, resulting in tonic limb posturing • Usually bilateral tonic contraction due to activation of the supplementary motor region • The consciousness is usually not altered
Tonic-clonic seizure	• Starting with a generalized tonic posturing, usually accompanied by an initial scream (caused by a tonic muscle contraction including the diaphragm and causing air to be pressed through the vocal folds) • Followed by generalized rhythmic convulsions (during the seizure clonic convulsions typically increase in amplitude and decrease in frequency)

	• Loss of consciousness, amnesia
	• Often associated with tongue bite, enuresis or encopresis
	• Postictally patients are confused (usually 10–30 minutes) and tired
	• These seizures are associated with a generalized epileptic brain activation
Atonic seizure	• Seizures with abrupt loss of muscle tonus
	• An atonic seizure caused by generalized brain activation lasts for about 1–2 minutes and is usually associated with drops
	• Short (30–400 ms) atonic seizures, called atonic myoclonic seizures, are usually initiated by an activation of the central region
	• Some atonic jerks can only be detected during muscle activation
	• Atonic seizures can be due to a generalized or focal epileptic brain activation, especially of the primary negative motor area or the supplementary negative motor area
Myoclonic seizure	• Seizures with short, isolated muscle contractions
	• They can be focal or generalized
	• Myoclonic seizures are most often caused by a generalized epileptic activation, but can also be due to frontal epileptic activity
Versive seizure	• Seizure with lateral eye and head movement, often accompanied by a tonic turning of the trunk
	• The eye turning can be saccadic or tonic
	• Versive movements are most likely caused by an activation of the contralateral frontal eye field

Complex Motor Seizure

- Involuntary complex motor action, differing from physiological movements just by their situative inappropriateness
- Consciousness is usually disturbed.

Automotor seizure	• Seizures with inappropriate repetitive, stereotypic movements
	▪ Automatisms are usually localized in the distal part of the limbs like manual automatisms
	▪ Most frequently orofacial and manual automatisms can be observed
	▪ These seizures are most often due to a temporal or frontal brain activation
Hypermotor seizure	• Seizures with complex, heavy and sometimes bizarre movements
	▪ Sometimes consciousness is unimpaired
	▪ Hypermotor seizures are usually caused by an epileptic activation of the frontal lobe

In focal epilepsies, certain clinical signs may help in correct lateralization and localization of the epileptogenic region (Tables 10.1 and 10.2). This is important while correlating the seizure etiology with MRI lesion(s) and in particular when planning epilepsy surgery in patients with bilateral lesions or no visible MRI lesions.

Table 10.1: Lateralizing signs in focal epilepsy.

Semiology	Lateralization
Unilateral clonic movement	Contralateral
Unilateral tonic movement	Contralateral
Unilateral paresthesia	Contralateral
Head and eye version	Contralateral
(Unforced) head turning	Ipsilateral
Asymmetric termination of tonic-clonic seizure	Ipsilateral to the last clonic jerk
Dystonic hand posturing	Contralateral
'Figure of 4' sign	Ipsilateral to flexed arm
Ictal eye blinking	Ipsilateral
Ictal nystagmus	Contralateral to the fast phase
Negative myoclonus	Contralateral
Unilateral akinesia	Contralateral
Unilateral piloerection	Ipsilateral
Aphasia	Dominant hemisphere
Ictal speech	Non-dominant hemisphere
Ictal spitting	Non-dominant hemisphere
Ictal vomiting	Non-dominant hemisphere
Peri-ictal water drinking	Non-dominant hemisphere
Peri-ictal urinary urge	Non-dominant hemisphere
Automatisms with preserved responsiveness	Non-dominant hemisphere
Postictal coughing	Non-dominant hemisphere
Postictal nose-rubbing	Ipsilateral
Postictal paresis	Contralateral

Table 10.2: Localizing signs in focal epilepsy.

Semiology	Localization
Epigastric aura	Temporal lobe
Simple visual aura	Occipital lobe
Complex visual aura	Temporo-occipital junction
Acoustic aura	Insular region
Gustatoric aura	Insular region
Olfactory aura	Amygdala, orbitofrontal region
Autonomic aura	Insular region
Aphasia	Dominant temporal lobe
Unilateral, distal jerks	Perirolandic region
Unilateral somatosensory aura	Paracentral region
Bilateral tonic posturing	Supplementary motor area
Epigastric aura → automatisms → generalized tonic-clonic seizure	Temporal lobe
Gelastic seizure	Hypothalamus

Methodology

Interictal: Epilepsy Specific Report

It is important to get information about seizure semiology and epilepsy characteristics by a structured patient report to classify the seizures and the epilepsy syndrome. **The following questions help in generating valuable information regarding the patient's seizures:**

- Can you remember your seizures?
- Do you feel something heralding a seizure? (aura, hints for a focal seizure origin)
- Have you found yourself in places and cannot recall how you came there?
- Can you understand/remember what people say to you during seizures? Can you respond or follow commands during a seizure?
- Can you influence/stop your seizures?
- Have you hurt yourself during seizures?
- Did you bite your tongue or did you have enuresis or encopresis during the seizures?
- Did your muscles ache the day after a seizure?
- How often do the seizures occur?
- In which occasions do the seizures occur? Any association to the sleep wake cycle (during sleep)?
- Did seizure frequency change with anticonvulsive medication?
- How old have you been when seizures started?
- Did you have febrile seizures, head trauma, encephalitis or a stroke? Do you have a brain tumor? Does someone else in your family have epileptic seizures?
- Has someone observed your seizures or is there any video recording (smart phone) of your habitual seizures?
- Ask family members or friends to describe what they observed during your seizures (duration, responsiveness, movements, falls, behavior)
- Assess handedness, for example with help of the Edinburgh handedness inventory.

Ictal Testing

- When you have the chance to observe a seizure, test the patient's responsiveness to get more localizing and lateralizing information about seizure semiology
- Aphasia can only be assessed if tested for it:
    1. Remember the test word ... (e.g. "banana")
    2. Tell me your first name
    3. Raise your arms with the palms turned upwards (let them hold 10s)
    4. Show objects and ask the patient to name them
    5. If the person fails to name objects ask to describe the use of the presented objects or to show their use. If no response is available, restart at 2. again

- During generalized tonic clonic seizures turn the patients into recovery position.

Observations and Interpretations

From a clinical point of view, epilepsy syndromes are classified based on age of onset, seizure semiology, additional signs and symptoms, test results and etiology. The most common epilepsy syndromes are listed below:

West syndrome: Pediatric syndrome with generalized tonic or myoclonic seizures starting between 3rd and 12th month of life, it can be symptomatic or of unknown etiology.

Lennox-Gastaut syndrome: Predominantly generalized tonic seizures, diverse seizure semiology with myoclonic, atonic, absence, generalized tonic-clonic and sometimes focal seizures, seizures start during first decade, high seizure frequency, patients are also mentally and physically retarded, higher incidence in boys.

Benign focal epilepsy of childhood: Rare focal seizures, especially during night, also generalized tonic-clonic seizures occur from time to time, seizures start during 5th and 14th year of life and are called benign, because they usually cease before adolescence.

Childhood absence epilepsy (CAE): High frequency of absence seizures, starting between 6th and 12th year of life, seizures can stop spontaneously, in adolescence generalized tonic-clonic seizures can start in addition, no neurological or cognitive deficit, high genetic predisposition. 80% remission rate.

Juvenile myoclonic epilepsy (JME): Morning myoclonic jerks of the shoulder girdle, absence seizures and generalized tonic-clonic seizures, usually provocation factors can be identified (stroboscopic light, emotions, sleep deprivation), seizures start during youth and persist over decades.

Grand mal epilepsy: Only generalized tonic-clonic seizures starting in the second decade of life, low seizure frequency, seizures typically occur in the first hours after getting up and can be triggered by sleep deprivation.

Temporal lobe epilepsy: Patients typically describe an epigastric, psychic or autonomic aura, followed by automotor seizures and/or generalized tonic-clonic seizures, seizures usually start in the second half of the first decade of life, interictally they usually show verbal (dominant) or visual/orientation (non-dominant) memory deficits depending on the side of the affected temporal lobe.

Frontal lobe epilepsy: Most often patients have sleep associated bilateral tonic, hypermotor, automotor or generalized tonic-clonic seizures of short duration, absence seizures can occur as well.

Paracentral epilepsy: Unilateral clonic seizures (mostly face and hand), eye/head version can occur, a "Jacksonian march" reflects the spread of the epileptic activity over the homunculus.

Parieto-occipital lobe epilepsy: Seizures are characterized by a visual aura which can evolve into focal versive, simple-motor or complex-motor seizures, parietal lobe seizures can be associated with somatosensory auras, neuropsychological symptoms such as aphasia (dominant hemisphere), often postictal headache.

Caveats

- Initial seizure description by the patient or relatives may be insufficient. Information for the relatives to enable them to provide better description of the observed seizures can be very helpful
- Nowadays, smartphone video recordings add considerable information on seizure semiology
- The differentiation between epileptic and non-epileptic seizures may be impossible without sufficient clinical information is discussed in Table 10.3.

Table 10.3: Differences between epileptic and non-epileptic seizures.

Criteria	Epileptic seizure	Non-epileptic seizure
Eyes	Open	Closed
Semiology	<ul><li>Stereotyped semiology</li><li>Rhythmic jerks</li></ul>	<ul><li>Variable semiology depending on interaction</li><li>Irregular movements with pauses</li></ul>
Controllability	No	Often
Duration	Up to a few minutes	Up to hours and days
Frequency	Irregular, from rare seizures up to several seizures a day, frequency can be higher after sleep deprivation (JME) and alcohol consumption	Varying seizure frequency with more seizures during working days and less during weekends, etc.
Occurrence	Unpredictable, sleep related seizures associated with frontal lobe epilepsy	Mostly with bystanders, stress triggered, rarely unobserved
Injuries	Associated with bruises, tongue bites, fractures	Usually no injuries
Psychic side-diagnosis	None	Usually depression, borderline/personality disorder
Suggestibility	No	Often triggered by suggestions, and manipulations (such as tuning fork stimulation, hyperventilation), providing opportunity to record and analyze the seizure from its onset

Etiologies for non-epileptic seizures include cardiogenic, psychogenic, or metabolic conditions. Migraine attacks may mimic epileptic auras.

ANSWERS TO THE PRETEST

Case 1

Semiology: Epigastric aura → automotor seizure → versive seizure to the left → generalized tonic-clonic seizure.

A sensation of discomfort in the epigastrium with a tendency to raise upward is typical for an epigastric aura. The dystonic posturing of the left hand with right hand automatisms (automotor seizure), the forced head and eye turning towards the left (i.e. version to the left) as well as the tonic posturing called "sign of 4" with the left arm stretched (Fig. 10. 1B red lines) suggest a right hemispheric seizure origin. The described seizure evolved into a generalized tonic-clonic seizure.

The sequence of epigastric aura, automotor seizure and generalized convulsions has a high association with temporal lobe seizure onset. In summary, the above mentioned seizure semiology is highly suggestive for seizures arising from the right temporal lobe.

MRI of this patient showed right mesial temporal sclerosis (Figs. 10.3A and B).

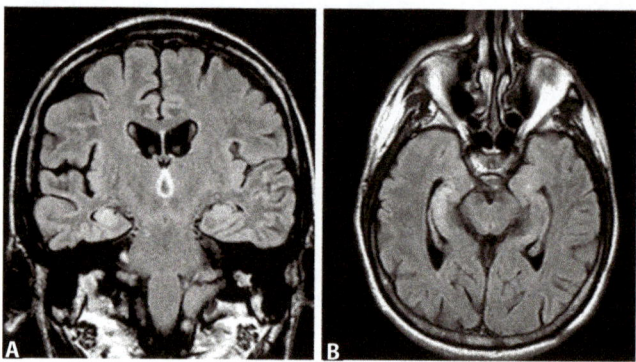

Figs. 10.3A and B: (A) MRI (FLAIR) showing right mesial temporal sclerosis in a coronal; (B) Axial image.

Case 2

Seizure semiology: Myoclonic jerks, absence seizures, generalized tonic-clonic seizures

The seizure onset age and seizure semiology with myoclonic jerks, absence seizures and generalized tonic-clonic seizures is typical for juvenile myoclonic epilepsy (JME). Most JME patients report triggering factors such as sleep deprivation, increased alcohol consumption, exposure to stroboscobic light or emotional or cognitive triggers. Conventional MR scans are usually normal.

Case 3

The late age of onset is suggestive of a symptomatic etiology. However, the very short duration of the episodes with subsequent rapid reorientation suggests a non-epileptic event. Stereotyped attacks characterized by nausea followed by loss of consciousness, atonic falls associated with some jerks of the limbs is suggestive of a convulsive syncope. During the seizure described above an asystole of 11 seconds was documented (without an EEG seizure pattern). ECG revealed an intermittent 3rd degree AV block. A pacemaker was implanted to prevent further cardiac syncopes.

BIBLIOGRAPHY

1. Fisher RS, van Emde Boas W, Blume W, et al. Epileptic seizures and epilepsy: definitions proposed by the International League Against Epilepsy (ILAE) and the International Bureau for Epilepsy (IBE). Epilepsia. 2005;46(4);470-2.
2. Lüders HO, Noachtar S. Atlas and classification of electroencephalography. WB Saunders: Philadelphia; 2000.
3. Noachtar S. Video analysis for defining the symptomatogenic zone. 2004;3:185-98.
4. Stoyke C, Bilgin O, Noachtar S. Video atlas of lateralising and localising seizure phenomena. Epileptic Disorders. 2011;13(2):113-24. doi:10.1684/epd.2011.0433.
5. Wyllie E. Wyllie's treatment of epilepsy: principles and practice. 6th edition. Lippincott, Williams & Wilkins: Philadelphia; 2015.

CHAPTER 11

Examination of a Patient with Vertigo

GRK Sarma, Thomas Mathew

The first step in performing the vestibular system examination is to mentally map the orientation of the semi circular (SC) canals in a given patient. This is especially useful while performing positioning maneuvers and in interpreting them correctly (Figs. 11.1A and B and 11.2). It is possible to test bedside each semicircular canal and the utricle separately. Assessment of saccule requires electrophysiological tests.

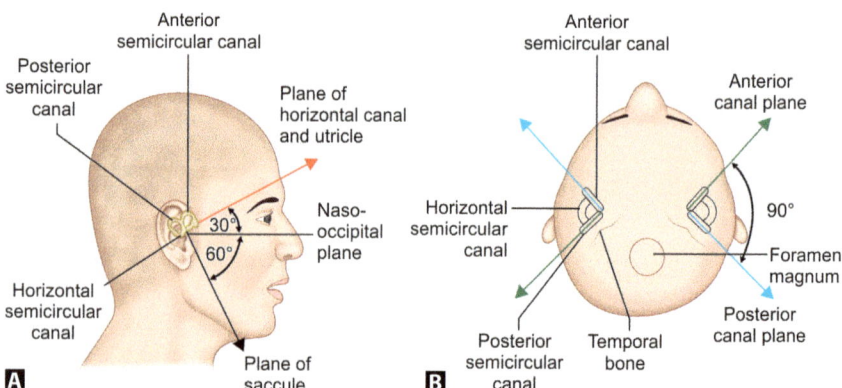

Figs. 11.1A and B: The plane of **horizontal** semicircular (SC) canals is approximately in the same direction as a line joining the **external auditory meatus to the superior orbital margin** in sagittal view. To test this canal, therefore, head is tilted forward by 30° and a NO-NO movement is produced; (B) The plane of the **posterior SC** canals can be visualized by joining **post-auricular area/mastoid on one side with the opposite orbit**. The **posterior SC canals** and the opposite anterior SC canals are coplanar, i.e. left anterior and right posterior canals are in same plane **(LARP)** while the right anterior and left posterior canals are in the same plane **(RALP)**. When head is turned 45° to right, backward tilt tests right posterior SC and forward tilt tests left anterior SC (YES-YES movement).

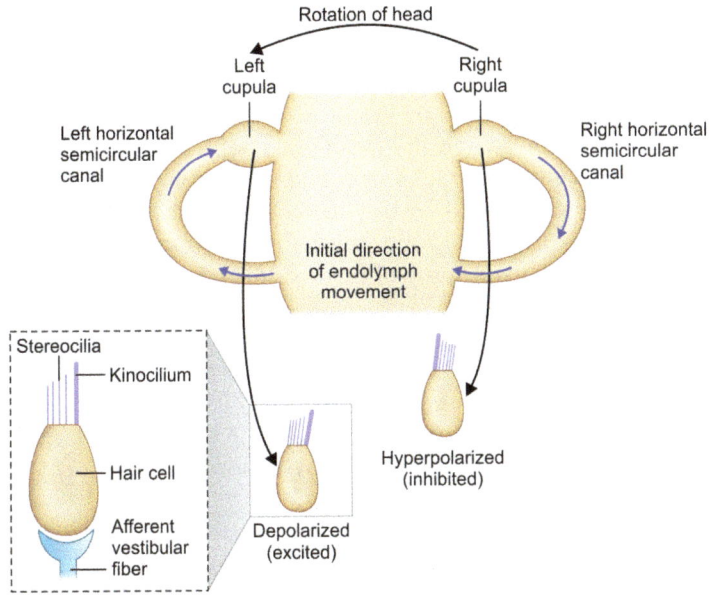

Fig. 11.2: Semicircular canal anatomy and physiology.

PHYSIOLOGIC BASIS

- Normally when the head is still, the left and right vestibular nerves and the neurons in the vestibular nucleus to which they project have equal resting discharge rates (vestibular tone)
- Each vestibular apparatus attempts to move the eyes to the opposite side, but, no net movement occurs as long as both sides are balanced
- If the vestibular tone is unequal, the side with higher tone pushes the eyes slowly to the opposite side which has the lesser tone and a corrective saccade to the intact side, resulting in nystagmus.
- Four laws help us in making nystagmus more prominent.
  1. **Ewald's first law**: A stimulation of the semicircular canal causes a movement of the eyes in the plane of the stimulated canal. This law is useful in understanding which SC canal is being stimulated, based on the observed nystagmus.
  2. **Ewald's second law**: In the horizontal semicircular canals, an ampullopetal endolymph movement causes a greater stimulation than an ampullofugal one. This law is put to use in head impulse and head heave tests.
  3. **Ewald's third law**: In the vertical semicircular canals, the reverse is true.
  4. **Alexander's law:** The intensity of nystagmus often depends on the position of the eye in the orbit.

- For example, in peripheral vestibular lesion on one side, if the eyes are looking to the healthy side, the available range of slow component is greater and nystagmus becomes more prominent (Alexander's law). On the contrary, on looking to the lesion side, the range of slow movement available is decreased and the nystagmus becomes less prominent (in central lesions, opposite phenomenon may be noted)
- The basic objective of all vestibular tests is to give certain tasks and demonstrate asymmetry in the vestibular function between right and left sides. The results of some of the tests also provide clue to a central vestibular dysfunction
- The more subtle the asymmetry, the more complex is the task required
- If the disease is more or less symmetric, a highly demanding (e.g. dynamic visual acuity) task is required
- The tasks commonly used areas listed below. A complete assessment of a dizzy patient requires utilization of most of the following:

Tests of utricular function	Tests of semicircular canal function	
	Vestibulo-ocular tests	Vestibulo-spinal tests
Ocular misalignment, ocular tilt reaction	Examination of eye movements	Standing (Romberg test)
Subjective visual vertical (bucket test)	Nystagmus to various stimuli	Walking (Fukuda test)
Head heave test	Vestibulo-ocular reflexes	Limb coordination (Past-pointing)

OCULAR ALIGNMENT AND OCULAR TILT REACTION

- Normally, both utricles provide similar information to the otolith-ocular and otolith-spinal connections regarding the position of the head in space. In unilateral utricular disease, asymmetry in this information induces certain changes in ocular and head position called the ocular tilt reaction (OTR) (Fig. 11.3).

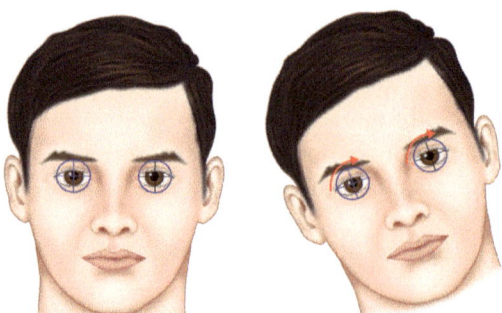

Fig. 11.3: Ocular response to head tilt in ocular tilt reaction (OTR).

- The ocular tilt reaction (OTR) refers to the **triad of lateral head tilt, ocular torsion, and skew** deviation. Head tilt and ocular torsion occur towards the lower eye
- While head tilt and skew deviation are easy to detect by simple observation, torsion is more difficult to appreciate
- There are ways to detect this:
  - By observing the orientation of bulbar conjunctival vessels (normally horizontal)
  - By observing the relation between the optic disc and the macula (normally at the same level) during ophthalmoscopy
  - In perimetry, by observing the relative positions of the blind spot and the fovea. Using these landmarks, intorsion and extorsion can be identified
- Pathway responsible for the OTR is known to cross the midline just above the abducens nucleus level and ascend in the contralateral medial longitudinal fasciculus (MLF)
- Peripheral vestibular damage or lesions within the vestibular nuclei in the medulla or caudal pons cause a head tilt toward the affected side (ipsilateral pathway involved)
- Lesions within the rostral pons and midbrain (commonly in the MLF) usually cause a head tilt away from the affected side (contralateral pathway involved). This implies that if there is a head tilt to one side, there is a possible ipsilateral caudal lesion or contralateral rostral lesion.

Caveats

- Skew deviation indicates a vertical misalignment of the eyes and can also be caused by anterior semicircular canal lesions or trochlear nerve palsy
- Patients with **trochlear nerve palsy** may be confused with OTR because of vertical misalignment and the head tilt. This can be differentiated with the following observations.

	Ocular misalignment	Trochlear nerve palsy
Torsion of the eye	Intorsion	Extorsion
Skew deviation comitance	Comitant	Non-comitant
Image orientation to the patient from both eyes	No torsional disparity (both images similarly oriented)	Torsional disparity (images titled in different angles)
Supine posture	Skew decreases	No change

SUBJECTIVE VISUAL VERTICAL (BUCKET TEST)

- A tilt of the subjective visual vertical (SVV) is a sensitive sign of a disturbance in the otolith-ocular pathway (Fig. 11.4)
- It often occurs together with the OTR.

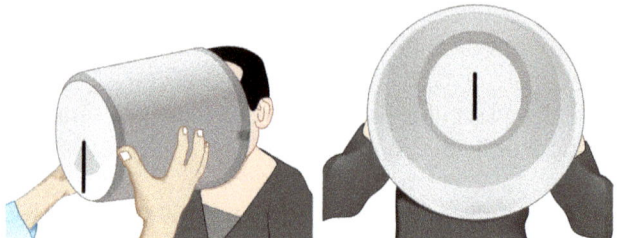

Fig. 11.4: The bucket test for the subjective visual vertical.

- Most patients with acute vestibular neuritis show a small and transient ipsilateral deviation of the SVV
- More central lesions can produce larger and more enduring tilts of the SVV
- In the rostral medullary tegmentum and caudal pons the tilt of the SVV is usually ipsilateral to the lesion; in the rostral pons and caudal mesencephalic tegmentum the tilt of the SVV is usually contralateral to the lesion
- The SVV can be measured at the bedside using the bucket method
- The subject estimates verticality by aligning a dark straight line visible on the bottom of a bucket that is rotated to the right or left by the examiner
- On the outside, there is a plumb line on the bottom of the bucket that originates from the center of a semicircle divided into degrees with the zero line adjusted to the dark line inside. In this way the deviation from true vertical can be measured by averaging a few trials.

HEAD HEAVE TEST

This is discussed along with rotational vestibulo-ocular reflex.

EXAMINATION OF EYE MOVEMENTS

Physiologic Basis

- A disturbance in vestibulo-ocular function results in some characteristic eye movement abnormalities
- These differ from eye movement abnormalities seen in central lesions. Therefore, it is important to do a complete eye movement examination in a patient with suspected vestibular disorder.

Methodology

- Examine gaze holding in straight ahead position for spontaneous nystagmus and other movements
- If no obvious nystagmus is observed, **Frenzel's glasses or Michael's glasses** need to be put on by the patient. These are high dioptre lenses that prevent visual fixation, which typically suppresses nystagmus of peripheral origin
- If these glasses are not available, a less optimal method is to observe the jerky movement of the corneal bulge when the eyes are gently closed
- Another method is to close one eye and examine the fundus of the other eye. As the visual fixation is removed, nystagmus is brought out and is seen as jerky movement of the optic disc **(occlusive ophthalmoscopy)**
- Examine gaze holding in eccentric positions for gaze evoked nystagmus (see below for discussion on this phenomenon)
- Examine saccades, pursuits (see detailed methods in "III, IV, VI Cranial Nerves" chapter)
- Examine convergence, specifically looking for its effect on spontaneous nystagmus.

Interpretation

- On gaze holding in straight position, spontaneous nystagmus may be seen and indicates a tone imbalance between the corresponding semicircular canals of the two sides. The slow phase is directed towards and the quick phase away from the side of the vestibular lesion
- If there is spontaneous nystagmus that subsides on head flexion to 30°, it is typical of horizontal SC canal disease. On head flexion to this angle, the effect of the gravity on the slightly up-tilted horizontal SC canal is removed and the canal stimulation ceases

- Nystagmus of peripheral origin is usually of small amplitude and high frequency. Central nystagmus is usually of large amplitude and low frequency
- If a strong downbeat nystagmus is brought out on convergence, it is suggestive of central nystagmus (central vestibular or cerebellar)
- Spontaneous down beat nystagmus is usually due to lesions in the flocculus of cerebellum, which has predominantly down gaze Purkinje cells. It is better in supine position and worse in prone position.

Caveats

- Saccadic oscillations like opsoclonus also become prominent on eye closure
- During occlusive ophthalmoscopy, the direction of fast phase and slow phase of the disc movements are opposite to those of the eye ball seen during gross examination. This is because the front and the back of the eye are at the opposite poles around the axis of rotation. Thus, the nystagmus direction should not be confused while reporting based on disc examination.

GAZE-EVOKED NYSTAGMUS

Physiological Basis

- Nystagmus that develops when patients take eccentric eye positions caused by impaired gaze-holding in those positions
- Gaze-evoked nystagmus (GEN) beats in the direction of gaze because it is a result of failure of gaze holding
- For the same reason, it changes in direction when gazing in different directions
- GEN is attributed to dysfunction of the common neural integrator
- The nucleus prepositus hypoglossi and medial vestibular nuclei are the main neural integrators for horizontal eye movements
- The interstitial nucleus of Cajal is the main contributor to neural integration for vertical and torsional eye movements
- GEN is one of the most sensitive ocular motor signs for central pathologies in patients with acute vestibular syndrome
- The most common cause of GEN is medications, usually sedatives, tranquilizers, or anticonvulsants, or alcohol
- GEN due to medication usually occurs in both the horizontal and vertical planes.

Methodology and Observations

- Ask the patient to look in different directions, avoiding extreme gaze (not more than 30°)
- Hold the gaze in each direction and observe the direction of nystagmus.

Interpretation

- If the nystagmus appears only on one direction of eccentric gaze, it is likely to be of peripheral vestibular origin (based on Alexander's law). If it has mixed torsional horizontal component, peripheral lesion is all the more likely
- If the nystagmus appears in all directions of eccentric gaze and the fast phase changes to the direction of the gaze, it indicates a gaze holding defect, seen in central lesions
- In some patients, a mixture of central and peripheral nystagmus is seen. They have large amplitude low frequency nystagmus in one direction and small amplitude high frequency nystagmus on the other (**Brun's nystagmus**). This is typical of large cerebellopontine angle lesion
- A strong down-beating component brought out on lateral gaze implies central vestibular or cerebellar dysfunction
- Periodic alternating nystagmus (PAN) changes its horizontal direction every few minutes and is a sign of abnormal function of the cerebellar nodulus. PAN reflects instability in the velocity-storage mechanism within the vestibular nuclei because of a loss of inhibition by Purkinje cells from the nodulus.

Caveats

- Gaze-evoked nystagmus should be differentiated from the end-point nystagmus that may be observed in extreme gazes even in normal subjects
- End-point nystagmus is mostly transient, with a low amplitude, and frequency.

HEAD-SHAKING NYSTAGMUS

Physiologic Basis

- Asymmetric vestibular inputs would be generated during head-shaking in peripheral vestibulopathies
- Since excitatory vestibular inputs are more effective than inhibitory ones (Ewald's second law), these asymmetric vestibular inputs are believed to accumulate in the central vestibular structures (velocity storage) during headshaking, and to discharge as contra lesional nystagmus after the headshaking.

Methodology

- Patient preferably wears Frenzel's or Michael's glasses
- Assessed using either a passive (by the examiner) or active (by the patient) headshaking maneuver
- The patient's head is tilted forward by approximately 20° to bring the horizontal semicircular canals (HCs) into the plane of stimulation, the

head is shaken horizontally in a sinusoidal fashion at a rate of about 2–3 Hz for 15 seconds
- An amplitude of 20° is sufficient
- After the headshaking is completed, observe for nystagmus for 1 minute
- This has to repeated in vertical direction also.

Observation

- In unilateral peripheral vestibulopathy, the typical pattern of Head shaking nystagmus (HSN) initially consists of contra lesional nystagmus (fast phase to opposite side and slow phase to the lesion side) that decays over 20 seconds and then goes through a weak reversal
- In central lesions, the patterns of HSN include unusually strong HSN elicited by weak head shaking, ipsilesional HSN, HSN in the direction opposite to the spontaneous nystagmus, and perverted HSN (i.e. vertical or torsional nystagmus developing in response to horizontal head-shaking)
- HSN from central causes usually is due to lesions involving the vestibulocerebellum, which is comprised of the flocculus/paraflocculus, nodulus and ventral uvula.

HYPERVENTILATION-INDUCED NYSTAGMUS

Physiologic Basis

- Hyperventilation produces "dizziness" in many subjects, especially anxious ones without objective signs
- In vestibular disease, hyperventilation can produce objective signs like nystagmus
- Hyperventilation is hypothesized to improve axonal conductance in partially demyelinatd vestibular nerve fibers. Thus, the "recovery nystagmus" will have a slow component to the healthy side and fast component to the diseased side.

Methodology and Observation

- Patient has to wear Frenzel's or Michael's glasses
- Subjects are asked to hyperventilate for about 30–60 seconds while seated in the darkness, taking an average of one deep breath per second.

Interpretation

- Nystagmus beating to the side of reduced caloric response or hearing loss may be a valuable sign for cerebellopontine-angle (CPA) tumors
- It is also seen in central as well as peripheral vestibular disorders, including compensated peripheral vestibulopathies, perilymph fistula, acoustic neuroma, lesions at the craniocervical junction, and cerebellar degeneration or with demyelination in central pathways (e.g. in multiple sclerosis)

- HV can produce nystagmus in cerebellar disease by altering the metabolism of Purkinje cells
- HV can also alter the intracranial pressure and produce nystagmus in craniovertebral junction disease and in perilymphatic fistula.

Caveats

The direction of nystagmus is variable and is not entirely reliable.
- The main use of this test may to bring out nystagmus which is not evident on routine tests.

VIBRATION-INDUCED NYSTAGMUS

Physiologic Basis

- The vibration impulses are transmitted throughout the skull and to both labyrinths nearly equally
- When both labyrinths respond equally to this stimulation in healthy individuals, no nystagmus occurs
- In unilateral vestibular disease, asymmetric response results in nystagmus with slow phase towards and fast phase away from the diseased side.

Methodology and Observation

- Patient has to wear Frenzel's or Michael's glasses
- Low frequency vibration (64Hz) applied to the forehead or mastoid
- Nystagmus is seen in various vestibular disorders
- In peripheral vestibulopathies, the direction of vibration-induced nystagmus (VIN) is mostly toward the healthy side, with an exception in some patients with Ménière's disease.

VALSALVA-INDUCED NYSTAGMUS

Physiologic Basis

- The Valsalva maneuver can induce nystagmus either by increasing intracranial pressure (straining against closed glottis as with lifting a heavy weight) or by increasing pressure in the middle ear (blowing out against pinched nostrils)
- Change in intracranial pressure and middle ear pressure is transmitted to the inner ear and stimulates the vestibular organ to produce vertigo and nystagmus.

Methodology and Observations

- Patient is asked to perform Valsalva maneuver against closed glottis (as in lifting heavy weight)
- Patient is asked to blow his cheeks against closed nostrils

- Compression of the tragus can also provoke nystagmus by changing the middle-ear pressure (Hennebert's sign).

Interpretation

- Seen in patients with craniocervical junction anomalies such as Arnold-Chiari malformation, with perilymph fistula, or superior canal dehiscence
- Tullio's phenomenon (noise-induced nystagmus and oscillopsia) often occurs in patients who have Valsalva-induced nystagmus and is commonly associated with a superior canal dehiscence, perilymph fistula, chronic middle ear disease, petrous meningioma, Ménière's disease.

POSITIONAL TESTING

- Positional nystagmus refers to the nystagmus that develops in association with changes in the dependent position of the head in the direction of gravity
- Positional nystagmus may be either paroxysmal or persistent. Both peripheral and central vestibular disorders may produce positional nystagmus.

Methodology and Observations for Posterior Semicircular Canal Testing (Figs. 11.5A to C)

All positional tests are better performed with patient wearing Frenzel's/Michaels glasses on.

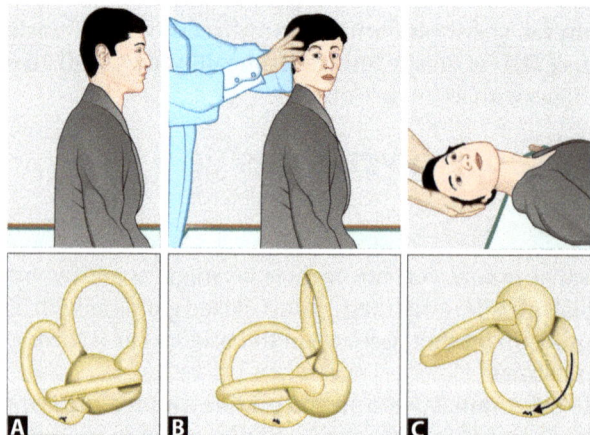

Figs. 11.5A to C: The Dix-Hallpike maneuver for benign paroxysmal positional vertigo involving the right posterior semicircular canal (PC). After seating the patient upright (A), the head is turned 45° in the direction of the involved ear (B: right ear in this figure). The patient is then moved from the sitting to the supine position, ending with the head hanging at 20° off the end of the examination table (C). The corresponding illustrations demonstrate the orientation of the semicircular canals and location of the otolithic debris in the PC (viewed from the patient's right side).

A. **The Dix-Hallpike Maneuver** is the gold-standard test for a diagnosis of benign paroxysmal positional vertigo (BPPV) involving the posterior semicircular canal (PC-BPPV).
   - While seated on the examination table, the patient's head is turned 45° toward the side to be tested
   - The patient is then moved en bloc to a supine position, ending with the head hanging 20° below the examination table
   - This maneuver places the PC in the most dependent position
   - In PC-BPPV the elicited nystagmus would be mixed up beat and torsional with the upper pole of the eyes beating toward the lower ear
   - When free-floating otolithic debris is present (canalolithiasis) in the PC being tested, nystagmus usually develops with a latency of several seconds (up to 30 seconds)
   - It resolves within 1 minute (usually within 30 seconds). It may reverse direction upon sitting and tends to habituate with repeated testing.
B. **Side-Lying Test (Fig. 11.6)**
   - If the Dix-Hallpike maneuver is contraindicated or not possible due to the presence of a cervical spine disease, (e.g. cervical spine instability, cervical disc herniation) the side-lying test may be performed
   - Patient sits on the cot with both legs hanging down, with the examiner standing infront of him
   - The head of the patient is turned 45° opposite to the side being tested
   - The patient is quickly laid toward the side being tested.

In rare cases the positional nystagmus is observed in patients with lesions involving the inferior cerebellar vermis. This central positional nystagmus (CPN) may be either paroxysmal or persistent. The nystagmus is mostly vertical

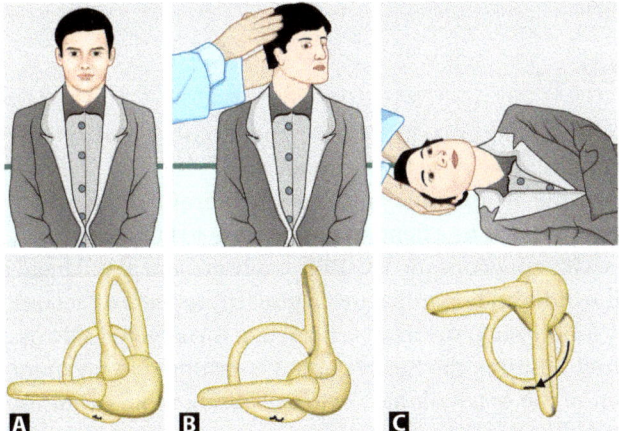

Figs. 11.6A to C: Side-lying test for diagnosis of right posterior canal benign proxysmal positional vertigo. After seating the patient on the examination table (A), the head is turned 45° away from the involved ear (B). The patient then lies on the side of the involved ear (C). The corresponding illustrations demonstrate the orientation of the semicircular canals and location of the otolithic debris in the posterior canal (viewed from the front).

or apogeotropic, and may change direction depending on the positional maneuver. Prominent positional nystagmus in the absence of dizziness also suggests a central pathology.

Methodology and Observations for Horizontal SC Canal Testing

Supine Roll Test (fast phase direction points to the lesion side)

- The HC can be maximally stimulated using the supine roll test
- In supine position, the patient's head is first flexed forward about 30°
- Then it is turned about 90° to each side
- Two types of nystagmus may be observed in BPPV involving the HC (HC-BPPV):
    1. Geotropic nystagmus beating toward the ground (lower ear) or
    2. Apogeotropic nystagmus beating toward the ceiling (upper ear).
- In both types of nystagmus, the direction of fast phase points to the side involved when the head is placed on the side where more intense nystagmus is elicited
- The nystagmus has a shorter latency, longer duration and more intense movement than posterior SCC BPPV
- With the above knowledge, we can work out the other details
- For example, in geotropic nystagmus, the fast phase is downward. This means that the lesion side is the lower one, i.e. when the head is turned to the lesion side, the nystagmus is stronger
- In contrast, if a patient exhibits apogeotropic nystagmus, the fast phase being directed upwards, the lesional side is the upper one, and healthy side is dependent, i.e. when head is turned to the healthy side, the nystagmus is stronger.

Interpretation

- Geotropic nystagmus indicates free floating debris in the canal (canalolithiasis) far away from cupula
- Apogeotropic nystagmus indicates adherent debris in the cupula (cupulolithiasis) or free floating debris close to cupula
- Patients with apogeotropic HC-BPPV may present a null head position in which the induced horizontal nystagmus disappears or becomes minimal (usually found when the head is turned to the affected side by 10–20°)
- At the null position, the heavy cupula is assumed to be aligned with the direction of the gravitational vector, resulting in no or minimal cupular deflection
- However, central positional nystagmus (CPN) should be considered, especially when the repeated canalith repositioning maneuvers fail to ameliorate the nystagmus and vertigo in apogeotropic positional nystagmus.

In this example, the right ear is the diseased side. In the Figure 11.7A, the debris is in the canal far away from the cupula. When head is turned to

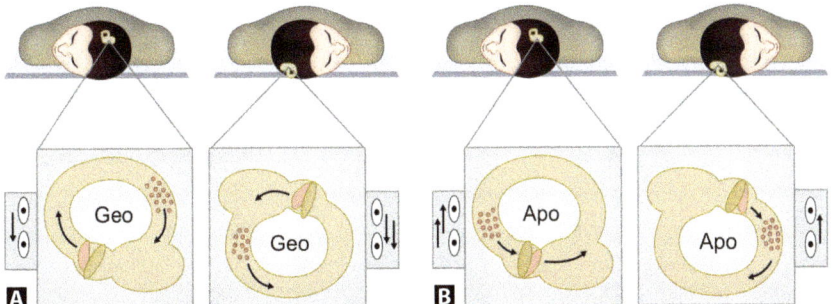

Figs. 11.7A and B: (A) Geotropic LSC BPPV pathophysiology, right side; (B) Apogeotropic nystagmus in LSC pathology. The direction of nystagmus is schematically shown in adjacent boxes.

the right side, the debris gravitates down towards the ampulla and generate an excitatory current. This causes slow eye deviation to the left and fast component to the right (the dependent ear). When the head is turned to the left side, the debris gravitate towards the utricular orifice and generate ampullofugal inhibitory current. This causes, slow eye deviation to the right and fast component to the left (again the dependent ear).

In the Figure 11.7B, the movement of the debris is reversed causing apogeotropic nystagmus when head is turned to either side.

Methodology and Observation in Anterior Canal BPPV

- Straight head hanging as well as the Dix-Hallpike maneuver on either side may elicit downbeat nystagmus with a small ipsitorsional component (i.e. with the upper poles of the eyes beating toward the affected side)
- While doing Dix-Hallpike maneuver, nystagmus is elicited when the normal ear is dependent, in contrast to posterior canal BPPV, where it is with diseased ear being dependent. This is because, one anterior canal is coplanar with the opposite posterior canal
- This differentiation (posterior canal Vs opposite anterior canal BPPV) on Hallpike maneuver is difficult unless the torsion is carefully observed. In posterior canal BPPV, the torsion of the upper pole is towards the dependent ear, while in anterior canal BPPV, it is towards the non-dependent ear
- For example, while doing a left Hallpike maneuver, if there is a torsional nystagmus with uppe pole beating to the left ear, it suggests left posterior canal BPPV. If the torsion of the upper pole is towards the right ear, it suggests right anterior canal BPPV
- AC-BPPV should be differentiated from CPN, especially when the torsional component is minimal and the downbeat nystagmus is persistent.

Bedside Evaluation of Dizziness

Table 11.1: Differentiation of peripheral and central nystagmus.

Characteristic	Central	Peripheral
Pattern	Variable	Mixed horizontal-torsional
Directional	Unidirectional may change direction	Unidirectional
Fixation effect	Variable	Suppression

*The pnemonic **HINTS** (**H**ead **I**mpulse, **N**ystagmus, **T**ests of **S**kew) along with examination of gaze (saccades and pursuits) is useful in bedside differentiation of central from peripheral nystagmus.*

THE VESTIBULO-OCULAR REFLEX

- Unilateral loss of vestibular function leads to a difference not only in **the tonic (static) discharges** between the vestibular nuclei on the two sides, but also a decreased **dynamic sensitivity** during rotation
- Loss of this dynamic sensitivity results in reduced vestibulo-ocular reflex (VOR) gain, which can be identified using bedside tests.

Head Impulse Test (Rotational VOR) (Figs. 11.8A and B)

- The head impulse test is the most effective method of detecting loss of dynamic vestibular function at the bedside
- If the patient's gaze is held steadily on the target during head rotation, it indicates that the VOR is working normally. This is accomplished by a slow, equal but opposite gaze deviation generated by the normal vestibular systems.

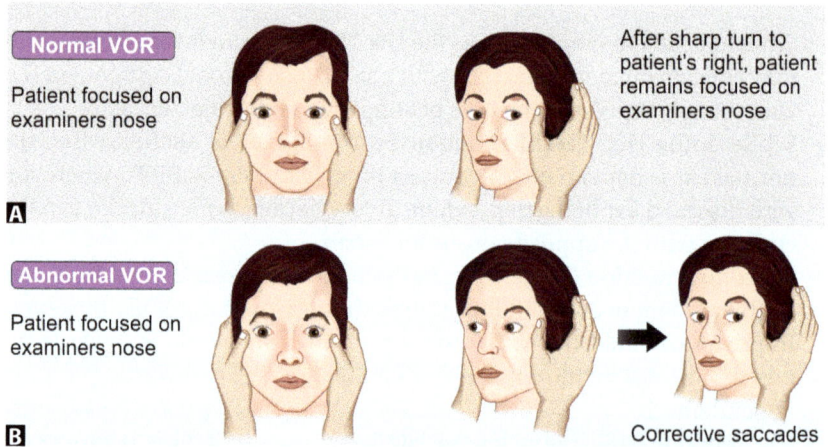

Figs. 11.8A and B: Head impulse test. (A) In healthy subjects, a head impulse normally induces a rapid compensatory eye movement in the opposite direction, and steady fixation is attained; (B) In patients with unilateral peripheral vestibular hypofunction, a head impulse toward the affected side produces a corrective saccade after head rotation since the eyes move with the head due to a defective vestibulo-ocular reflex, and lose the target with the head rotation.

Methodology and Observations

- The examiner asks the patient to fixate upon a target in front of the eyes (like the tip of the examiner's nose) and then briskly turns the patient's head horizontally
- The head rotation can be initially slow (0.5 Hz/s). If corrective saccades are not detected at this frequency, more quicker movements can be tried
- The head movements should be unpredictable with a low amplitude (10–20°) and a high acceleration
- Examiner watches for corrective saccades in the direction of head rotation or in an opposite direction
- The function of the vertical semicircular canals can also be assessed with vertical head impulses, in which the patient's head is rotated vertically in either the right-AC left PC or left-AC-right-PC plane
- If the head impulse test is positive, re-look for skew deviation and gaze-evoked nystagmus (GEN) as these help in differentiating central from peripheral lesions.

Interpretation

- If the head impulse test is **negative** in a patient with an acute vestibular syndrome, it suggests **central** lesion. However, a **positive** head impulse test can occur in **both peripheral and central lesions**. Further localization depends on the quality of the positive response
- If there is a **corrective saccade in a direction opposite to the head rotation**, it indicates a **vestibular lesion (peripheral or central)** on the side towards which the head is rotated. This occurs as the diseased vestibular system fails to produce the equal and opposite slow movements required to fixate on the target (reduced VOR gain). As the fovea moves away from the target in the direction of the rotation, a corrective saccade in opposite direction is produced to re-fixate the target
- If there is a **corrective saccade in the direction of head rotation**, it indicates that there is excessive VOR gain as in **cerebellar lesion**. Here, the compensatory slow movements overshoot the target in a direction opposite to head rotation. To refix the target on the fovea, the corrective saccades produced are in the direction of head rotation
- A central lesion is also suggested if the direction of corrective saccades is inappropriate to the direction of head rotation (e.g. during horizontal rotation, corrective saccades in vertical direction)
- A positive head impulse test with presence of skew deviation and bilateral GEN argues in favor of central lesion.

Caveats

- A bedside head impulse test may be negative when the vestibular deficits are partial. Therefore, only in a severely symptomatic patient, a negative head impulse test points to a central lesion.
- In chronic unilateral vestibular lesions, compensatory mechanisms may completely mask the abnormalities and head impulse test may be negative.

HEAD HEAVE TEST (TRANSLATIONAL VOR)

- It is analogous to the head impulse test, but evaluates the translational VOR
- It is a test of the function of the utricle
- An abrupt, high-acceleration lateral movement of the head (along the interaural axis) is produced while the patient fixes his vision on a close target such as the nose of the examiner
- The lateral excursion of the head need be no more than 3–4 cm
- corrective catch-up saccade indicates the tVOR is hypoactive
- Normal individuals usually show symmetrically hypoactive VOR with a corrective saccade in either direction
- Thus, only an asymmetric response is significant
- Positive head heave test becomes rapidly compensated unlike rotational VOR, which persists a long time (mostly permanent).

Visual Cancellation of the VOR

Physiologic Basis

- When the head is in motion and the VOR is in action, the latter has to be adequately inhibited in order to shift the direction of gaze to a target
- Structures that are concerned with smooth pursuit and eye-head tracking, which includes the flocculus/paraflocculus and the medial superior temporal area, frontal eye field, and dorsal pontine nuclei are involved in this VOR suppression/cancellation.

Methodology and Observations

- While seated on a rotating chair, subjects are asked to outstretch the arm forward with the thumb up and maintain fixation on the thumb
- Examiner initiates rotation of the chair and hence also the subjects' body from side to side
- If the VOR cancellation is impaired, the eyes will be continually taken off the target by slow phases of the VOR and corrective saccades will be made.

Interpretation

VOR cancellation is impaired in lesions involving structures listed above.

Dynamic Visual Acuity Test

Physiologic Basis

- The dynamic visual acuity test is especially useful for diagnosing bilateral vestibular failure. Here, most other tests may be inconclusive due to bilaterality of disease
- During headshaking, if there is bilateral vestibular dysfunction, VOR suppression may not adequate. Hence, the visual acuity deteriorates markedly during headshaking

- Specificity and sensitivity of DVA for detecting unilateral and **especially bilateral loss** is quite high.

Methodology and Observations
- Visual acuity is noted at rest using Snellen chart
- The examiner then manually oscillates the patient's head horizontally, vertically and laterally (ear to shoulder) at about 2 Hz, while the patient reads a Snellen visual acuity chart.

Interpretation
- If the visual acuity drops **by more than 2 lines**, it is abnormal
- This indicates that the VOR gain is abnormal
- DVA is degraded more during horizontal rotations toward the paretic than toward the healthy ear.

Caveats
- Patient may slow down at the end of each movement and be able to read the smaller letters, giving a false impression of good acuity. This must be prevented by instructing them not to slow down at any phase of the to and fro movement
- Normal individuals may lose up to one or two lines and this should not be overinterpreted as abnormal.

Box 11.1: Key maneuvers to elicit unilateral labyrinthine hypofunction.
- Subjective visual vertical (SVV) with bucket test: Deviation toward the side of lesion
- Eliminate fixation to look for spontaneous nystagmus: Slow phases directed toward the affected ear
- Head impulse test: There is an impaired slow phase when rotating toward the affected ear requiring a corrective saccade (opposite to the head movement)
- Horizontal head shaking: There is a horizontal nystagmus afterward (usually with a torsional component) with slow phases directed toward the affected ear
- Vibration over skull (mastoids and vertex): There is a nystagmus with slow phases directed toward the affected ear

Box 11.2: Lateral canal benign paroxysmal positional vertigo.
- Geotropic nystagmus: When supine with right of left ear down, nystagmus beats toward the ground (usually canalolitiasis)
- Apogeotropic nystagmus: When supine with right of left ear down, nystagmus beats away from the ground (cupulolithiasis or canalolithiasis)
- Side of pathology: When lying on the side is which the nystagmus is most intense the nystagmus will be beating toward the affected ear (i.e. geotropic with affected ear down and apogeotropic with affected ear up)
- Bow and lean test: When head upright or tilted straight back (bow), there is a spontaneous horizontal nystagmus which beats to normal side in geotropic and beats toward affected side in apogeotropic nystagmus. When head pitched forward (lean) the spontaneous nystagmus reverses direction

BIBLIOGRAPHY

1. Bertholon P, Bronstein AM, Davies RA, et al. Positional down beating nystagmus in 50 patients: cerebellar disorders and possible anterior semicircular canalithiasis. J Neurol Neurosurg Psychiatry. 2002; 72: 366-72.
2. Bronstein AM. Vestibular reflexes and positional maneuvers. J Neurol Neurosurg Psychiatry. 2003;74:289-93.
3. Fife TD, Tusa RJ, Furman JM, et al. Assessment: vestibular testing techniques in adults and children: report of therapeutics and technology assessment subcommittee of the American academy of Neurology. Neurology. 2000;55:1431-41.
4. Halmagyi GM, Cremer PD. Assessment and treatment of dizziness. J Neurol Neurosurg Psychiatry. 2000;68:129-34.
5. Kerber KA, Baloh RW. Dizziness, vertigo and hearing loss. In: Bradley WG, (Eds). Neurology in clinical practice. Butterworth Heinemann publishers, 5th edition; 2008.
6. Rinne T, Bronstein AM, Rudge P, et al. Bilateral loss of vestibular function. Acta Otolaryngol Suppl. 1995;520:247-50.
7. Young-Eun Huh, Ji-Soo Kim. Bedside evaluation of dizzy patients. J Clin Neurol. 2013;9:203-13.
8. Zee DS. Ophthalmoscopy in examination of patients with vestibular disorders. Ann Neurol. 1978;3:373.

CHAPTER 12

Autonomic Nervous System

GRK Sarma

PICTORIAL PRETEST

This young lady presented with recurrent episodes of syncope.

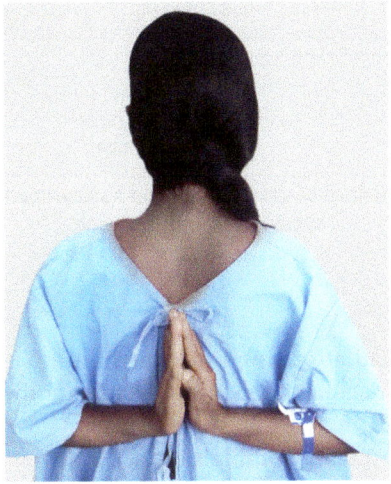

Questions

1. What is the sign that is demonstrated here?
2. What is its significance in a patient with syncope?

(Answers are discussed at the end of the chapter)

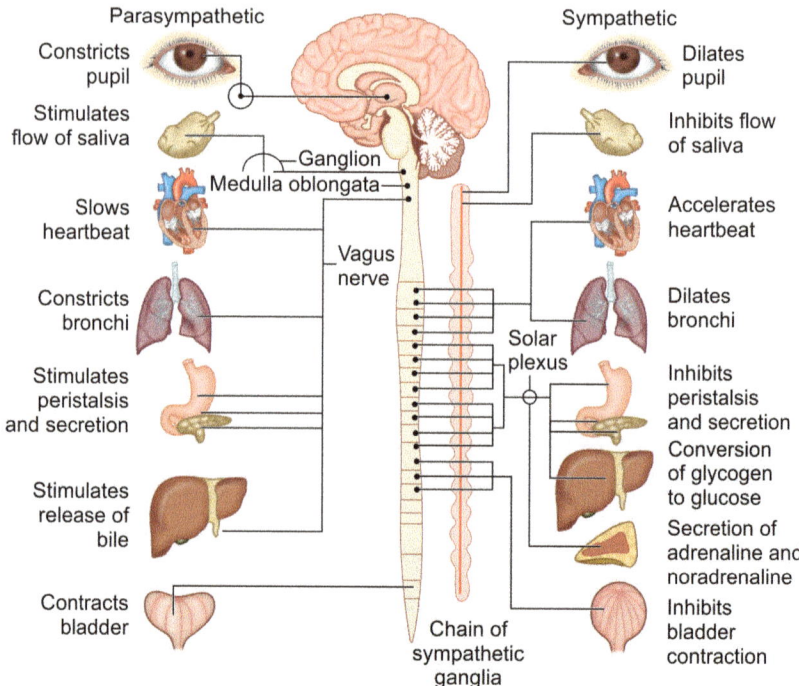

Fig. 12.1: Functions of sympathetic and parasympathetic nervous systems in various organs.

INTRODUCTION

- Techniques to evaluate autonomic function are numerous but only a limited number are considered to be suitable for routine bedside clinical application.
- Bedside screening tests complement a clinical evaluation in various neurological disorders, but are often ignored by clinicians.
- The role of the clinician is to perform a thorough evaluation of clinical autonomic symptoms, perform a bedside autonomic examination, and determine if there are any indications for formal autonomic function studies.

Methodology

The clinical methods of evaluation of autonomic system will be described under the following sections:
- History
- General physical examination
- Bedside autonomic tests

Historical Clues to Autonomic Dysfunction

- Many of the following symptoms are usually volunteered by patients, but dismissed as non-specific symptoms or psychogenic symptoms if the clinician is not tuned to keep autonomic disorders among the list of differential diagnoses.
- Conversely, sometimes, these symptoms are reported only when a direct question is asked by the clinician, as the patients attribute many of them to "general weakness".
- Thus, it is important to have a checklist of autonomic symptoms and try to elicit them in appropriate cases. A formal questionnaire like COMPASS 31 (composite autonomic symptom scale) includes these symptoms and has been found useful in autonomic nervous system assessment.
- A formal questionnaire like COMPASS 31 (composite autonomic symptom scale) includes these symptoms and has been found useful in autonomic nervous system assessment.

- Orthostatic intolerance:
  - Light headedness
  - Visual blurring
  - Coat hanger distribution pain
  - Confusion
  - Slurred speech
  - Nausea
  - Palpitations
  - Tremulousness
  - Loss of consciousness
  - Nocturia
- Orthostatic symptoms precipitated by:
  - Food intake (especially heavy carbohydrate meal)
  - Exercise
  - Prolonged bed rest
  - Hot water bath
  - Fever
  - Hot environment
  - Hyperventilation
  - Alcohol
- Skin:
  - Anhydrosis
  - Hyperhydrosis
  - Pain (glove and stocking type or patchy)
  - Loss of hair
  - Shininess and excess smoothness
  - Edema
  - Color change
  - Gustatory sweating
- Thermoregulatory:
  - Hypothermia
  - Hyperthermia
- Eyes:
  - Dry eyes
  - Foreign body sensation in the eyes
  - Visual blurring (accommodation difficulty)
- Mouth:
  - Dry mouth
  - Dental caries
- Gastrointestinal:
  - Constipation
  - Diarrhea
  - Postprandial bloating
  - Anorexia, weight loss
  - Fecal urgency, incontinence
- Genitourinary:
  - Urgency, incontinence
  - Retention
  - Nocturia
  - Recurrent urinary tract infection
  - Erectile dysfunction
  - Retrograde ejaculation
  - Vaginal dryness
- Non-autonomic symptoms relevant in autonomic disorders
  - Weight loss, cachexia (paraneoplastic syndrome)
  - Parkinsonism symptoms
  - Unsteadiness, falls (MSA)
  - Dysphagia, dysarthria (MSA)
  - Sleep disorder, REMBD (MSA)
  - Family history (familial dysautonomia)

General Physical Examination

- A thorough general examination often discloses relevant physical signs in autonomic disorders.

Skin:
- Dryness
- Reduced hand wrinkling
- Pallor
- Loss of hair on extremities
- Shininess of legs
- Edema of feet
- Abnormal sweating (increased or decreased)

Eyes:
- Dry eyes (more formally assessed by the Schirmer's test)
- Impaired pupillary reflexes
- Ptosis

Cardiovascular:
- Resting tachycardia
- Bradycardia
- Hypo/ hypertension

Gastrointestinal system:
- Dry mouth
- Dental changes (caries)
- Abdominal bloating
- Reduced anal tone

Genitourinary:
- Urinary urgency, incontinence
- Atonic bladder

Non-autonomic features relevant in autonomic dysfunction:
- Parkinsonism
- Ataxia
- Abnormal eye movements
- Joint hyperextensibility (association of Ehlers-Danlos syndrome with syncope)

- The following tests are elaborated further:
    - Schirmer's test
    - Joint hyperextensibility
    - Specific autonomic tests.

Schirmer's test

- The Schirmer test is used to test tear production
- The test is performed by instilling a topical anesthetic and then placing a thin strip of filter paper in the inferior cul-de-sac
- The corners of soft tissue may be used to wick all liquid from the inferior fornix by capillary attraction (i.e. without any wiping) before the paper is placed
- The patients' eyes are closed for 5 minutes, and the amount of wetting in the paper strip is measured
- Less than 5 mm of wetting is abnormal; 5-10 mm is equivocal
- The Schirmer's test is performed in 2 different ways
- The Schirmer I test, which measures both basic and reflex tearing, consists of the same test without the use of a topical anesthetic agent
- Less than 10 mm of wetting after 5 minutes is abnormal. The test is relatively specific, but it is poorly sensitive
- The Schirmer II test, which measures reflex tearing, may be done if the initial Schirmer test yields abnormal results
- It is similar to the basic secretion test, but with the addition of nasal mucosal irritation induced with a cotton tip applicator
- Wetting of less than 15 mm after 5 minutes is consistent with abnormalities of reflex secretion
- A positive Schirmer's test indicates xerophthalmia, which may be a component of Sjogren's syndrome.

Joint hyperextensibility
- An association between postural orthostatic tachycardia syndrome (POTS) and joint hypermobility has been reported.
- Causes of joint hypermobility include Ehlers-Danlos syndrome (EDS) and benign joint hyperextensibility syndrome (both with genetic basis)
- Thus, it is important to identify joint hyperextensibility in patients with dysautonomia, especially syncopes.
- A standard method of assessing joint hyperextensibility is to estimate the Beighton score.

The Beighton score

The Beighton score consists of a series of five tests, the results of which can add up to a total of nine points.

The score is worked out as follows:
- One point if the patient can place his palms on the ground while standing with legs straight
- One point for each elbow that bends backwards ≥15°
- One point for each knee that bends backwards
- One point for each thumb that touches the forearm when bent backwards
- One point for each little finger that bends backwards beyond 90°

If the Beighton score is four or more, it is likely that the patient has joint hypermobility. But, true joint hypermobility syndrome requires associated clinical symptoms and signs in addition to the score.

Specific bedside autonomic function tests
- The following categories of autonomic function tests are routinely performed in the laboratory, but only the first two categories will be elaborated, as they can be tested to a reasonable extent bedside:
    1. **Tests of cardiovagal innervation** (parasympathetic innervation): heart rate (HR) response on deep breathing, Valsalva ratio, and HR response to standing (30:15 ratio)
    2. **Tests of adrenergic innervation**: Beat-to-beat blood pressure (BP) responses to the Valsalva maneuver, sustained hand grip, and BP and HR responses to tilt-up or active standing.
    3. **Sudomotor tests**: QSART, SSR, TST
- Thus, three tests can be performed bedside:
    1. **Deep breathing**: Assess heart rate variation
    2. **Active standing**: Assess heart rate and blood pressure variation
    3. **Valsalva maneuver**: Assess heart rate and blood pressure variation

HEART RATE RESPONSE TO BREATHING

Methodology
- Heart rate variability is simple to record and measures are sensitive indicators of parasympathetic function.

- Cyclic deep breathing is the best validated stimulus; both afferent and efferent pathways are vagally mediated and blunted by anticholinergic agents
- Connect standard electrocardiography (ECG) leads to the patient and start recording
- Ask the patient to breathe deeply and slowly. The effect is maximal with 6 breaths per minute for 1–2 minutes (longer duration blunts the variability)
- At the end of the test, analyze the ECG and measure the longest and the shortest RR interval, and calculate the maximal and minimal heart rates
- A simple measure is the ratio of the minimal to maximal R-R interval differences (E: I ratio)
- One can also calculate the difference between maximum and minimum heart rates.

Interpretation

- Normally, the heart rate increases in inspiration and decreases in expiration
- The normal E: I ratio is ≥1.2 :1
- The normal difference between maximum and minimum heart rates is ≥15 beats per minute
- Reduced values of the above parameters indicate cardiovagal neuropathy.

BEDSIDE ORTHOSTATIC TEST (ACTIVE STANDING)

Physiological Basis

- Consensus group of the American Autonomic Society has defined OH as a reduction of SBP of at least 20 mm Hg or diastolic blood pressure (DBP) of at least 10 mm Hg within 3 minutes of standing
- With the assumption of an upright posture, there is a downward shift of approximately 500 mL of blood to the dependent areas (mainly abdomen and legs)
- This gravitational shift in blood results in decreased venous return, decreased cardiac output, and eventually decreased BP
- It is interesting to consider that standing BP at the level of the brain is near the lower limit of cerebral autoregulation
- This "unloads" the baroreceptors, both high-pressure baroreceptors in the aortic arch and carotid sinus, and low-pressure receptors in the heart and lungs
- These changes trigger a reflex sympathetic activation with a resultant increase in heart rate (HR) and systemic vasoconstriction (countering the initial decline in BP)
- In a healthy individual, the net effect of assumption of upright posture is an increase in HR of 10 to 20 bpm, a minimal change in systolic BP, and an approximately 5 mm Hg increase in diastolic BP

- In patients with orthostatic hypotension, the efferent limb of the baroreflex cannot be adequately engaged. This can result in a lack of sympathetically mediated vasoconstriction (and increase in vascular resistance) and a fixed HR, instead of the expected increased HR
- Together, this physiology results in a lack of counterregulation and a drop in BP and syncope or presyncope result.

Methodology

- Patient is made to rest in supine position for at least 5–10 minutes
- Heart rate and blood pressure are noted in this position. An ECG machine may be connected for measuring the respiratory rate (RR) interval variation, but is optional
- Patient assumes standing position with sphygmomanometer cuff in place
- Heart rate and blood pressure are noted immediately, 1 minute and 3 minutes after standing. Ideally, a recording after 5 minutes is also needed
- In some patients with Parkinsonism, it may be necessary to wait longer to demonstrate the autonomic insufficiency (up to 30 minutes in some)
- If the patient develops orthostatic intolerance during the active standing, the test is aborted and patient is placed in supine position again, after noting the heart rate and blood pressure.

Interpretation

- Normally, there is a slight or no fall in blood pressure (≤20 mm Hg SBP/10 mm Hg DBP) along with a slight increase in heart rate (11–30 beats per minute)
- 30:15 ratio (R-R interval at beat 30)/(R-R interval at beat 15) ≥ 1.04 indicates normal cardiovagal function
- In early autonomic dysfunction, there is a marked increase in heart rate that prevents a fall in blood pressure
- In moderate dysfunction, there is tachycardia and slight fall in blood pressure
- In severe dysfunction, the hypotension is progressively greater and the heart rate may fail to change much from the resting rate (cardiac denervation)
- In contrast, patients with POTS have excessive HR increases, commonly defined as a 30 beats per minute increase usually with a rate exceeding 120 beats per minute
- In autonomic failure, the BP and HR changes occur quickly, within 5 minutes
- In contrast, in vasovagal syncope, prolonged standing is often required, following which, there is an abrupt fall in BP along with reproduction of symptoms of presyncope/syncope

- If there is no orthostatic hypotension on standing, but the suspicion is strong for dysautonomia, the patient is re-tested soon after (within 1 hour of) a large meal or after 10 squats. If this is negative, clinically significant autonomic dysfunction is unlikely
- If these are all negative in a patient with suspected autonomic disorder, a formal autonomic laboratory testing is indicated.

VALSALVA MANEUVER

This provides information for both parasympathetic and sympathetic function if beat-to-beat HR and BP data are recorded.

Methodology

- Devices that noninvasively monitor continuous BP are typically used
- The subject blows into a closed tube at 40 mm Hg for 15 seconds while HR and BP are recorded. At bedside, patient may be asked to blow the mercury column of sphygmomanometer to 40 mm Hg, with the cuff tied over the arm
- If continuous BP measurement is not available, at least the post Valsalva overshoot in BP can be captured using the bedside sphygmomanometer. The valve is minimally opened so that active blowing of air is maintained
- For this, record the SBP just before the Valsalva maneuver, and without deflating the cuff, initiate the Valsalva. As the BP initially increases, inflate the cuff further to capture the maximum SBP. Inflate the cuff over and above this by 10 mm Hg and continue to auscultate over the brachial artery
- Just after the valsalva maneuver concludes, normally, the SBP overshoots the previous SBP to produce audible sounds
- Valsalva ratio: This ratio is derived from the maximal HR generated by the Valsalva maneuver divided by the lowest HR following the Valsalva maneuver.

Normal Response

The blood pressure waveform in response to Valsalva maneuver is divided into 4 distinct phases (I-IV).

Phase	Phase event	Major mechanism
I	Beginning of maneuver	Mechanical compression of great vessels
Early II	Blood pressure decreases	Reduced venous return, countered by vagal release
Late II	Blood pressure recovers Heart rate increases	Peripheral sympathetic vasoconstriction, vagal release
III	Brief fall in BP (<3 sec)	Decreased mechanical pressure
IV	Sustained BP overshoot	Maintained vasomotor and cardiac sympathetic tone

Abnormalities

- Abnormal responses may involve phase II or phase IV or both. Each has a different clinical significance
- If phase II is blunted, it suggests α-adrenergic insufficiency (phase II is primarily mediated by α-adrenergic activity). Phase IV also get blunted as the normal overshoot of BP cannot be produced by reduced peripheral vasoconstriction. The typical example for such a response is autonomic neuropathy of amyloidosis
- If phase IV is reduced, with no overshoot of BP, it suggests β-adrenergic insufficiency. This is the typical response seen in patients with orthostatic intolerance
- If the heart rate responses are impaired, it suggests parasympathetic insufficiency.

Caveats

- Leg muscle contraction necessary for active standing triggers an exercise reflex that transiently reduces BP that can mimic true, sustained orthostatic hypotension
- Pressure normally returns to baseline levels within 1 to 2 minutes but recovery can be delayed for 3 to 15 minutes in patients with mild orthostatic intolerance
- Some individuals have a robust exercise reflex with a marked acute, often symptomatic, BP decline that rapidly recovers without other abnormality; these patients are sometimes misdiagnosed to have orthostatic hypotension. Formal testing can separate these phenomena.

ANSWERS TO THE PRETEST

1. The sign demonstrated is one of joint hyperextensibility. The patient was able to internally rotate and extend the shoulders beyond the normal limits when asked to imitate 'namaste' posture behind her back. She also had hyperextensibility of thumbs, wrists and elbows.
2. Now, there is an increasingly recognized association between autonomic dysfunction, especially POTS, and joint hyperextensibility disorders (particulary Ehlers-Danlos syndrome). In one study, nearly 20% of patients with POTS had features of EDS.
   Nearly 30% of POTS patients are found to be positive of anti-ganglionic acetylcholine receptor (gAchR) antibodies, suggesting an autoimmune basis and treatment implications.

BIBLIOGRAPHY

1. Chowdhury D, Patel N. Approach to a case of autonomic peripheral neuropathy. JAPI. 2006;54:726-32.
2. Hollister A. Orthostatic hypotension—causes, evaluation, and management. Western J Med. 1992;157:652-57.

3. Lanier JB, Mote MB, Do; and Clay EC. Evaluation and management of orthostatic hypotension. Am Fam Physician. 2011;84(5):527-36.
4. Sletten DM, Suarez GA, Low PA, Mandrekar J, Singer W. COMPASS 31: a refined and abbreviated Composite Autonomic Symptom Score. Mayo Clinic Proceedings. 2012; 87(12):1196-201.
5. The Consensus Committee of the American Autonomic Society and the American Academy of Neurology. Consensus statement on the definition of orthostatic hypotension, pure autonomic failure, and multiple system atrophy. Neurology. 1996;46:1470.
6. Wallman D, Weinberg J, Hohler AD. Ehlers-Danlos syndrome and postural tachycardia syndrome: a relationship study. J Neurol Sci. 2014;340(1-2):99-102.
7. Watari M, Nakane S, et al. Autoimmune postural orthostatic tachycardia syndrome. Ann Clin Transl Neurol. 2018; 5(4): 486-92.
8. Weimer LH. Autonomic testing: common techniques and clinical applications. The Neurologist. 2010;16:215-22.

CHAPTER 13

Examination of a Patient with Neck Pain

GRK Sarma

PICTORIAL PRETEST

A 65-year-old man presented with chronic neck pain in the following distribution (Fig. 13.1). The pain was mild to moderate and is brought on and increased after walking for 10 minutes, and relieved by rest. Mostly, he is forced to rest because of the pain. There was no associated chest pain or diaphoresis.

He is a known to have poorly controlled diabetes mellitus with end organ involvement including nephropathy and peripheral neuropathy. His cervical spine was non-tender, with nearly normal range of movements. There were no neurological deficits to suggest cervical radiculopathy or myelopathy. His MRI cervical spine showed mild disc bulges at multiple cervical levels without significant root or cord compression. His cardiac evaluation was normal including electrocardiography (ECG), echocardiography and treadmill test. In the latter, the patient developed the habitual neck pain without ECG changes.

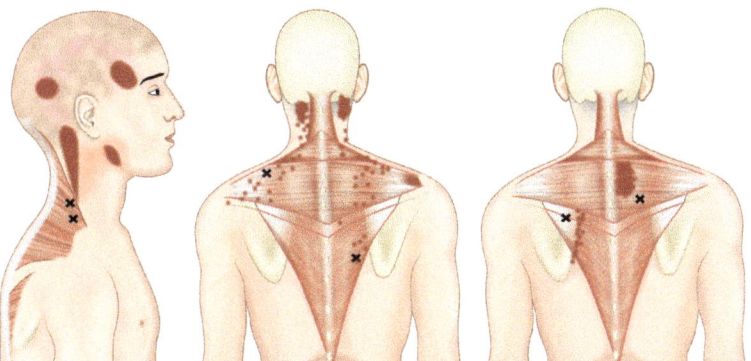

Fig. 13.1: Pain distribution in a 65-year-old man, precipitated by walking.

Questions

1. What is the source of the neck pain in this patient?
2. What is this distribution of pain known as?

3. Which bedside or laboratory test may confirm the diagnosis?
(Answers are discussed at the end of the chapter)

EXAMINATION OF A PATIENT WITH NECK AND ARM PAIN (FIGS. 13.2 TO 13.5)

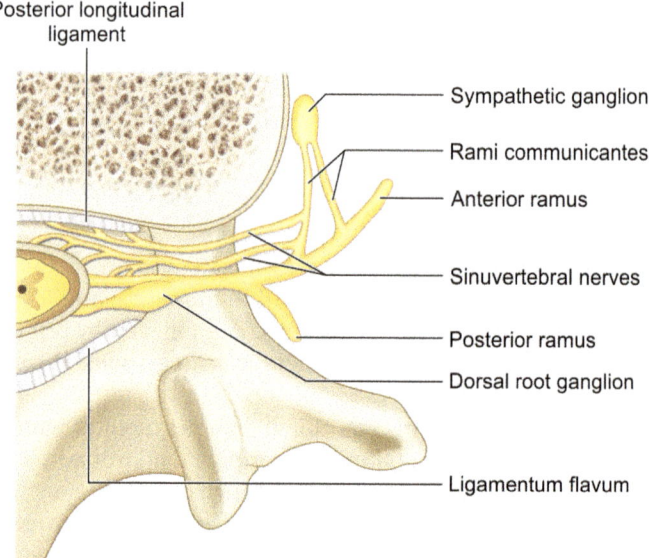

Fig. 13.2: Spinal nerve roots and their branches.

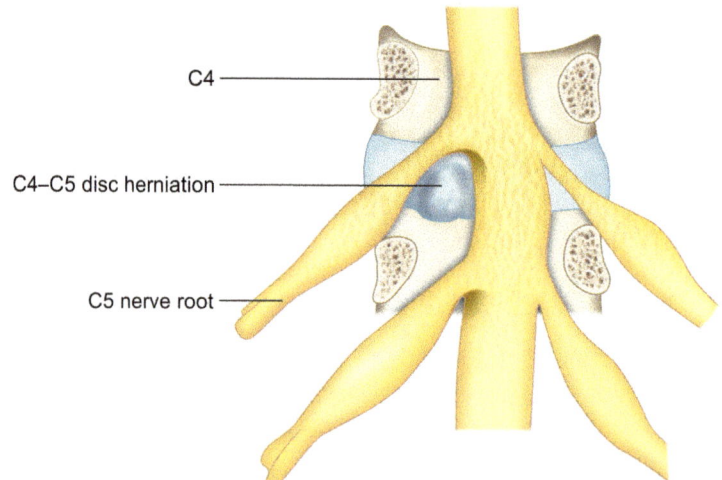

Fig. 13.3: Relation between the vertebral level and the root level in the cervical spine.

Examination of a Patient with Neck Pain

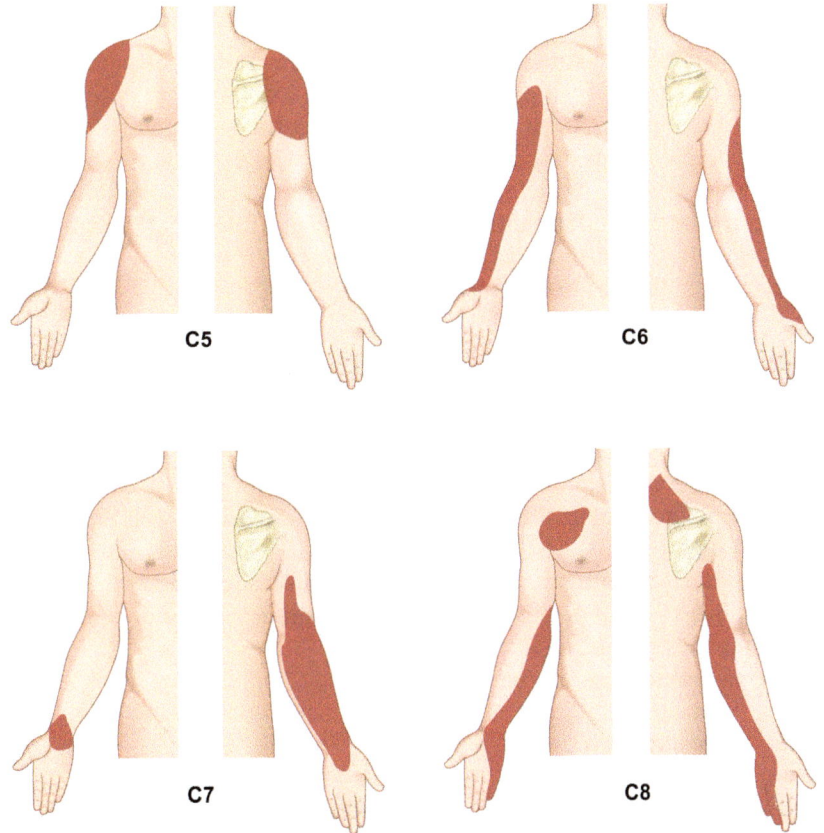

Fig. 13.4: Distribution of radiating pain in radiculopathy at various levels.

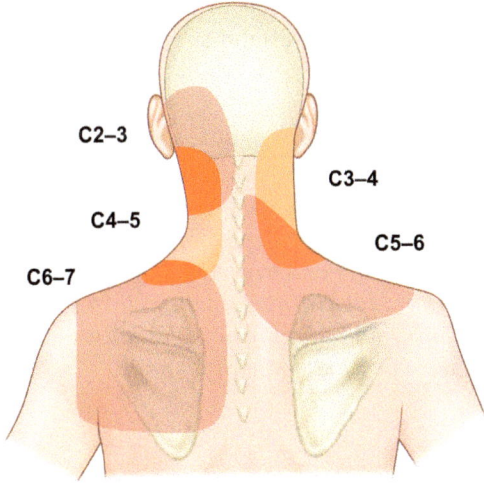

Fig. 13.5: Local pain distribution in disc disease at various levels.

Physiologic Basis

Certain anatomical factors are important in understanding the pathogenesis of spinal disease as well as the variability in its clinical manifestations. Some of the more important anatomical factors are described below. For a comprehensive review of spinal anatomy, please see the references.
- The mid-sagittal diameter of the cervical spinal canal is an important parameter in understanding pathogenesis of cervical compressive myelopathy. Its normal values are as follows:
  - C1-3: 21 mm (16–30 mm)
  - C4-7: 18 mm (14–23 mm)
  - The cervical cord occupies 40% of the diameter of the spinal canal.
- With neck extension, the diameter decreases by 2–3 mm and can cause cord compression in the already diseased spine (e.g. spondylosis/congenital canal stenosis).
- Neck hyperextension can also compromise the anterior spinal artery by the same mechanism and cause ischemic cord injury as well as vertebral artery dissection.
- Neck pain is a common symptom of various disease processes that involve the spine. To evaluate this symptom in a systematic way, understanding its pathogenesis is important.
- The pain sensitive structures of spine are:
  - Skin
  - Subcutaneous tissue
  - Adipose tissue
  - Ligaments (longitudinal spinal, interspinous, flaval)
  - Periosteum
  - Epidural fibrofatty tissue
  - Dura
  - Arterioles
  - Veins (epidural and paravertebral)
  - Paravertebral muscles
  - Nerve roots
  - Diseases involving any of the above structures can cause neck pain.

Notably absent from the list is the inter-vertebral disc, which has no significant nociceptive fibers. When the herniated disc comes into contact with ventral root, painless weakness can result. When it contacts the sinuvertebral nerves in the posterior ligaments and the dura of the nerve root sleeve, pain is produced. This explains why a prolapsed disc can: (a) be painless, (b) cause non-radiating pain, (c) cause radicular pain, and (d) cause radicular weakness with or without pain.

Classifications

Neck pain may be classified as **radiating, non-radiating and referred pain**. Each of these pain types has a different source and a different nerve supply.

Non-radiating Neck Pain

- It is presumed to be due to musculoligamentous injury and degenerative changes.
- It is mediated by the **posterior primary ramus** and the recurrent meningeal nerves (**sinuvertebral nerves**) (Figure 13.2).
    - The **posterior rami** provide sensory fibers to fascia, ligaments, periosteum and facet joints.
    - The **sinuvertebral nerves** innervate the degenerated intervertebral discs, anterior and posterior longitudinal ligaments, dura mater and blood vessels.
- The usual areas where non-radiating pain is reported by patients with disc lesions at various levels are depicted in the Figure 13.4.
- Salient differences between the non-radiating pain and radiating pain are listed in the (Table 13.1).
- Another important cause of neck pain (the so called "**coat hanger**" pain) is orthostatic hypotension. The mechanism is ischemia of the cervical structures in erect posture. It is often mistaken for "spondylotic pain" with unsuccessful management strategies. It is brought on by prolonged standing or exercise in patients with autonomic insufficiency.

Radiating Neck Pain

- It is mediated by the spinal nerves
- It originates from mechanical compression or inflammation
- Inflammation is partly immunologic (due to exposure of the herniated nucleus pulposus to immune system) and partly neurogenic
- The distribution of radiating pain with root compression at different levels is shown in the Figure 13.4.

Table 13.1: Differences between radicular and musculoskeletal pains.

Parameter	Radicular pain	Musculoskeletal pain
Quality of pain	Sharp, lancinating	Deep aching pain
Location	Along dermatomal distribution	Paraspinal region
Spread	Along dermatomal pattern	Shoulder, scapula, upper arm only
Duration	Lasts days to weeks	Lasts 1–3 months
Diurnal variation	Worse on waking up	Worse as the day passes
Effect of Valsalva	Worsens or reproduces	Remains localized
Neurological deficits	Often present	Absent

Referred Pain

- It is poorly defined and often cramping type of pain
- Its precipitating and relieving factors provide a clue to the organ that is generating the pain.
- It is usually referred to midback or low back, and rarely to cervical level.
- Some possible causes include: Myocardial ischemia, aortic dissection, etc.

Methodology

The clinician must aim to find physical tests that reproduce each of the patient's symptoms.

Inspection

The following signs may be looked for:
- Head tilt
- Neck deformity
- Restricted neck movements
- Visible spasm of the paraspinal muscles
- Long droopy neck

Note the distribution pattern of pain as described by the patient as it has a localizing value (Table 13.1).

Palpation

- Tenderness
- Range of neck movements
- Trigger points.

Neuromechanical Tests

Spurling test (formainal compression test)(Fig. 13.6):
- Tilt the head to the side of the arm pain
- Compress the head downwards
- Pain and paresthesia radiating down the ipsilateral arm suggest its root compression.
- The sensitivity of this test is reported as 40–60% while specificity is 90–100% for cervical radiculopathy.
- Caveats:
  - This test does not indicate the etiology, though prolapsed disc is the most common one
  - In some patients, pain and paresthesia may radiate down the contralateral limb due to stretching of the compressed root on that side.

Arm abduction test (Relief sign): It was also described by Spurling.
- Reduced nerve root tension is the possible cause for symptom relief with shoulder abduction
- Method: Active abduction of symptomatic arm, placing patient's hand on head.
- Positive test is relief or reduction of ipsilateral cervical radicular symptoms.
- Sensitivity of 40–50%, specificity of 80–100% for cervical radiculopathy have been reported.

Traction test (opposite of the Spurling test):
- Patient is usually placed in supine position
- Hold the patient's head in both hands, with one hand under the chin and the other below the occiput
- Gently lift the head away from the fixed trunk
- Relief of pain and paresthesia suggests root compression
- Sensitivity of 40% and specificity of 80% have been reported.

Valsalva test: Increase in pain on Valsalva maneuver suggests that the intrathecal pressure is being transmitted to the compressed/inflamed nerve root.

Lhermitte's test:
- Patient is seated comfortably
- Flex the neck of the patient as much as possible
- Pain and paraesthesia radiating down the back or to the arms is abnormal
- Positive Lhermitte's test suggests posterior column disease as in B_{12} deficiency and multiple sclerosis. It is also seen in compressive lesions of the cord
- The sensitivity and specificity of this sign have not been systematically evaluated.

Trigger points:
(See the chapter on Trigger Points)

Facet joint:
Cervical facet syndrome includes following symptoms and signs:
- Axial neck pain (rarely radiating past the shoulders), most common unilaterally
- Pain with and/or limitation of extension and rotation
- Tenderness upon palpation
- Palpate along the paravertebral regions and directly over the transverse processes because the facet joints are not truly palpable.

Adson's test:
- Has been described as a sign of cervical rib or scalenus anticus syndrome
- Its utility has been discussed in Adson's review of 169 surgically treated cases
- However, there are no other studies on the sensitivity or specificity of this test.

Method:
- The patient's head is rotated to face the tested shoulder
- The patient then extends the head
- The examiner laterally rotates and extends the patient's shoulder
- The examiner locates the radial pulse, and the patient is instructed to take a deep breath and hold it.

- A disappearance of the pulse is indicative of a positive test
- About 80–90% of patients with positive Adson's test had good relief after surgical treatment in the above series.

Neurological Examination

i. Muscle power in myotomal pattern
ii. Sensory examination in dermatomal pattern
iii. Sensory level and sacral sparing or involvement
iv. Deep tendon reflexes
v. Abdominal reflexes, plantar reflexes, cremasteric reflexes (see respective chapters)
vi. Autonomic signs
vii. Signs that indicate additional supraspinal or extraspinal lesion: Even in a patient with neck pain and a clear radicular pain, it is useful to check the following signs. Sometimes, there could be an unrelated brain lesion (multi-infarct state in an elderly man with neck pain due to spondylosis) or a related brain lesion (demyelinating plaques in brain in addition to cord lesion).
    - Jaw jerk
    - Palmomental reflex
    - Snout reflex
    - Pout reflex
    - Extrapyramidal signs
    - Scalp tenderness
    - Temporal artery tenderness
    - Temporomandibular joint tenderness.

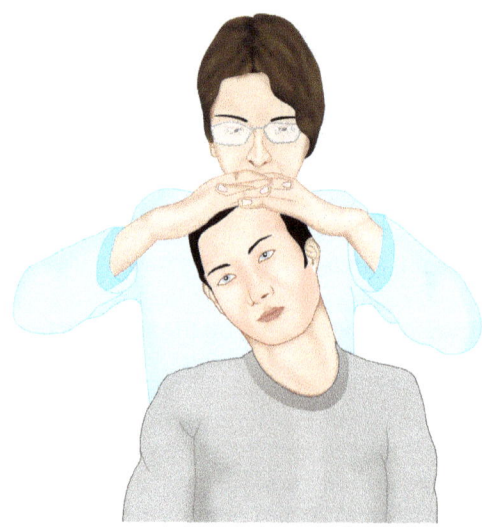

Fig. 13.6: Spurling test.

Caveats

In many instances, the pain may not be clearly localized to the source of its origin, inspite of various clinical symptoms and signs. In such cases which are not improving with therapy, a neuroimaging is warranted.

ANSWERS TO PRETEST

The pain distribution is called "coat hanger" headache. It is described in orthostatic hypotension and is believed to be due to ischemia of the cervical and cranial structures in erect position and walking. In this patient, local causes were excluded by clinical examination and normal MRI. Referred pain from myocardial ischemia is a concern, but a treadmill test was negative for inducible ischemia, inspite of pain reproduction.

Bedside measurement of BP and pulse rate are the initial steps in the diagnosis. Formal autonomic function tests with head up tilt may be very informative. His autonomic function studies revealed significant postural drop of blood pressure and a failure of compensatory tachycardia. He improved significantly with elastic compression stockings and fludrocortisone.

BIBLIOGRAPHY

1. Adson AW. Cervical ribs: symptoms, differential diagnosis, and indications for section of the insertion of the scalenus anticus muscle. J Internat Coll Surg. 1951; 16:546-59.
2. Devereaux MW. Anatomy and examination of the spine. Neurol Cli. 2007;25:331351.
3. Fast A, Parikh S, Marin EL. The shoulder abduction relief sign in cervical radiculopathy. Arch Phys Med Rehabil. 1989;70:402-3.
4. Malanga GA, Landes P, Nadler SF. Provocative tests in cervical spine examination: Historical basis and scientific analyses. Pain Physician. 2003;6:199-205.
5. Sandmark H, Nisell R. Validity of five common manual neck pain provoking tests. Scand J Rehab Med. 1995;27:131-6.
6. Viikari-Juntura E, Porras M, Laasonen EM. Validity of clinical tests in the diagnosis of root compression in cervical disease. Spine. 1989;14:253-7.
7. Viikari-Juntura E. Interexaminer reliability of observations in physical examinations of the neck. Phys Ther. 1987;67:1526-32.

CHAPTER 14

Examination of a Patient with Low Back Pain

GRK Sarma

PHYSIOLOGICAL BASIS

A thorough knowledge of the anatomy and physiology of the lumbosacral spine is essential in the diagnosis and treatment of patients with low back pain.

Vertebrae (Fig. 14.1)

- Lumbar vertebrae are large because of their weight bearing function
- Central spinal canal is small and triangular
- Unlike the cervical vertebrae, they lack the foramina in the transverse processes (meant for the vertebral artery)
- Unlike the thoracic vertebrae, they lack the articulating facets (meant for the ribs)
- The intervertebral foramen is bounded by the pedicles of the superior and inferior vertebrae at that level
- Facet joints are synovial joints formed by the superior and inferior facets of the adjacent vertebrae. Facet joint disease is an important cause of low back pain and is clinically and radiologically under-diagnosed (Fig. 14.2).
- The intervertebral disc acts as a shock absorber and dissipates the mechanical stress.

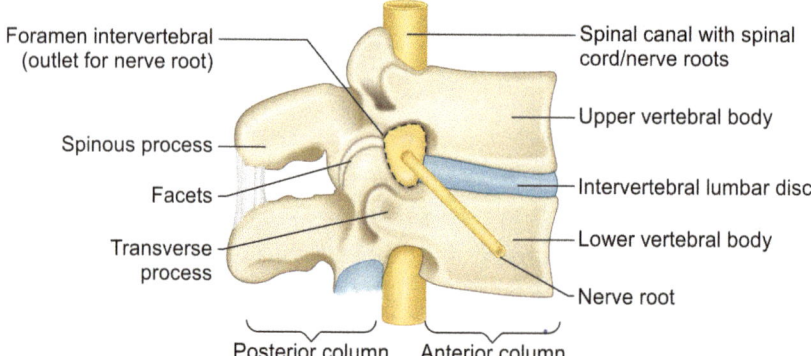

Fig. 14.1: Normal motion segment (two adjacent vertebrae, disc and ligaments) of the lumbar spine.

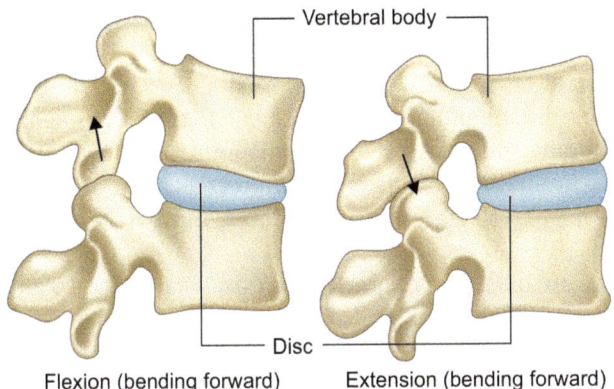

Fig. 14.2: Facet joints in motion.

Note the size of the intervertebral foramen during flexion and extension to understand the reflex guarding posture adopted by patients with disc prolapse. However, flexion increases the intradiscal pressure and extension reduces it. These changes contribute to the aggravation or relief of pain in various spinal disease processes (see Table 14.1).

Ligaments

- A strong anterior longitudinal ligament is attached to the anterior surface of the vertebral bodies
- A weaker posterior longitudinal ligament runs along the posterior surface of the vertebral bodies
- The ligament flava (yellow ligaments) connect the lamina
- The supraspinal ligament connects the tips of the spinous processes
- The intraspinal ligaments connect the adjacent spinous processes from their roots to their tips.

Nerve Roots and Spinal Cord in Relation to Vertebrae (Fig. 14.3)

- At birth, the tip of the cord is at the upper border of L3 vertebra
- By age 5 years, it is at the level of L2 vertebra
- By 12 years, it is at the lower border of L1 vertebra
- Each nerve root travels in a slanted manner to reach the intervertebral foramen below its corresponding vertebral body level. For example, L4 root exits between L4 and L5 level, while L5 root exits between L5 and S1 level
- The direction of the disc herniation (lateral/far lateral/medial/extrusion-migration) determines which root(s) will be compressed.
- In lateral disc herniation at a particular level, the root of the lower level will be compressed. For example, L4-5 disc herniation will compress the L5 root, while L5-S1 disc herniation involves S1 root.

- In far lateral herniation, the upper level root can also be compressed. Thus, a disc herniation at L4-5 level will compress both L5 and L4 roots. A disc herniation at L5-S1 level will compress both S1 and L5 roots. Failure to remember this anatomic relation may lead to erroneous decision making in the operative treatment of disc herniations
- In medial herniation, the disc can compress all the roots below that level. For example, L5-S1 disc herniation can compress S1 as well as S2, 3, 4 roots
- If a disc is extruded and migrates upwards, it can trap two adjacent roots at that level. For example, L4-5 disc herniation and upward migration can involve L4 and L5 roots.

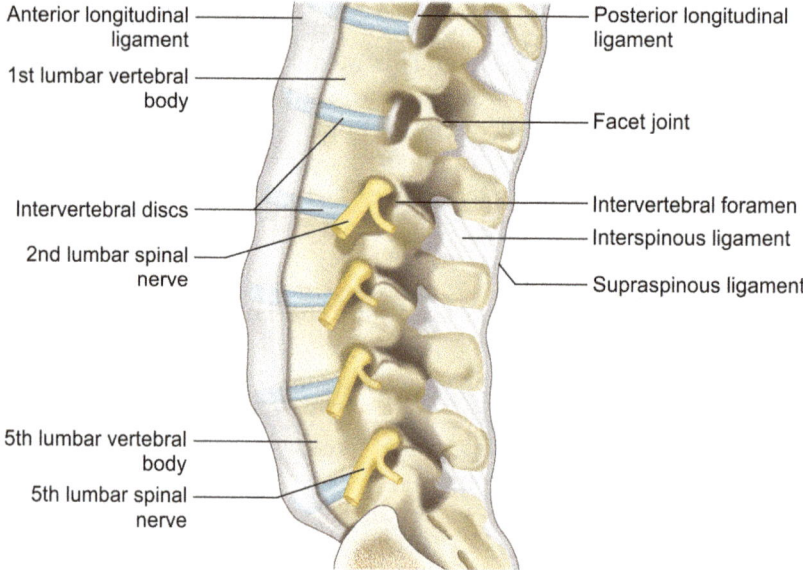

Fig. 14.3: Left lateral view of lumbar spine.

Myotomes

Certain general principles are extremely useful in remembering the apparently complex myotomes of the lower limbs. If one remembers that hip flexion is innervated by L2, 3, one can synthesize the innervations of the entire lower limb (Fig. 14.4).
- Each joint movement is innervated by two adjacent myotomes (e.g. hip flexion, adduction, internal rotation by L2, 3)
- The opposite movement at that joint is by the next two segments (e.g. hip extension, abduction, external rotation: L4, 5)
- Movement at the next joint is by **one** lower segment than the proximal joint (e.g. hip flexion L2, 3; knee extension: L3, 4)

- The following table can be worked out in this systematic fashion:

Table 14.1: Organization of myotomes of the lower limb.

Joint	Agonist movement	Myotomes	Antagonist movement	Myotomes
Hip	Flexion	L2, 3	Extension	L4, 5
	Adduction	L2, 3	Abduction	L4, 5
	Internal rotation	L2, 3	External rotation	L4, 5
Knee	Extension	L3, 4	Flexion	L5, S1
Ankle	Dorsiflexion	L4, 5	Plantar flexion	S1, 2
Great toe	Dorsiflexion	L5	Plantar flexion	S1, 2
Other toes	Intrinsic muscles	S1, 2, 3		

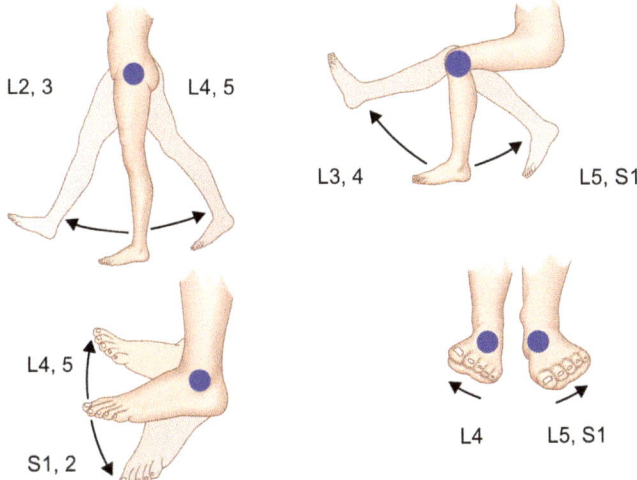

Fig. 14.4: Complex myotomes of the lower limbs. Each joint movement consists of 4 consecutive spinal nerves.

Dermatomes

- The dermatomes of the human body have been well known (Fig. 14.5A)
- Often, the sensory loss does not match entirely with the whole dermatome due to overlap of adjacent dermatomes
- A knowledge of "autonomous" sensory zones (i.e. areas innervated exclusively by a particular dermatome) helps in better localization (Figs. 14.5A and B).

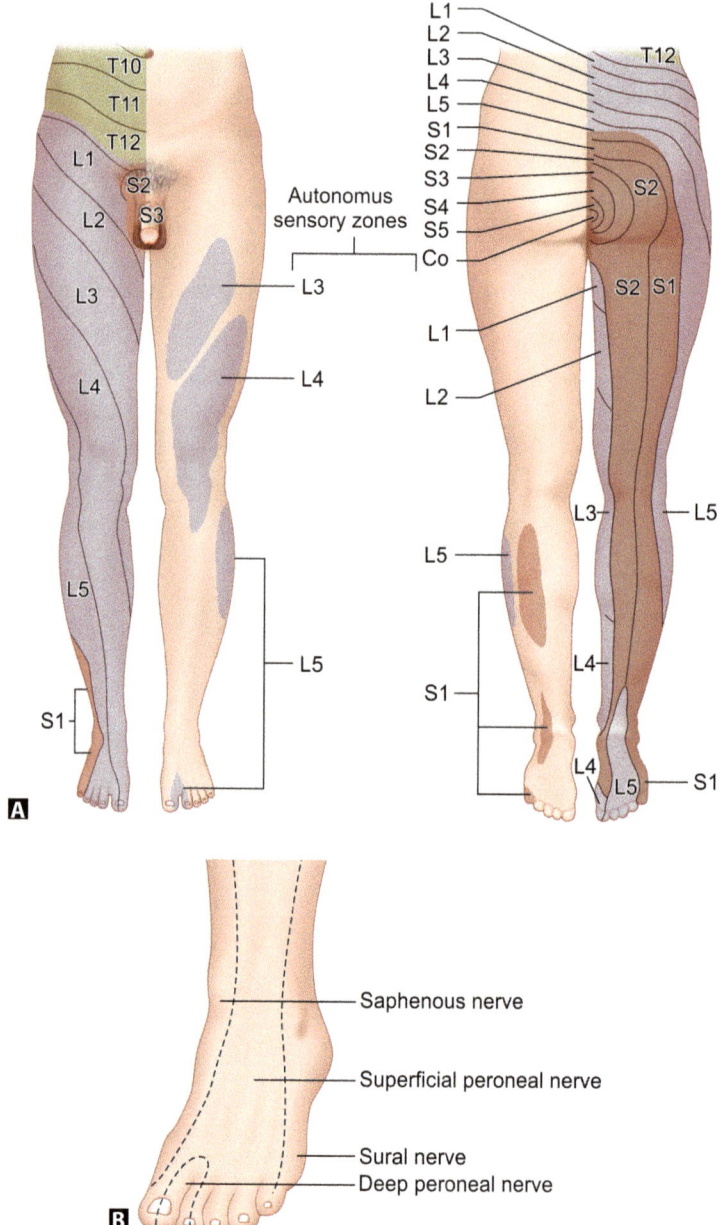

Figs. 14.5A and B: Dermatomes. (A) Schematic demarcation of dermatomes (according to Keegan and Garrett) shown as distinct segments in the right lower limb. There is actually considerable overlap between any two adjacent dermatomes. An alternative dermatomes map is that provided by Foerster is shown in the left lower limb; (B) Peripheral nerve innervation of the foot.

EXAMINATION

Posture

Examine in standing, sitting, supine and prone positions.

Standing

- Body build
- Posture
    - *Kyphosis*: Typically seen in chronic spinal canal stenosis due to degenerative spinal disease. Flexion of the spine increases the spinal canal diameter (Fig. 14.7)
    - *Loss of lordosis*: Secondary to paraspinal muscle spasm
    - *Scoliosis*: Lateral flexion increases the diameter of intervertebral foramen. Thus, the spine is lateral-flexed to the side opposite to the herniated disc that causes formainal compromise.
- Deformities
    - Gibbus
    - Step sign of listhesis
    - Spine alignment
- Percuss over the spinous processes for tenderness as in disc prolapse.
- Palpate for muscle spasm
- Trigger zones
- Myofascial nodules
- Sacroiliac tenderness
- Walking on heels
- Walking on toes detects mild weakness of gastro-soleus muscle that cannot be identified by the manual testing of plantar flexion
- Trendelenburg sign assesses hip abductors (gluteus medius, L5, S1 roots, superior gluteal nerve): Patient is asked to stand on one leg. Normal pelvis remains at level or tilts upwards on the unsupported side. Its tilting downwards indicates ipsilateral hip abduction weakness
- Test spinal movement for flexion, extension, rotation, lateral flexion: Passive extension of spine reproduces pain of IVDP. Lateral flexion to the side of the disease reproduces the pain.

Sitting

Straight leg raising in sitting position (methodology described below).

Supine

- Straight leg raising test: Flex the hip and then extend the knee with foot dorsiflexed. Painful limitation of the knee extension beyond 60° is abnormal, indicative of sciatic nerve stretch
- Measure the leg length
- Palpate the peripheral pulses.

Prone

- Examine the spine extension
- Palpate for muscle spasm and local tenderness.

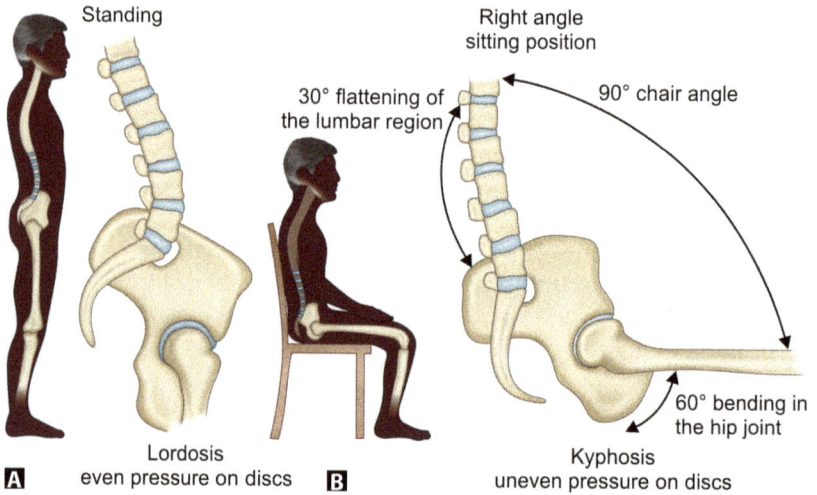

Figs. 14.6A and B: Pain arising from a herniated disc worsens on sitting and is better on standing.

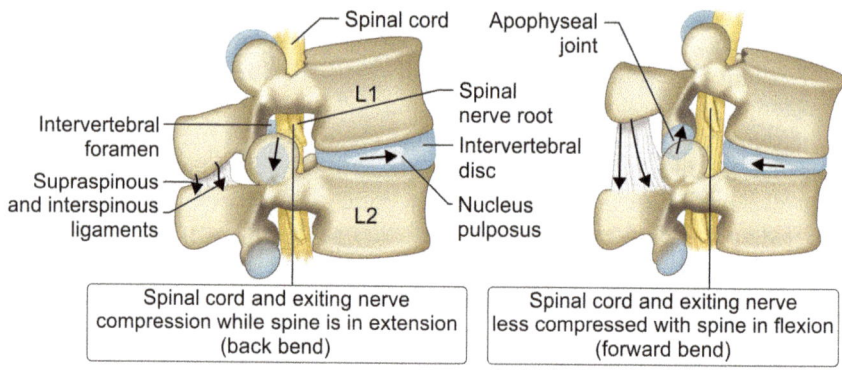

Fig. 14.7: Pain in chronic degenerative spinal canal stenosis behaves in opposite way, decreasing on sitting (due to spinal flexion) and increasing on standing (due to spinal extension).

Supine Straight Leg Raising Test

- Patient in supine position, with knee extended
- Slowly raise one leg, with knee extended, until pain is reported along the back and radiating pain along the leg.

- At this point, dorsiflex the foot or the great toe to stretch the lumbar roots as evidenced by aggravation of the pain (Spurling's sign).

INTERPRETATION

- Ability to raise the leg beyond 70° is considered normal in most individuals
- Pain at less than 30° is unusual and may raise suspicion of non-organic pain
- Inability to raise to less than 70° indicates either lumbar disc disease or hip joint disease
- These two are differentiated by raising the leg with knee in flexed position. This is still limited with hip disease but not with lumbar root disease.
- Crossed SLR, i.e. pain on diseased side when the healthy leg is raised, is highly suggestive of root disease.

Seated Straight Leg Raise

- Patient is seated in a chair with knees flexed and feet on the ground
- One knee is slowly extended until pain is reported in the back and radiating along the leg
- In true radicular pain, the supine and seated SLR reproduce the radiating pain
- If patient reports pain in supine SLR but can perform seated SLR, it suggests non-organic pain.

Reverse Straight Leg Raise

- Patient in prone position
- Move the knee gradually to maximum flexion
- Alternatively, pull up the extended knee to passively extend the hip
- Pain in the back or in the femoral nerve distribution indicates ipsilateral upper lumbar root disease.

INTERPRETATION

Pain suggestive of claudication can be of vascular or neurogenic origin. These can be differentiated clinically as shown in Table 14.2 (see Nadeau et al. for a detailed validation study). This is important because, presence of lumbar spinal stenosis on MRI correlates poorly with clinical picture. Similarly, all patients with abnormal indices on arterial Doppler do not necessarily have vasogenic claudication. Some patients can have both types of pain. Hence, clinical correlation is of utmost importance. Comparison of pain from herniated disc, lateral recess stenosis and spinal canal stenosis is discussed in Table 14.3.

Table 14.2: Similarities and differences between neurogenic and vasogenic claudication.

Feature	Neurogenic claudication	Vasogenic claudication
Location of pain	Above knees, up to buttocks, often bilateral	Below knees
Standing	Triggers pain	Relieves pain
Bending forward (shopping cart sign)	Relieves pain	No effect
Trigger	Standing/walking	Walking
Relief	Sitting	Standing
Claudication distance	Variable	Constant
Subjective weakness	May be present	May be present
Cramping pain	May be present	May be present

Table 14.3: Comparison of pain from herniated disc, lateral recess stenosis and spinal canal stenosis.

	Herniated disc	Lateral recess stenosis	Spinal canal stenosis
Age	30–50 years	>60 years	>60 years
Maneuvers aggravating the pain	Sitting, spinal flexion, coughing, straining	Standing, walking, spinal extension or ipsilateral flexion	Standing, walking, spinal extension
Maneuvers relieving the pain	Standing, lying down, spinal extension	Sitting, spinal flexion, lying down	Sitting, spinal flexion, stooping, lying down
SLR	Usually positive	Usually negative	Usually negative

- In a patient with foot drop, it is important to clinically localize the possible lesion to the peroneal nerve or sciatic nerve or L5 root lesion (Table 14.4).

Table 14.4: Differential diagnosis of foot drop.

	Peroneal neuropathy	Sciatic nerve palsy	L5 radiculopathy
Back pain	No	May be	May be
Radiating pain	No	May be	May be
Foot dorsiflexion	Weak	Weak	Weak
Foot plantar flexion	Normal	Weak / normal (partial injuries)	Normal
Foot eversion	Weak	Weak	Weak
Foot inversion	Normal	Weak	Weak
Hip abduction	Normal	Normal	Weak
Sensory loss	Dorsum of the foot	Dorsal and plantar aspect of the foot and leg (below knee)	Dorsum of foot and lateral shin

BIBLIOGRAPHY

1. Borczuk P. An evidence-based approach to the evaluation and treatment of low back pain in the emergency department. Emerg Med Pract. 2013;15(7):1-23.
2. Brazis PW, Masdeu JC, Biller J. Localization in clinical Neurology, 6th edition. Philadelphia: Wolters Kluwer/ Lippincott Williams & Wilkins, 2011.
3. Campbell WW. DeJong's The Neurologic examination, 7th edition. Wolters Kluwer/ Lippincott Williams & Wilkins; 2013.
4. Golob AL, Wipf JE. Low back pain. Med Clin North Am. 2014;98(3):405-28.
5. Kinkade S. Evaluation and treatment of acute low back pain. Am Fam Physician. 2007;75(8):1181-8.
6. Manusov EG. Evaluation and diagnosis of low back pain. Prim Care. 2012;39(3):471-9.
7. Nadeau M, Patricia Rosas-Arellano M, et al. The reliability of differentiating neurogenic claudication from vascular claudication based on symptomatic presentation. Can J Surg. 2013;56(6):Vol. 56, No. 6, December 2013: 372-77.
8. Patrick N, Emanski E, Knaub MA. Acute and chronic low back pain. Med Clin North Am. 2014;98(4):777-89.
9. Wheeler AH. Diagnosis and management of low back pain and sciatica. Am Fam Physician. 1995;52(5):1333-41.

CHAPTER 15

Examination of Other Joints

GRK Sarma

SHOULDER JOINT

Introduction
- Shoulder joint pain often overlaps with neck pain due to cervical spine disease
- It may be perceived over a distance away from the source and can cause errors in diagnosis
- In this chapter, some methods of examining the shoulder joint are described to minimize these errors.

Physiologic Basis
- The shoulder is composed of the humerus, glenoid, scapula, acromion, clavicle and surrounding soft tissue structures.
- The shoulder region includes the glenohumeral joint, the acromioclavicular joint, the sternoclavicular joint and the scapulothoracic articulation.
- The glenohumeral joint capsule consists of a fibrous capsule, ligaments and the glenoid labrum.
- Static joint stability is provided by the joint surfaces and the capsulolabral complex, and dynamic stability by the rotator cuff muscles and the scapular rotators (trapezius, serratus anterior, rhomboids and levator scapulae) (Fig. 15.1).

Examination scheme includes:
   A. Inspection
   B. Palpation
   C. Range of movement assessment
   D. Rotator cuff testing
   E. Provocative testing

A. Inspection
The following observations need to be made:
- *Atrophy:* Supraspinatus and infraspinatus atrophy suggests rotator cuff tear or suprascapular nerve lesion

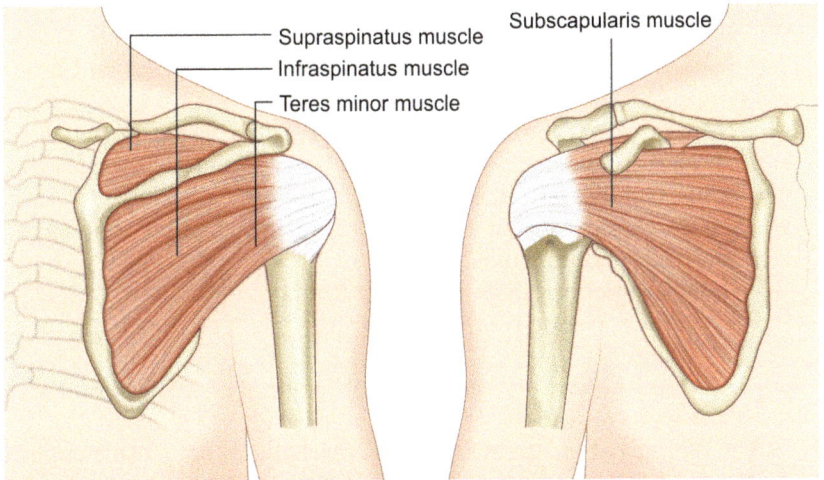

Fig. 15.1: Muscles of the rotator cuff.

- *Change in contour:* Squaring of the shoulder suggests anterior dislocation.
- *Swelling:* Suggests inflammation.
- *Winging of scapula:* Suggests trapezius or serratus weakness, but is also seen in shoulder instability.
- Range of movements in cardinal directions should be assessed.

B. Palpation

- *Palpate the following structures and look for tenderness or deformity:*
    - Acromioclavicular joint
    - Sternoclavicular joints
    - Glenohumeral joint
    - Coracoid process
    - Acromion
    - Scapula
    - Cervical spine
    - Biceps tendon.
- *Drop-arm sign:* Abduct the shoulder to 90° and release the arm, asking the patient to lower it gradually. This elicits severe pain in supraspinatus tendonitis
- *Rent test to feel the torn rotator cuff through the deltoid:*
    - Patient is seated and relaxed
    - Examiner stands behind patient
    - Elbow to be flexed to 90°
    - Palpate anterior margin of the acromion through the deltoid
    - Grasp the patient's arm one hand at the elbow/forearm and bring into extension
    - Passively internally and externally rotate patients arm to palpate rotator cuff tendons
    - Feel for prominent eminence of greater tuberosity or a sulcus (rent)
    - Either of these findings suggest full-thickness tear.

C. Range of Movement Assessment

- Test in flexion, extension, abduction, adduction, medial and lateral rotation, circumduction
- Check the range of movement in both active and passive movements. If active range of movements is less than the passive range, it is suggestive of neuromuscular disease rather than a joint disease
- Watch for excessive scapular motion during arm abduction. This suggests restriction of glenohumeral joint
    - Apley's scratch test (Figs. 15.2A and B):
        - Patient tries to reach the opposite shoulder to touch it from the front
        - From behind the neck to reach the upper vertebral border of the opposite scapula
        - From behind the lower back to reach the lower tip of the opposite scapula.

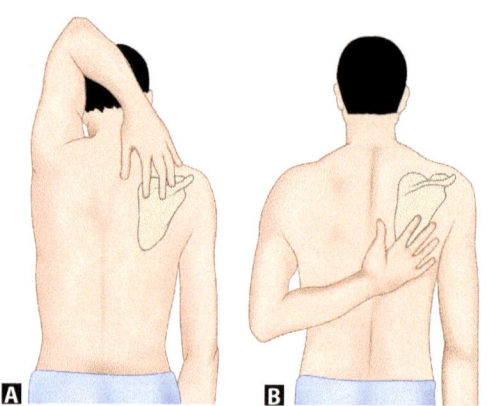

Figs. 15.2A and B: Apley scratch test. The patient attempts to touch the opposite scapula to test range of motion of the shoulder. (A) Testing abduction and external rotation. (B) Testing adduction and internal rotation.

D. Rotator Cuff Testing

This is described in the section on muscle power assessment.

E. Provocative Testing

Neer's test: Pain in this maneuver suggests subacromial impingement (Fig. 15.3).

Hawkins test: Pain in this maneuver suggests subacromial impingement or rotator cuff tendinitis (Fig. 15.4).

Cross-arm test: This isolates the acromioclavicular junction, which may mimic shoulder impingement (Fig. 15.5).

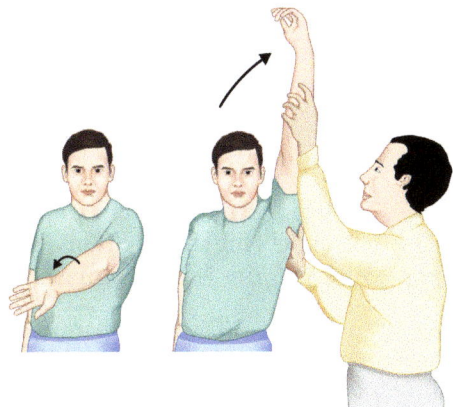

Fig. 15.3: Neer's test for impingement of the rotator cuff tendons under the coracoacromial arch. The arm is fully pronated and placed in forced flexion.

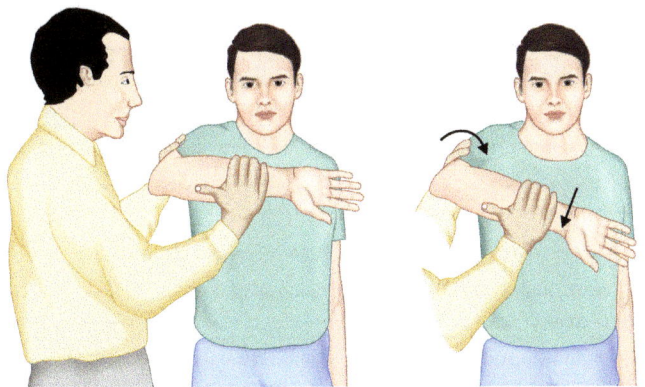

Fig. 15.4: Hawkins test for subacromial impingement or rotator cuff tendonitis. The arm is forward elevated to 90°, then forcibly internally rotated.

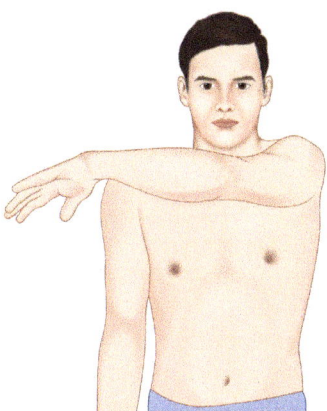

Fig. 15.5: Cross-arm test for acromioclavicular joint disorder. The patient elevates the affected arm to 90°, then actively adducts it.

Pain elicited in this maneuver suggests acromioclavicular disease rather than shoulder impingement.

Painful arc sign: Ask the patient to elevate the arm in abduction through 180°, or passively abduct his arm through 180°. Pain felt between 60–120° is suggestive of impingement syndrome.

Empty can test: Internally rotate the arm and hyperpronate the forearm, flex the shoulder by 30° and then abduct the shoulder. This resembles the posture of upper limb as if emptying a can. This isolates supraspinatus action.

Yergason's test: Flex the elbow to 90° with forearm pronated. From this position, supinate the forearm against examiner's resistance. Pain reproduced is bicipital tendinitis.

Lippman's test: Move the biceps tendon back and forth in the bicipital groove (just below anterior deltoid fibers). Reproduction of pain indicates biceps tendonitis.

Table 15.1: Key findings in the history and physical examination.

Finding	Probable diagnosis
Scapular winging, trauma, recent viral illness	Serratus anterior or trapezius dysfunction
Seizure and inability to passively or actively rotate affected arm externally	Posterior shoulder dislocation
Supraspinatus/infraspinatus wasting	Rotator cuff tear, suprascapular nerve entrapment
Pain radiating below elbow, decreased cervical range of motion	Cervical disc disease
Shoulder pain in throwing athletes, anterior glenohumeral joint pain and impingement	Glenohumeral joint instability
Pain or 'clunking' sound with overhead motion	Labral disorder

SACROILIAC JOINT

Introduction

- Sacroiliac joint (SIJ) disease causes pain in the posterior region (buttock) that may radiate to the posterior thigh
- Sacroiliac joint pain is often misinterpreted as lumbosacral disk or root-related pain, because of the overlap in the pain distribution
- *The following tests may help in the correct diagnosis:*
    - Gaenslen's test (Fig. 15.6)
        - Patient in supine position
        - One hip and knee are flexed to stabilize the pelvis
        - Patient positioned at the edge of the cot so that the buttock is partially off the cot, allowing the leg to drop down
        - This hip extension reproduces the pain of SI joint disease

- *Alternate method:* Patient in lateral decubitus, examiner forcefully extends the leg to cause hip extension. Pain is reproduced in SI joint disease
- *Distraction test (Fig. 15.7):*
  - Patient in supine position
  - Vertically-oriented pressure is applied over both the anterior superior iliac spines
  - Distraction of sacroiliac joints reproduces the pain.
- *Compression test (Fig. 15.8):*
  - Patient in lateral decubitus

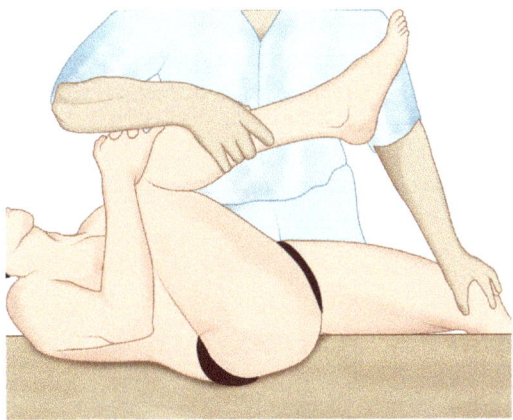

Fig. 15.6: Gaenslen's test (testing the right SIJ in posterior rotation and the left SIJ in anterior rotation).

Note: The pelvis is stressed with a torsion force by a superior/posterior force applied to the right knee and a posteriorly directed force applied to the left knee.

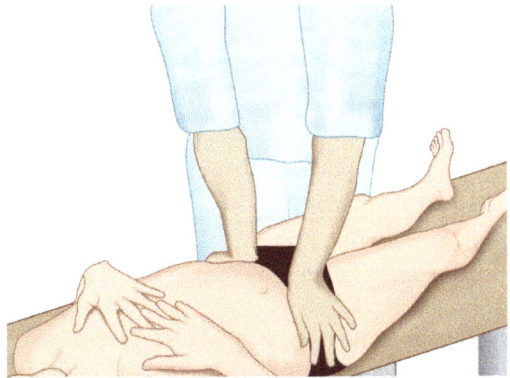

Fig. 15.7: The distraction test (testing right and left SIJ simultaneously).

Note: Vertically oriented pressure is applied to the anterior superior iliac spinous process directed posteriorly, distracting the sacroiliac joint.

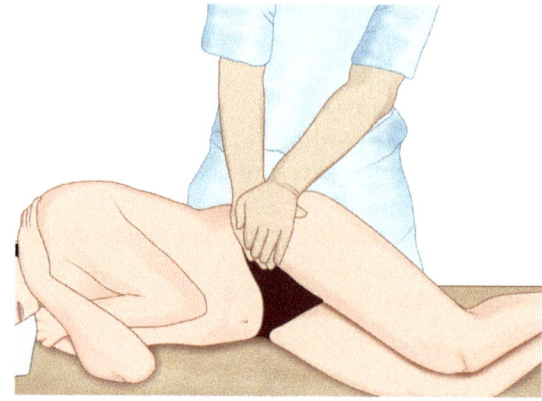

Fig. 15.8: The compression test (testing right and left SIJ).

Note: A vertically directed force is applied to the iliac crest directed towards the floor, i.e. transversely across the pelvis, compressing the SIJs.

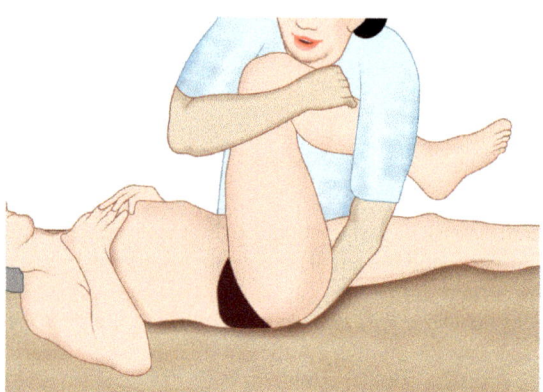

Fig. 15.9: The thigh thrust test (testing the right SIJ).

Note: The sacrum is fixated against the table with the left hand, and a vertically oriented force is applied through the line of the femur directed posteriorly, producing a posterior shearing force at the SIJ.

- ♦ Pressure is applied over the iliac crest towards the floor to compress both SI joints
- ♦ Reproduction of pain indicates SI joint disease.
- Drop test (Fig. 15.10):
  - ♦ Patient raises one heel, supporting the entire weight on the toes
  - ♦ Then he suddenly drops the heel to the floor, producing a cranially directed force at the SI joint (knee must be kept extended during the test)
  - ♦ SI joint pain is reproduced.

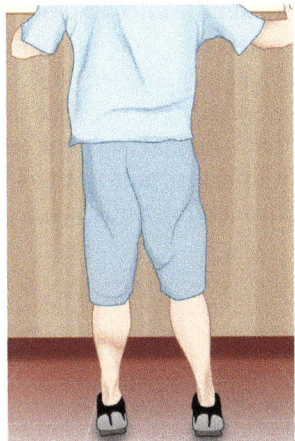

Fig. 15.10: The drop test (testing the left SIJ).

Note: The patient raises the heel from the floor taking near full bodyweight, then drops the heel to the floor with a bump, retaining the knee in extension at all times, producing a cranially directed shear force at the left SIJ.

KNEE JOINT

Introduction

A proper knee joint examination is very important in neurological practice because of the following reasons:
- Pain of lumbosacral root compression is sometimes reported in the back of the knee. This needs to be differentiated from pain of knee joint disease
- Many patients report "knees giving way" while walking. This has to be correctly categorized as neuromuscular or orthopedic in origin
- Patients with knee joint disease report pain radiating down the leg and this is misinterpreted as neuropathic pain.

Physiological Basis

- Ligaments in and around the knee keep it in a stable position
- The medial collateral ligament (MCL) provides medial stability. It runs from the medial femoral epicondyle to the tibia where it fans out on the medial side
- The lateral collateral ligament (LCL) provides lateral stability and runs from the lateral femoral epicondyle to the fibular head
- The anterior cruciate ligament (ACL) prevents anterior displacement of the tibia with respect to the femur and the posterior cruciate ligament (PCL) prevents posterior displacement of the tibia with respect to the femur
- The cruciate ligaments are also important for internal rotation stability of the knee. The posterolateral corner (PLC) is a complex stabilization unit

on the posterolateral side of the knee and prevents dorsal displacement of the lateral tibial plateau (i.e. exorotation of the tibia with respect to the femur, lateral instability, and hyperextension)
- Stability testing is based on trying to mobilize the tibia with respect to the femur in the direction that is limited when the tested ligament is intact
- When ligament rupture is present, larger excursions are seen. Comparison with the contralateral knee is always mandatory.

Methodology

Physical examination starts with:
1. Inspection
2. Active mobilization
3. Passive mobilization
4. Palpation
5. Neurovascular examination
6. Specific tests
7. Isometric muscle testing

Inspection

Supine position
- Observe for swelling, redness, hematoma, scar tissue, quadriceps atrophy.
- Swelling can be intra-articular or extraarticular
- Intra-articular effusion can be seen as a swelling in the region proximal of the patella. The normal aspect of the distal quadriceps is not visible anymore
- Extra-articular swelling is more locally present
- Swelling in the anterior aspect of the patella is usually due to a prepatellar bursitis
- When redness is present, infection must be excluded
- Abnormalities of the patellar ligament or Hoffa's fat tissue can also be observed.

Standing

Front view
- The load axis of the leg is normally neutral, meaning that the leg is straight
- If an O configuration is seen, a varus load axis is present
- If an X configuration is seen, a valgus load axis is present.

Lateral view
- Look for flexion deformity when the knee cannot be fully extended
- A recurvatum deformity when the knee can be hyperextended beyond neutral position.

Walking
- Step and stride length
- Symmetry

- Limb loading (left versus right)
- Flexion and extension of the knee during walking.

Active Mobilization
- Assess range of motion, smoothness of motion, pain on movement, occurrence of crepitus, and lateralization of the patella
- Range of motion is tested for extension, flexion, medial and lateral rotation
- The patient is asked to fully extend and flex the knee
- Normal range from full extension to a flexion is 140°. Comparison with the contralateral side is advised
- When the knee cannot be fully extended (0 degrees), an extension deficit or a flexion contracture is present
- When the knee can extend beyond full extension, hyperextension is present
- Rotation in the knee is checked with the knee flexed to exclude hip rotations
- Exorotation is approximately 40° and endorotation is approximately 30°. Again, comparison with the contralateral side is advised (Figs. 15.11A and B).

Passive Mobilization
- Passive mobilization assesses range of motion, smoothness of motion, pain on movement, occurrence of crepitus, and lateralization of the patella.
- The endpoints of movement should be evaluated. They can be fixed or resilient and may be painful or not. During movement of the knee, crepitus or patellar clunking can be palpated.
- When an extension deficit is noticed during active mobilization and full extension is possible during passive mobilization, an extension lag is present.
- Passive flexion usually exceeds active flexion of the knee and can be up to 160°.
- Passive range of rotation of the knee is larger than active range of rotation (Figs. 15.12A to D).

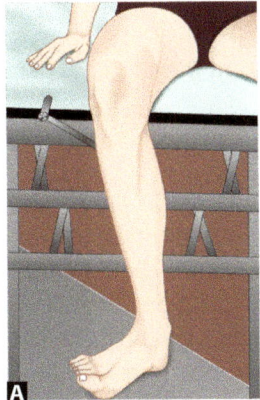 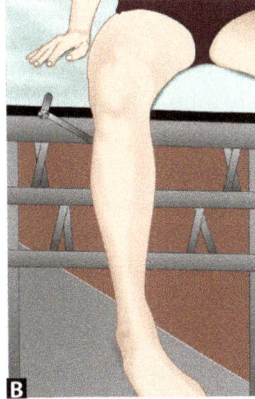

Figs. 15.11A and B: (A) Checking 'exorotation' of the knee in active mobilization; (B) Checking 'endorotation' of the knee in active mobilization.

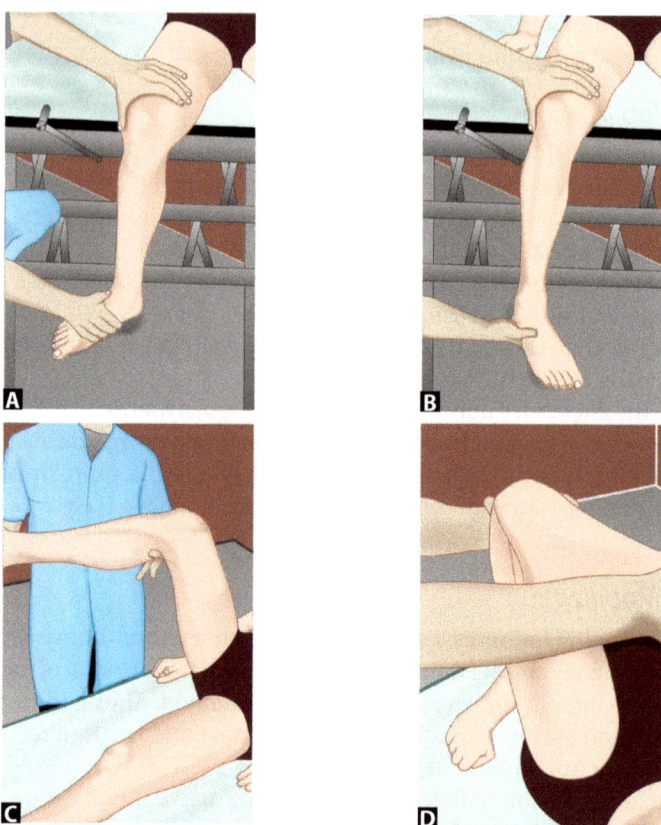

Figs. 15.12 A to D: (A) Checking exorotation of the knee in passive mobilization; (B) Checking endorotation of the knee in passive mobilization; (C and D) Checking rotation of the hip in passive mobilization.

Palpation

- Palpation is performed to determine the point maximum of pain, assess muscle tone, and qualify the swelling
- Palpation of the anterior or posterior joint line is tender when a meniscal tear is present
- When the tenderness extends more to proximal or distal regions, the collateral ligament can be the cause of pain instead of the meniscus
- Normal anatomic landmarks such as the patella, the epicondyles, the joint lines, the tibial plateau, tibial tuberosity, and proximal fibula can be palpated and tenderness of anatomic structures should be assessed
- Soft tissues like the quadriceps muscle, anserine bursa, Hoffa's fat pad, iliotibial tract, patellar ligament and lateral and medial collateral ligaments have to be assessed by palpation.

Neurovascular Examination

Neurovascular examination is performed to briefly check neurovascular status of the limb.

Specific Tests

These are directed at
- *Menisci:*
  - Medial meniscus
  - Lateral meniscus
- *Ligaments:*
  - Medial collateral ligament
  - Lateral collateral ligament
  - Anterior cruciate ligament
  - Posterior cruciate ligament
  - Patellar stability.
- With patient in supine position with knee **semiflexed**, passively extend the knee. If the knee cannot be extended beyond a certain angle with a resilient stop, it suggests bucket handle rupture of a meniscus
- In the same position, passively flex the knee to the maximum. A resilient stop to this movement indicates a posterior horn lesion of the meniscus
- With knee **flexed fully**, apply **varus stress, external rotation** and then slowly extend the knee. Paiful snap during this movement indicates medial meniscal lesion
- With the knee **fully flexed**, apply **valgus and internal rotation** force to the knee and then slowly extend it. Painful snap in this movement suggests lateral meniscal lesion
- With knee **flexed to 30°**, apply **abduction force** with one hand at the ankle, while stabilizing the thigh with the other hand. This tests the medial collateral ligament. An excess movement indicates instability
- With the knee **flexed to 30°**, apply **adduction force** with one hand at the ankle while the other hand stabilizes the thigh. This tests the lateral collateral ligament
- For the **anterior drawer test** for the **anterior cruciate ligament**, the patient is in a supine position. The hip is flexed 45°, the knee is passively held in 90° of flexion with the tibia in neutral rotation, and the patient is asked to relax. The examiner stabilizes the lower extremity by gently sitting on the foot. The hamstrings are checked for slackness and a gentle anterior force to the proximal tibia is applied
- For the posterior drawer test for the posterior cruciate ligament, in the same position as above, a backward gentle force is applied and any laxity is noted.

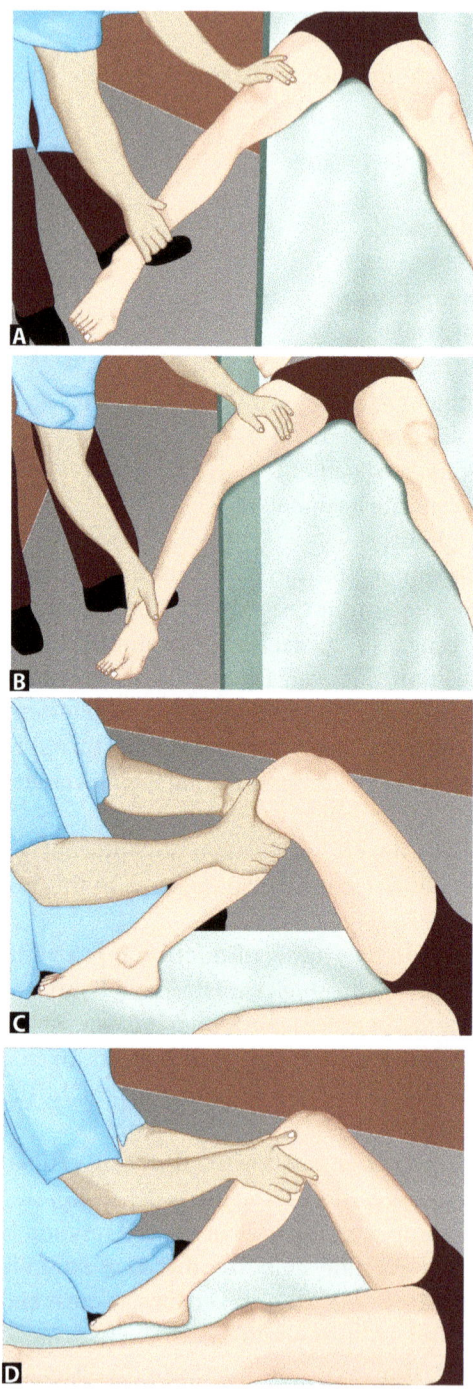

Figs. 15.13A to D: (A) Valgus stress test for medial instability; (B) Varus stress test for lateral instability; (C) Anterior drawer test for anterior instability; (D) Posterior drawer test for posterior instability.

Patellar Instability

- When the patella is not seen or palpated at its normal position in the femoral trochlea but more lateral, a luxation is present. It spontaneously reduces when the leg is passively extended
- Intra-articular effusion is often present due to laceration of the medial retinaculum
- The medial side of the patella is often tender also due to this laceration, but the lateral part of the patella can also be tender due to trauma of the bony lateral restraints
- *Q Angle* is defined as the angle between the line from the anterior superior iliac spine to the center of the patella and the patellar tendon in the frontal plane
- A normal Q angle is between 10 and 15°. Increased Q angle predisposes to patellar subluxation
- *Patellar subluxation test:*
    - The patient is in the supine position and asked to relax
    - The knee is flexed 20° and a gentle force in lateral direction is applied to the medial side of the patella (Fig. 15.10)
    - When subluxation is imminent, the patient will respond with quadriceps spasm as a guarding reflex.
- *Rabot test/patellofemoral grinding test/patellofemoral compression test*
    - The patient is in the supine position and asked to relax
    - The knee is in extension
    - The patella is palpated on the proximal side and held in position
    - The patient is asked to contract the quadriceps (Fig. 15.14)
    - The test is positive when this quadriceps contraction is painful.

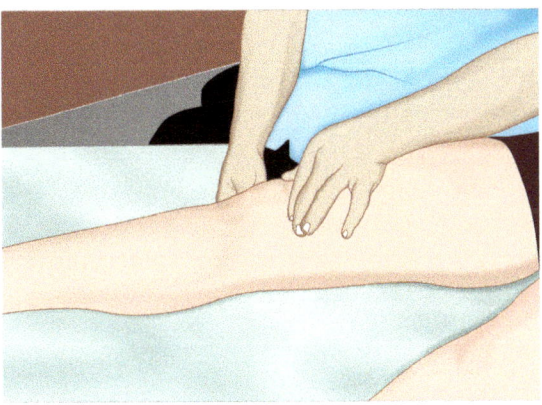

Fig. 15.14: Patellofemoral compression test.

BIBLIOGRAPHY

1. Deutsch A, Altchek DW, Veltri DM, et al. Traumatic tears of the subscapularis tendon: clinical diagnosis, magnetic resonance imaging findings, and operative treatment. Am J Sports Med. 1997;25:13-22.

2. Gerber C, Krushell RJ. Isolated rupture of the tendon of the subscapularis muscle: clinical features in 16 cases. J Bone Joint Surg [Br]. 1991;73B:389-94.
3. Hawkins RJ, Kennedy JC. Impingement syndrome in athletes. Am J Sports Med. 1980;8:151-7.
4. Mark Laslett. Evidence-based diagnosis and treatment of the painful sacroiliac joint. J Man Manip Ther. 2008;16(3):142-52.
5. Miniaci A, Salonen D. Rotator cuff evaluation imaging and diagnosis. Orthop Clin North Am. 1997;28:43-58.
6. Neer CS. Impingement lesions. Clin Orthop. 1983;173:70-7.
7. Woodward TW, Best TM. The painful shoulder: part I. Clinical evaluation. Am fam Physician. 2000;61(10):3079-88.

CHAPTER 16

Examination of Trigger Points

GRK Sarma

MYOFASCIAL PAIN

- Myofascial pain is a very common cause of neck and back pain, that can be successfully treated, if correctly identified.
- It includes pain that originates from taut muscle bands and trigger points (Figs. 16.1A and B).
- It is a great imitator that can mimic joint pains, bursitis, radiculopathies, migraine, autonomic cephalalgias and even visceral disorders.
- Muscles in spasm can also compress the adjacent neural structures to cause truly neurogenic pain. For example, brachial plexus (by taut scalene muscles) and sciatic nerve (by taut piriformis muscle), can be involved in the process
- Some authors include fibromyalgia in myofascial pain syndromes, while others do not.
- Acute trauma or repetitive, microtrauma, lack of exercise, prolonged poor posture, vitamin deficiencies, sleep disturbances, joint diseases, occupational overuse may all predispose to the development of trigger points.

Definitions

- Fibromyalgia: It is a chronic disorder with diffuse muscle pains and symmetric tender points as defined by the American College of Rheumatology. These spots are distributed below and above the waist in a symmetric fashion.
- Tender point: An area in a muscle that on palpation causes local pain, but not radiating pain, muscle twitch or autonomic features. These usually occur at the **insertion zone** of the muscle.
- Taut band (TB): A linear area in the muscle which is firmer than the rest of the muscle and is tender to palpation.
- Trigger point (TrP): Trigger points are discrete, focal, painful, tender, in a taut band of skeletal muscle that on palpation produce referred pain, referred tenderness, motor dysfunction, and autonomic phenomena. These are usually located in the **muscle belly**.

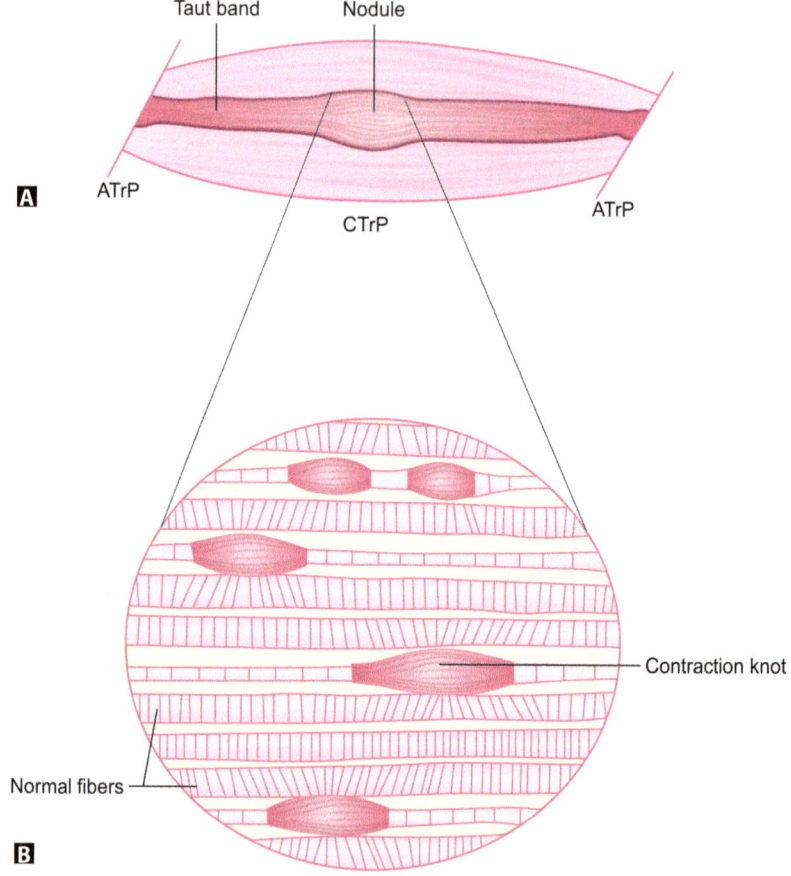

Figs. 16.1A and B: Trigger point complex.

- Satellite trigger point: When myofascial pain (MFP) persists for some time without treatment, adjacent structures may also evolve their own TrP called satellite TrP.
- Active TrP: An active trigger point causes pain at rest. It is tender to palpation with a referred pain pattern that is similar to the patient's pain complaint.
- Latent TrP: A point that does not cause spontaneous pain, but may restrict movement or cause muscle weakness.

Examination Method (Figs. 16.2 to 16.7)

Inspection

Look for asymmetry of posture and restriction of active and passive range of motions. Abnormal movement pattern as a result of myofascial pain and tightness should also be noted.

Examination of Trigger Points 453

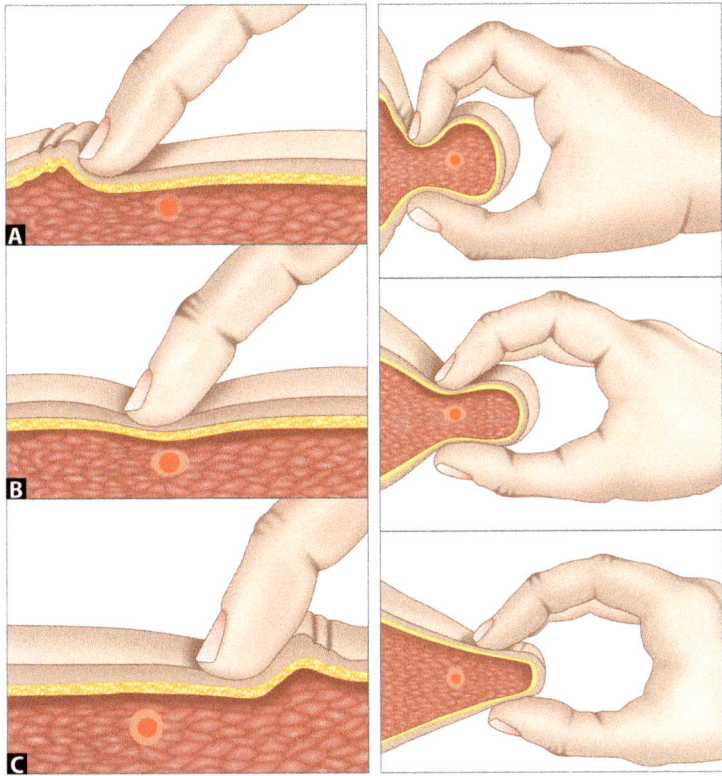

Figs. 16.2A to C: Rolling and pinching techniques to locate the trigger point in a taut band. When the same movements are performed rapidly and vigorously, it is called snapping palpation and elicits a twitch response in a patient with trigger point (TrP) pain.

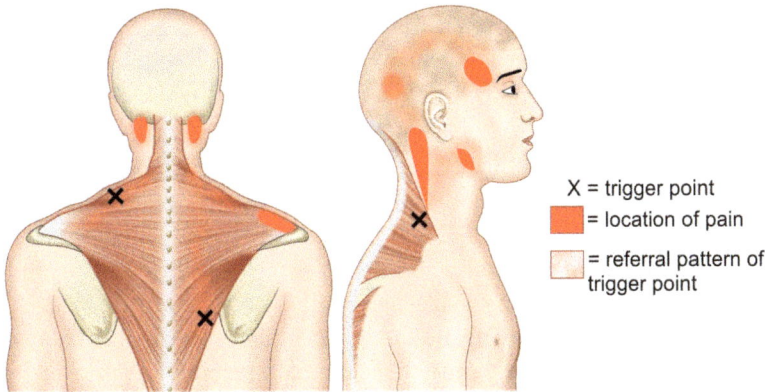

X = trigger point
▬ = location of pain
☐ = referral pattern of trigger point

Fig. 16.3: Pain in the upper trapezius muscle.

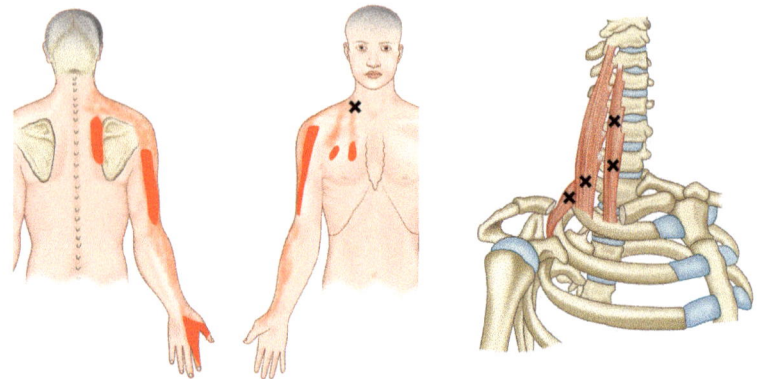

Fig. 16.4: Scalene trigger points and referred pain pattern.

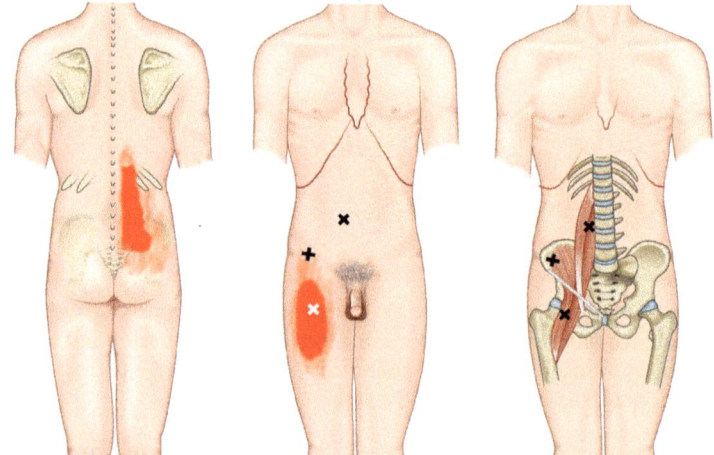

Fig. 16.5: Iliopsoas trigger points and referred pain patterns. Pattern of pain (bright red) referred from palpable myofascial trigger points (Xs) in the right iliopsoas muscle (deep red). The essential pain reference zone is solid red; the spill-over pattern is stippled.

Palpation

- First relax the muscle by passively approximating its origin and insertion
- Feel the muscle with finger pulp, finger tip and pincer grasp depending on the muscle size and accessibility. For large muscles, flat of the hand may be used
- Feel the taut band within the muscle.
- Further probe the TB for the trigger point.
- Confirm the trigger point by sudden snapping across the band to reproduce the pain, radiation and by the muscle twitch response. A muscle twitch produces transient visible contraction or dimpling

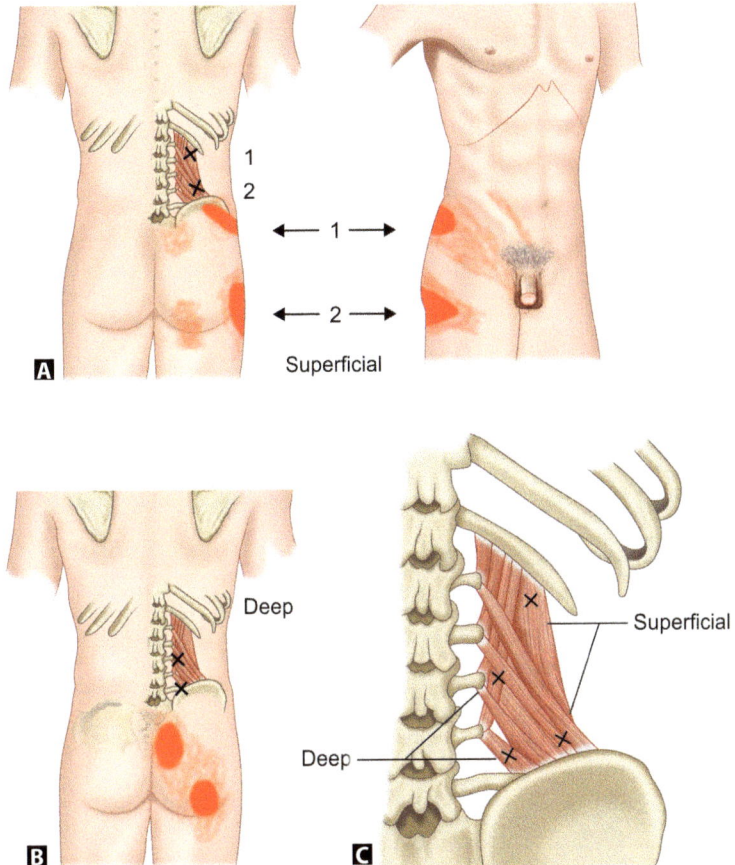

Figs. 16.6A to C: Trigger points in quadratus lumborum muscle.

- Roll the overlying skin between thumb and forefinger to notice skin edema that commonly occurs in TrP pain (autonomic dysfunction)

Thorough neurological and orthopedic examination is needed to rule out more ominous causes.

- Once TrP are identified, identify the precipitating and aggravating postures like poor physical conditioning, non-ergonomic posture at work, repetitive stress injury, etc. Unless these are corrected, the TrP will recur even after successful treatment
- A number of therapeutic options exist for TrP pain including massage, muscle stretching, ultrasonic massage, electrical stimulation, dry needling, injection of local anesthetic into the TrP and a spray and stretch technique (coolant anesthetic agent is used). In experienced hands, a gratifying and quick response can be achieved. A detailed discussion of these treatments is beyond the scope of this book.

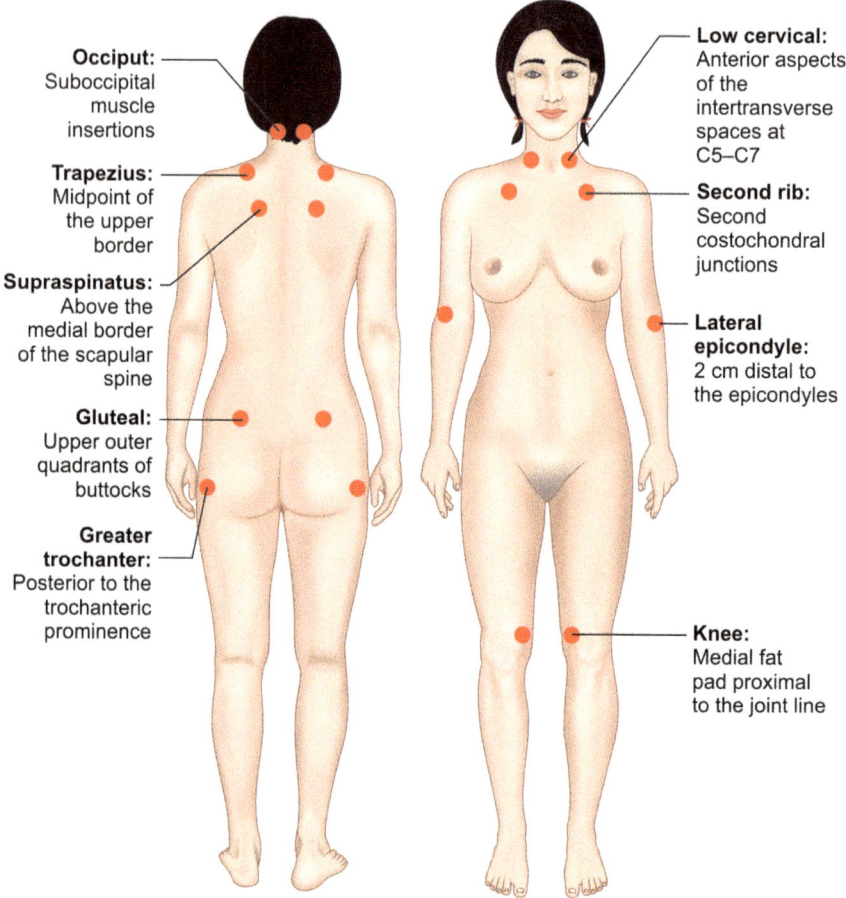

Fig. 16.7: Tender spots in fibromyalgia.

Interpretation

- It is important to differentiate TrP from tender points (Table 16.1)

Table 16.7: Differences between trigger points and tender points.

Feature	Trigger points	Tender points
Local tenderness	+	+
Taut band	+	–
Local twitch response	+	–
Referred pain	+	–
Location	Muscle belly	Muscle insertion zone
Distribution	Usually asymmetric	Symmetric in fibromyalgia

- Tender points are typically seen in fibromyalgia
- Trigger points occur in a wide variety of conditions (see physiologic basis section).

BIBLIOGRAPHY

1. Alvarez DJ, Rockwell PG. Trigger points: diagnosis and management. Am Fam Physician. 2002;65:653-60.
2. Bron C, Dommerholt JD. Etiology of Myofascial Trigger Points. Curr Pain Headache Rep. 2012;16:439-44.
3. Eduardo Vázquez-Delgado, Jordi Cascos-Romero, Cosme Gay-Escoda. Myofascial pain associated to trigger points: A literature review. Part 2: Differential diagnosis and treatment. Med Oral Patol Oral Cir Bucal. 2010;15(4):e639-43.
4. Yap EC. Myofascial pain—An overview. Ann Acad Med Singapore. 2007; 36:43-8.

CHAPTER 17

Neurological Examination of a Neonate

Chandrakala BS

INTRODUCTION

- The neurologist is usually consulted by the neonatologist/pediatrician in the following scenarios:
    - Neonatal seizures
    - Neonatal encephalopathy (drowsy/irritable)
    - Neonatal weakness (e.g. floppy infant syndrome)
    - Other neurological deficits (e.g. poor vision/hearing, etc.)
- A basic knowledge of neonatal neurological examination is invaluable in proper assessment and management of such conditions.
- Neonatal examination is a dynamic process. Examination cannot be conducted systematically as in adults, as it leads to crying and fussing which gives only minimal information. Experience of the examiner and serial examination are necessary for the reliable diagnosis
- The objectives of neonatal neurological examination are:
    - To identify a neurologic abnormality and it's likely etiology
    - To assess the severity and duration of the insult
    - To detect those at risk of future developmental delay so early intervention can be started
- The first neurological examination of the newborn begins in the delivery room with observation of the alertness, activity, and tone. The neonatalogist's record would provide this important information to the neurologist.
- In addition, one must review the antenatal records regarding fetal growth and movement, α fetoprotein levels, ultrasonography and if performed, fetal magnetic resonance imaging.
- A review of history emphasizing the following aspects may be relevant in the individual case:
    - Maternal anesthesia
    - Maternal narcotics use
    - Maternal medications
    - Prenatal exposure to licit and illicit drugs
    - Placental insufficiency
    - Neonatal illness

- Antepartum screening
- Family history about potential congenital disorders or genetic syndromes
- Previous birth outcomes
- Consanguinity
- Maternal infections
- Maternal neuromuscular illnesses (e.g. myasthenia, myotonia dystrophica, etc.)
- Maternal epilepsy.

Tools Required

For examination of the newborn, the following are needed:
- Bell/rattle (or a pleasant ring tone of cellular phone!)
- Red colored ball
- Torch
- Ophthalmoscope
- Reflex hammer
- Cotton
- Measuring tape.

Timing of the Examination

- It is important to assess the baby in its best state of quiet wakefulness which is usually **between** feeds
- Immediately after a feed, the infant may be drowsy. Towards the next feed, he may be irritable.

Examination Scheme

- A number of neonatal neurological examination schemes are available in the literature, but the general principles that underlie these techniques are same
- A simple and practical scheme by Dubowitz, et al. is mainly discussed here. Ballard scheme also is widely used. Other neuro assessment schemes are Amiel-Tison, Hammersmith's neonatal neurological assessment
- The examination time using the Dubowitz scheme was 10–15 minutes and the inter-rater agreement was 96% in the authors' experience
- It may be appropriate to complete all examinations that require only inspection, before handling the infant as in the following order:
    - General examination
    - Posture
    - Involuntary movements
    - Neurobehavioral items
    - Fontanelles and head circumference
    - Tone of the limbs
    - Tone of the trunk
    - Reflexes
- This chapter follows the above scheme.

The mnemonic "PRE-INFANT" may come handy for the beginner to remember all the items, though not in the order of actual performance.
- **P**osture
- **RE**flexes and Tone
- **I**nvoluntary movements
- **N**eurobehavioral items
- **F**ontanelles and head circumference
- **A**ll **N**eurological **T**ests (e.g. cranial nerves, sensory tests, etc.).

GENERAL EXAMINATION

Observe the Infant for

- Dysmorphic features of the face and hands
- Other congenital malformations
- Spinal deformities
- Joint contractures
- Fisting (hypoxic brain injury)
- Evidence of any trauma
- Abnormal pattern of movements of the respiratory muscles
- Contractures, skin dimpling, and poor dermatoglyphic patterns are all indicators of poor fetal movements, are highly suggestive of a neuromuscular disease
- Encephalocele
- Cutaneous lesions such as port-wine stains, hemangiomas
- Sacral dimples, tuft of hair or sinuses
- Cafe au lait spots
- A nevus flammeus, or port-wine stain.

POSTURE

Gently uncover the infant and loosen the diaper to note the predominant posture.

Note the posture of each of the limbs.

	28 weeks	32 weeks	36 weeks	Term	Abnormal response
Posture Infant supine, look mainly at position of legs but also note arms. *Score predominant posture*	Arms and legs extended or very slightly flexed	Legs slightly flexed	Leg well-flexed but not adducted	Leg well flexed and adducted near abdomen	Opisthotonus

Interpretation

- A 28-week infant will lie with minimally flexed limbs
- At 32 weeks, the newborn develops flexor tone at the hips and knees

- This progression correlates with increasing myelination of the subcortical motor pathways originating in the brainstem
- By 36 weeks, the infant develops flexion at the elbows
- By term, the infant is flexed in all extremities.

INVOLUNTARY AND SPONTANEOUS MOVEMENTS

Physiological Basis

- A 28-week infant will have writhing movements of the extremities (like **athetoid** movements)
- By term, the movements are of large amplitude "swatting" movements (**jerky**).

Examination

Inspect the infant for:
- Spontaneous movements (smooth vs. jerky, wide amplitude)
- Presence or absence of antigravity movements
- Abnormal movements:
    - Tremors
    - Startles
    - Twitching
    - Jitteriness
    - Abnormal eye movements.

Interpretation

- A 28-week infant with jerky movements is abnormal and drug withdrawal should be suspected
- Conversely, a term infant with choreoathetoid movements should be evaluated for a number of potential structural or metabolic abnormalities
- Relative sparing of antigravity movements in an otherwise floppy infant suggests central cause
- In neuromuscular causes of floppy infant, antigravity movements are also diminished
- Tremors, startles, myoclonus like movements and jitteriness are often seen in premature infants
- Jitteriness may also be a manifestation of hypoglycemia or seizure (Table 17.1)
- Persistent symmetric eye deviation suggests epileptic seizure.

Table 17.1: Differences between jitteriness vs seizures.

	Jitteriness	Seizures
Dominant movement	Tremor	Clonic
Stimulus sensitive	Yes	No
Suppressibility	Yes by holding the moving limb	No
Autonomic changes	No	May be seen
EEG abnormality	No	May be present

NEUROBEHAVIORAL ITEMS

Neurobehavioral assessment includes five types of items which are discussed below:

Alertness

- Arousal is defined by the duration of eye opening and spontaneous movement of the face and extremities.
- Tested as response to visual stimuli.
- If there is severe visual impairment, the nature of spontaneous movements provides a measure of level of alertness.

Irritability and Consolability

- Normal infants respond by crying for at least 3 seconds to stimuli like undressing, turning prone and pulling to sit. They tend to calm down soon after the stimulus ceases
- If the infant does not cry to any stimulus, he is considered apathetic
- If he is constantly crying even when not handled, he is considered irritable
- If the infant is inconsolable, it suggests a hyperactive state.

Nature of the Cry

Feeble cry may be seen in neuromuscular diseases.

Visual Orientation

- A red ball is shown to the infant and moved across in various directions
- Infant's ability to focus on the target and track it, is observed
- Even prior to 32 weeks' gestation, some preterm infants can focus on a target but they are usually not yet able to track
- After 32 weeks many of them are able to track horizontally or vertically and by 36 weeks many of them can track even in an arc.

Auditory Orientation

- A rattle is held 10–15 cm from the infant and sound stimulus is provided
- In normal term infants, a smooth head turning towards the stimulus and searching with eyes is noted
- A response to an auditory stimulus can be elicited from 27 to 28 weeks' postmenstrual age and becomes stronger with increasing gestational age.

FONTANELLES, SUTURES AND HEAD CIRCUMFERENCE

Physiologic Basis
- The birth process may result in an asymmetry of the skull caused by overlapping or overriding of the sutures (molding).
- On palpation, a bony ridge over the suture line may be appreciated (If this persists beyond age 1 week, craniosynostosis should be suspected).

Methodology
- Note the shape of the skull, any bulges or swellings
- Palpate the sagittal, coronal, lambdoid, and metopic sutures of the skull
- Palpate the fontanels for openness and any bulge (when the infant is calm)
- Measure the head circumference from above the eyebrows to the back of the head across the occipital protuberance (the measuring tape should go above the ears)
- Auscultate the fontanelles for bruits.

Interpretation
- Normal head circumference at term is 35 +/- 2 cm.
- It increases at the following rate:

Postnatal week	Rate of head growth (cm/week)
First	−0.60
Second	0.50
Third	0.75
After third	1.0

- Microcephaly or macrocephaly may point to an underlying infectious, metabolic, or genetic disorder
- A large anterior and posterior fontanel is found in neonates with hydrocephalus, hypothyroidism, and intrauterine growth restriction
- A bulging fontanel is seen in cases of increased intracranial pressure such as hydrocephalus, meningitis, and subdural hematoma
- A small anterior fontanel may be seen in cases of microcephaly and hyperthyroidism
- Abnormal head shape beyond 1 week may be due to extradural fluid collections, premature closure of the skull sutures, and underlying intracranial pathology
- A bruit over a fontanelle suggests a high flow state like vein of Galen malformation.

TONE

Physiologic Basis

- Posture and tone are age dependent, reflecting the increase in flexor tone in the limbs and in axial tone with increasing maturity
- Good extensor tone in the neck muscles often cannot be demonstrated until term
- Preterm infants tend to have less flexor tone in the limbs than full-term infants especially in the upper limbs
- A 28-week infant will lie with minimally flexed limbs and have minimal resistance to passive movement of all extremities
- In contrast, at 32 weeks, the newborn develops flexor tone at the hips and knees, with some resistance to manipulation of the lower extremities. This progression correlates with increasing myelination of the subcortical motor pathways originating in the brainstem. By 36 weeks, the infant develops flexion at the elbows, and by term, the infant is flexed in all extremities.

Methodology

- Tone has to be assessed in the upper limbs, lower limbs, trunk and neck by various maneuvers
- It is important to **keep the head in midline** to avoid asymmetries in tone related to the **asymmetric tonic neck reflex**
- The general principle underlying these tests is that with increasing maturity, tone of the flexor muscles becomes greater
- The flexor tone is tested by **phasic** (i.e. **stretch and leave** or "recoil" tests) and **tonic** (i.e. **stretch and hold** or "traction") methods.
- Flexor and extensor tone of neck muscles is assessed by putting them to work against gravity
- The examination may proceed in a systematic way in the upper limb (wrist, elbow, shoulder) and then the lower limb (knee, pelvic girdle).

The Angle of the Square Window

When the neonate's wrist is flexed, the angle formed progresses from 90° to 0° with advancing gestational age. At term, the hand should touch the wrist forming a 0° angle (Fig. 17.1).

Arm Recoil

- This tests the tone of the biceps brachii muscle
- Place the neonate in supine position
- Support his elbow with one hand beneath it
- With the other hand, hold the neonate's hand
- First fully flex the elbow
- Then quickly (but gently) extend the elbow fully and immediately release the hand

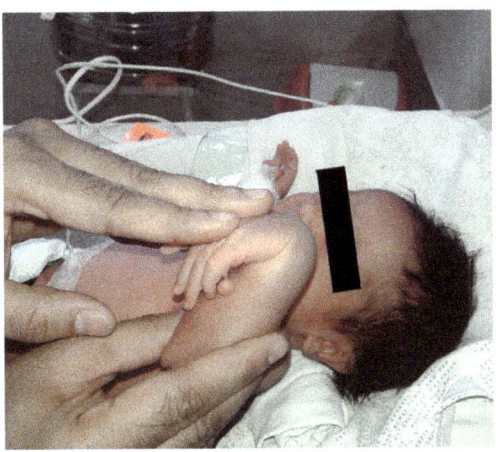

Fig. 17.1: Angle of the square window.

- Watch the angle to which, the elbow flexes back after release
- In immature neonate, there is no recoil at all
- In term neonates, the hand almost touches the face
- In hypertonic states, the extension itself may be restricted
- Caveats: After extending the elbow, if it is held in that position for long, the degree of recoil is reduced even in normal neonates. This is falsely interpreted as evidence of immaturity.

The Scarf Sign (Fig. 17.2)

- Assesses the tone of posterior shoulder girdle muscles
- Position the neonate in semi-reclining position instead of supine
- With one hand, hold the neonate's hand and place it on his chest

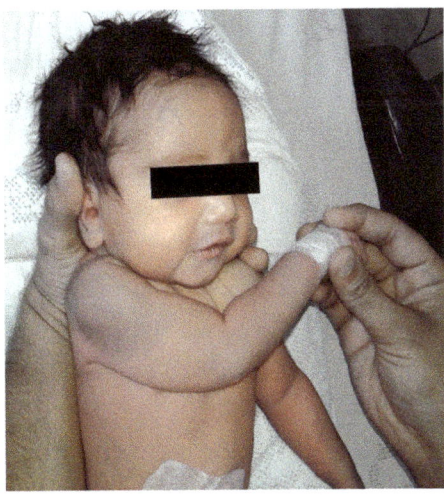

Fig. 17.2: The scarf sign.

- With the thumb of the other hand, apply gentle pressure and push the elbow across the chest until a clear resistance is felt.
  - The landmarks used to record the extent of this maneuverability are:
    - Contralateral axillary line
    - Contralateral nipple line
    - Xiphisternum
    - Ipsilateral nipple line
    - Ipsilateral axillary line
  - In mature neonates, the resistance is felt at the ipsilateral axillary line.

Arm Traction

- Test each side separately
- Hold the wrist and pull the arm upwards and hold there
- Normally, the arm flexes and shoulder is lifted from the bed and maintains in flexion
- A response less than the above is abnormal and indicates hypotonia.

Popliteal Angle (Fig. 17.3)

- This assesses the tone of the knee flexors
- Place the neonate is supine relaxed position
- Gently flex the thigh to reach the abdomen, with the knee fully flexed
- Wait until the baby stops kicking and is relaxed
- Hold the foot with one hand, and fix the thigh with the other
- Gently extend the knee until a clear resistance is felt
- The angle at which the resistance is felt is the popliteal angle
- This will progress from 180° to less than 90° with increasing gestational age
- With dorsiflexion of the ankle, the angle progresses from 90° to 0° with advancing gestational age
- A popliteal angle less than 90° indicates hypertonia.

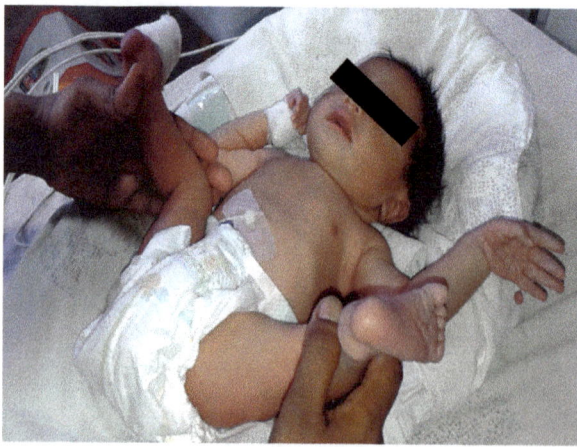

Fig. 17.3: Popliteal angle.

Heel-to-Ear Maneuver

- It tests the tone of posterior hip muscles
- Place the neonate in supine position
- With one hand, hold the foot of the neonate and bring it as close to the ipsilateral ear as possible. With the other hand, support the flexed thigh
- Landmarks noted in order of increasing maturity include resistance felt when the heel is at or near the:
    - Ear
    - Nose
    - Chin level
    - Nipple line
    - Umbilical area
    - Femoral crease

Leg Recoil (Fig. 17.4)

- Hold both ankles in one hand
- Flex the hips and knees
- Quickly extend the limbs fully and release
- A fast and complete flexion is the normal response
- Incomplete or slow flexion indicates hypotonia
- Difficulty in extending the limbs indicates hypertonia.

Leg Traction

- Test each side separately
- Hold ankle in one hand and pull upwards and hold
- Normally, the leg flexes as the buttock is pulled upwards and remains so

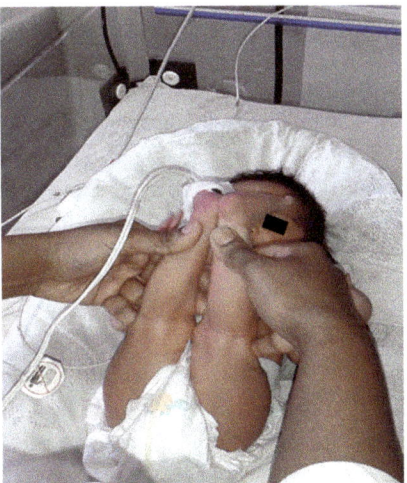

Fig. 17.4: Leg recoil.

- A response less than this is suggestive of hypotonia
- If the buttock remains flexed even after the trunk gets lifted off the bed, it suggests hypertonia.

Head Lag (Fig. 17.5)

- Infant in supine position
- As in arm traction test, pull the arms upwards towards a sitting posture
- Normally, the infant lifts the head in line with the body
- If the head lags behind the body, it suggests hypotonia
- If the head moves ahead of the body, it indicates flexor hypertonia.

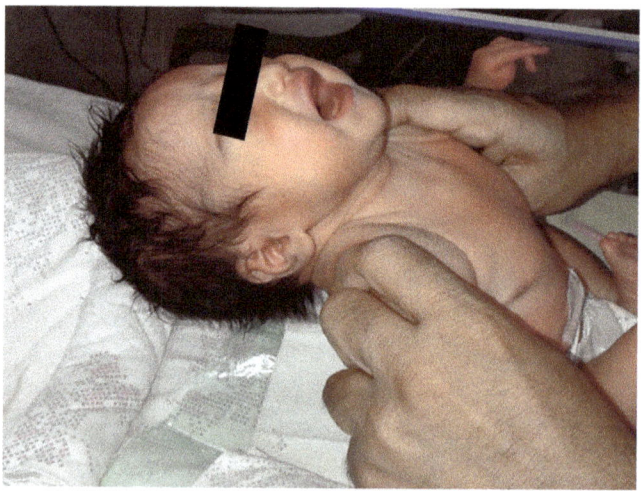

Fig. 17.5: Head lag.

Ventral Suspension

- Hold the infant in the hand in a prone position
- Normally, the back straightens, head comes in line with the back and limbs flex
- If the back remains curved, even slightly, it suggests hypotonia
- If the limbs hang down straight, instead of flexing, it indicates hypotonia
- If the head raises above the trunk level, it suggests hypertonia.

Interpretation

- Generalized hypotonia is nonspecific and is seen in a variety of insults
- Predominant axial hypotonia is more typical of CNS lesion
- Hypotonia of central cause suggests a recent insult. Later on, hypertonia emerges
- Hypertonia represents more chronic injury to the corticospinal tracts

Neurological Examination of a Neonate

Table 17.2: Assessment of maturation of head control up to term.

	28 weeks	32 weeks	36 weeks	Term	Abnormal response
Head control (1): *(extensor tone)* Infant sitting upright; Encircle chest with both hands holding shoulders. Let head drop forward	No attempt to raise head	Infant tries: Effort better felt than seen	Raises head but drops forward or back	Raises head: Remains vertical: it may wobble	
Head control (2): *(flexor tone)* Infant sitting upright; Encircle chest with both hands holding shoulders. Let head drop backward	No attempt to raise head	Infant tries: Effort better felt than seen	Raise head but drops forward or back	Raise head: remains vertical: it may wobble	Head upright or extended; cannot be passively flexed
Head lag Pull infant to towards sitting posture by traction on both wrists and support head slightly. Also note arm flexion	Head drops and stays back	Tries to lift head but it drops back	Able to lift head slightly	Lifts head in line with body	Head in front of body
Ventral suspension Hold infant in ventral suspension; observe back, flexion of limbs and relation of head to trunk	Back curved, head and limbs hang straight	Back curved head hangs down limbs slightly flexed	Back slightly curved, limbs flexed	Back straight, head in line, limbs flexed	Back straight, head above body

- Predominance of extensor tone compared to flexor tone (ventral suspension versus head lag) is often associated with hypoxic—ischemic lesions, meningitis or increased intraventricular pressure
-ABnormal patterns of leg tone in a quiet infant should raise the suspicion of CNS pathology like intraventricular hemorrhage, periventricular leukomalacia, hypoxic ischemic encephalopathy with basal ganglia lesions
- A disproportionately tight popliteal angle compared with the rest of the leg tone is frequently found in association with germinal matrix or intraventricular hemorrhages.

Table 17.3: Assessment of tone of upper and lower limbs up to term.

	28 weeks	32 weeks	36 weeks	Term	Abnormal response
Arm recoil: Take both hands, quickly extend arms parallel to the body, count to three. Release. Repeat x 3	Arms do not flex	Arms flex slowly, not always; not completely	Arms flex slowly; more complete	Arms flex quickly and completely	Arms difficult to extend; snap back forcefully
Arm traction: Hold wrist and pull arm upwards. Note flexion at elbow and resistance while shoulder lifts off table. Test each side separately	Arms remain straight; no resistance felt	Arms flex slightly or some resistance felt	Arms flex well till shoulder lifts, then straighten	Arms flex at approx 100° and maintained as shoulder lifts	Flexion of arms <100°; mantained when body lifts up
Leg recoil: Take both ankles in one hand, flex hips+knees. Quickly extend. Release. Repeat x 3	No flexion	Incomplete or variable flexion	Complete but slow flexion	Complete fast flexion	Legs difficult to extend; snap back forcefully
Leg traction: Grasp ankle and slowly pull leg upwards. Note flexion at knees and resistance as buttocks lift. Test each side separately	Legs straight - no resistance felt	Legs flex slightly or some resistance felt	Legs flex well till bottom lifts up	Knee flexes remains flexed when bottom up	Flexion stays when back + bottom up
Popliteal angle: Fix knee on abdomen, extend leg by gentle pressure with index finger behind the ankle. Note angle at knee. Test each side separately	180°	-150°	-110°	-90°	<90°

REFLEXES

Various reflexes, subserved in different segments of the body have to be examined:
- Cranial: Sucking reflex
- Upper limb: Palmar grasp
- Lower limb: Placing reflex
- Axial: Moro reflex, asymmetric tonic neck reflex
- Deep tendon reflexes

Types of Reflex

Sucking Reflex

- Elicited by the little finger in the mouth with the pulp facing upwards
- A good regular sucking movement is the normal response
- It is observed from 28 weeks of age and becomes stronger over next 4 weeks.

Palmar Grasp Reflex (Fig. 17.6)

- Examiner places his index finger in the hand and gently presses the palmar surface
- Normally, a good grasp is elicited
- Excessively strong response, in which, the whole infant can be lifted from the bed is abnormal
- Weak flexion of fingers and poor grasp are also abnormal
- Palmar grasp is present from 28 weeks post menstrual age and becomes stronger with maturity, disappears by 2–3 months (replaced by voluntary grasp).

Placing Reaction

- Infant is picked up and his dorsum of foot is brought into contact with the edge of the table or cot
- Normally, the limb flexes fully and the sole of the foot is placed on the surface of the table or cot
- This response is elicited from 34 weeks of age and becomes stronger over the next 4 weeks
- Asymmetry in the placing reflex indicates basal ganglia/brainstem/spinal cord lesion.

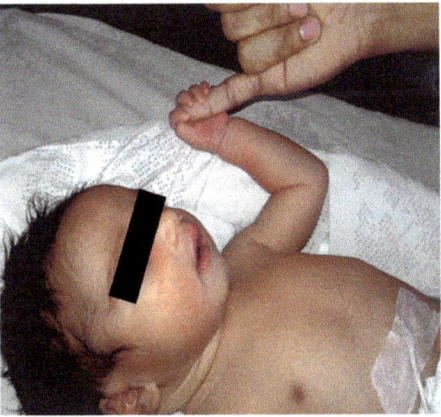

Fig. 17.6: Palmar grasp reflex.

Moro Reflex

- The infant is placed one hand of the examiner. The other hand supports the head
- The infant is tilted slowly to 45° with the infant relaxed
- Infant's head is allowed to drop by 10° while observing the response
- Minimal response of only opening of hands is seen at 27 weeks
- A normal complete response includes initial abduction at shoulder, extension of the upper limb followed by adduction of the shoulder. This is seen from 34 weeks of age onwards.

Asymmetric Tonic Neck Reflex (Fig. 17.7)

- Elicited by turning the head to one side with infant in supine position
- Normally, the infant responds by extending one arm toward the side to which the head was turned and flexing the arm on the side of the occiput forming a fencing posture
- This is present from 35 weeks' gestation to 6 months.

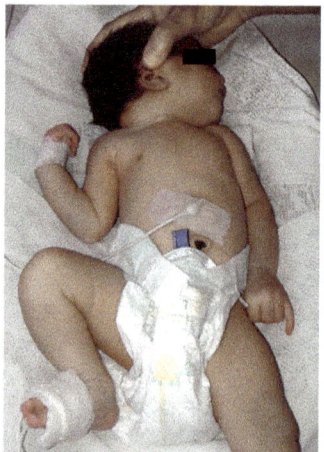

Fig. 17.7: Asymmetric tonic neck reflex.

Deep Tendon Reflexes

- Performance of the tendon reflexes in a normal newborn only requires tapping of a couple fingers placed over the tendon rather than using a tendon hammer
- In a hypotonic infant, it may be necessary to use a hammer to confirm areflexia
- Biceps, knee and ankle jerks can be tested as in adults
- Cross adductor responses and unsustained clonus may be normal in the normal newborn
- Brisk reflexes in a hypotonic infant suggest central cause, whereas absent reflexes suggest lower motor neuron lesion.

CENTRAL VERSUS NEUROMUSCULAR HYPOTONIA

Central and neuromuscular hypotonia is discussed in Table 17.4.

Table 17.4: Differences between central and neuromuscular hypotonia.

	Central	Neuromuscular
Weakness	Not prominent	Prominent
Distribution of hypotonia	Axial	Generalized
Antigravity muscles	Spared	Not spared
Deep tendon reflexes	Exaggerated	Diminished
Visual and auditory responses	May be reduced	May be spared
Alertness	May be reduced	Preserved
Poor dermatoglyphics	Not a feature	Suggestive
Contractures	Not a feature	Suggestive

Patterns of Weakness and their Usual Etiologies

- **Parasagittal cerebral injury:** Weakness involves lower limbs and shoulders (infarcts in the arterial border zones of the cerebral hemispheres).
- **Periventricular leukomalacia** and paraventricular/intraventricular hemorrhage. Weakness involves only lower extremities.
- **Spinal cord injury:** Symmetric lower extremity paralysis with sparing of the face and cranial nerves and possible involvement of the sphincters.
- **Peripheral nerve:** In the most common peripheral nerve injury, Erb's palsy there is paralysis of shoulder abduction, elbow flexion, and finger extension, so that the arm is held in a waiter's tip posture. There is loss of biceps reflex and loss of sensation in the lateral aspect of the arm.
- **Congenital myopathies:** Global hypotonia, proximal extremity weakness and limb deformities and contractures are the typical features.
- **Thumb in fist appearance:** It is seen in central nervous system insults.

CRANIAL NERVE EXAMINATION

Cranial nerve examination is ideally done before tone assessment. It is interesting to note that using only a torch, a bell and a pacifier, most of the cranial nerves can be reasonably examined.
- Torch: II, III, IV, VI nerves and the optic media
- Bell: VIII
- Pacifier: V, VII, IX, X, XII nerves

Cranial Nerve I

Infant's response to odorous substances like cinnamon can be noted. However, it is not a routine to test the smell function of an infant.

Cranial Nerves (CN) II and III, IV, VI

- Test the pupillary reflex which appears at 32 to 35 weeks gestation. A 28-week infant will blink to light shone into the eyes, testing CN II and VII
- The infant's optic disc should appear pale whitish-gray
- Absence of the red reflex should raise concerns for retinoblastoma or cataract
- Beginning at 34 weeks of gestation, an infant will be able to fix and follow on an object, thus testing CN II, III, IV, and VI
- After 25 weeks of gestation, doll's eyes maneuver can be elicited, by turning the head slowly to each side and holding in the position for few seconds, eyes will turn to the same side
- Vestibulo-ocular reflex can be tested by holding the baby underneath the axilla and slowly spinning 90° to each side, while noting the eye movement
- Optokinetic nystagmus can be elicited as early as 36 weeks
- Spontaneous roving eye movements are common at 32 weeks gestation, as are dysconjugate eye movements in the term infant when not fixing on an object.

Cranial Nerve V

- Tested by touching the skin and by observing facial grimace or change in sucking
- Though pin prick stimulus is described, it is not often required
- Sucking on a pacifier demonstrates V nerve motor function.

Cranial Nerve VII

- Facial symmetry and movement should be observed in both the quiet state and during active movement, including crying
- Blink in response to light or sound demonstrates symmetry or otherwise of facial muscles
- Sucking on a pacifier demonstrates facial muscle activity.

Cranial Nerve VIII

- Tested with a bell/by clapping and noting the response of the infant
- The newborn may have a very subtle response to auditory stimulus and respond with only a blink
- By 28 weeks' gestation, an infant should blink, startle, or turn toward the loud noises
- If these responses are absent consider genetic deafness and TORCH infections.

Cranial Nerve IX, X

- Wasting and fasciculations of sternomastoid may be noted in severe cases of anterior horn cell disease

- Sucking and swallowing without choking indicates integrity of IX, X innervated muscles
- Gag reflex may be observed while suctioning the neonate
- The 28-week infant can suck and swallow but the synchrony of breathing and feeding is not well developed
- As the brainstem matures, coordination improves by the 32nd to 34th week.

Cranial Nerve XII

- Tongue fasciculations may be noted on its margin
- The tongue should protrude in the midline during sucking the pacifier.

SUMMARY OF AGE RELATED NEUROLOGICAL EXAMINATION FINDINGS IN NEONATES

	28 weeks	32 weeks	34 weeks	40 weeks	Red flags
Mental status	Needs gentle rousing to awaken	Opens eyes spontaneously sleep wake cycles apparent		At 36 weeks↑ alertness, cries when awake	Irritable or lethargic infant
Cranial nerves					
Pupils	Blinks to light	Consistent pupillary reflex	Fix and follow		
Hearing	Pauses, no orientation to sound			Head + eyes turn to sound	• No response to auditory stimulus
Suck + swallow	Weak suck, no synchrony with swallow	Stronger suck, better synchrony with swallow		Coordinated suck + swallow at 37 weeks	Chomp suck: Clamps down on pacifier but no suck (bulbar dysfunction)
Motor	Minimally flexed	Flexed hips and knees	↑ Flexed in all hips + knees	Flexed in all extremities	• Hypotonia • Hypertonia • 28 weeks infant with jerky movements • Full-term infant with writhing movement
Reflexes					
Moro	Weak, incomplete hand opening	Complete extension + abduction		Full moro (with anterior flexion)	• Asymmetry
Asymmetric tonic neck reflex				ATNR appears at 35 weeks	• If obligatory or sustained, suggests pyramidal or extrapyramidal motor abnormal
Palmar grasp	Present but weak		Grasp stronger	Strong grasp able to be lifted out of bed	• Fixed obligate grasp (suggests bihemispheric dysfunction)

BIBLIOGRAPHY

1. Aicardi J. Preface to first edition. In: Aicardi J, (Ed). Diseases of the nervous system in Childhood. 2nd edition. High Holborn, London: Mac Keith Press; 1998: PP. ix–x.
2. Amiel-Tison C. Possible acceleration of neurological maturation following high-risk pregnancy. Am J Obstet Gynecol. 1980;138(3):303-6.
3. Ballard JL, Khoury JC, Wedig K, et al. New Ballard Score, expanded to include extremely premature infants. J Pediatr. 1991;119(3):417-23.
4. Bax M. Neurological examination of newborn. Dev Med Child Neurol. 1998;40:651.
5. Dayton GO Jr, Jones MH, Aiu P, et al. Developmental study of coordinate movements in the human infant. I. Visual acuity in the newborn human: A study based on induced optokinetic nystagmus recorded by electrooculography. Arch Ophthalmol. 1964;71:865-70.
6. Dubowitz L, Ricci D, Mercuri E. The dubowitz neurological examination of the full-term newborn. Mental retardation and developmental disabilities research reviews. 2005;11:52-60.
7. Dubowitz LM, Dubowitz V, Goldberg C. Clinical assessment of gestational age in the newborn infant. J Pediatr. 1970;77(1):1-10.
8. Farr V, Kerridge DF, Mitchell RG. The value of some external characteristics in the assessment of gestational age at birth. Dev Med Child Neurol. 1966;8:657-60.
9. Finnstrom O. Studies on maturity in newborn infants. II. External characteristics, Acta Paediatr Scand. 1972;61:24-32.
10. Fletcher MA. Physical assessment and classification. Fletcher MA. Textbook on Physical diagnosis in Neonatology. 1998;441-503.
11. Gould JB, Gluck L, Kulovich MV. The relationship between accelerated pulmonary maturity and accelerated neurological maturity in certain chronically stressed pregnancies. Am J Obstet Gynecol. 1977;127(2):181-6.
12. Kelley KR, Koenigsberger MR. Neurology. In: Polin RA, Spitzer AR, eds. Fetal & Neonatal Secrets, 2nd ed. Philadelphia, PA: Mosby Elsevier; 2006:345-72.
13. Khan OA, Rebecca Garcia-Sosa, Hageman JR, et al. Core concepts: neonatal neurological examination. Neoreviews. 2014;15;e316-24.
14. Swaiman KF. Neurological examination of the term and preterm infant. In: Swaiman KF, (Ed). Pediatric Neurology Principles & Practice, 4th edition. Philadelphia, PA: Mosby Elsevier; 2006:47-64.
15. Usher R, McLean F. Intrauterine growth of live-born Caucasian infants at sea level: Standards obtained from measurements in 7 dimensions of infants born between 25 and 44 weeks of gestation. J Pediatr. 1969;74:901-10.
16. Volpe JJ. Neurological examination: normal and abnormal features. In: Volpe JJ, (Ed). Neurology of the Newborn, 5th edition. Philadelphia, PA: Saunders Elsevier. 2008:121-48.
17. Yang M. Newborn neurologic examination. Neurology. 2004;62(7):E15-7.

CHAPTER 18

Pediatric Neurological Examination

Sushma K, Ranjini Srinivasan

INTRODUCTION

- The neurological examination of the infant and toddler poses a tough challenge to the clinician
- It is imperative that the child is willing to be examined and remains calm and cooperative for most part of the examination
- Hence, examination of a young child cannot follow the same format as that of an older child or adult and should begin with methods that are least disturbing to the child.

GENERAL PRINCIPLES OF PEDIATRIC NEUROLOGICAL EXAMINATION

- Observe the child while conversing with the parent to note his temperament, behavior, physical development, involuntary movements
- Plan the sequence of examination based on the observations and cooperativeness
- Establish a rapport with the child
- Let the parents undress the child and make him sit in the parent's lap
- Provide age appropriate toys to the child for motor system examination and coordination
- Drawings give information about the visual spatial abilities of the child and may reveal the child's attention span
- Once the child is at ease with the doctor, one can proceed with subsequent detailed examination of the child in the parent's presence in the order determined by the child's level of comfort
- The pediatric neurological examination may be organized as follows:
    - General physical examination
    - Neurological examination
        - Motor system
        - Reflexes
        - Higher mental functions
        - Cranial nerves

- Coordination
- Sensory system.

GENERAL PHYSICAL EXAMINATION IN PEDIATRIC NEUROLOGY

The importance given to the general examination of the child as part of neurological evaluation cannot be underplayed. One has to pay more attention to certain aspects of general physical examination which may be invaluable while arriving at a diagnosis. These may be discussed under the following headings:

- Vital signs: Heart rate rhythm, pulse volume and quality of pulse, blood pressure, respiratory rate and pattern of breathing, temperature
- Anthropometry: Weight, height, weight for height/BMI, midarm circumference
- Head: A detailed examination of the head forms an important component of any pediatric neurological exam. Although estimation of the head circumference is important, it can be disturbing to the child and may be done later. A systematic examination of the head of a child includes:
    - Shape of the skull: Observation for asymmetry/protruberances/indentations
    - Examination of fontanels/sutures—dimensions of fontanels, sutural overriding/separation/bulging fontanel/pulsations of fontanel (normally pulsates with heart beat)
    - Auscultation of cranium for intracranial bruits (Caution: bruits can be normal in children)
    - Transillumination (positive in hydranencephaly, porencephaly, subdural effusion, hydrocephalous, caput succedaneum)
    - Occipitofrontal circumference: Ideally measured three times and the largest measured circumference should be recorded and plotted on a graph.
- Eyes: Cataract, refractive errors, visual acuity, squint, chorioretinitis, cherry red spot, vasculitis, papilledema, retinal angiomas
- Ears: Abnormal dysplastic ears, abnormal placement of ears, evaluation of hearing
- Skin and hair: Adenoma sebaceum, ashleaf macules, café au lait spots, shagreen patches, angiomas, axillary freckling, hemangiomas, telangiectasia, light colored hair in phenylketonuria, signs of vasomotor instability like tachycerebrale, palmar erythema
- Midline of neck and back: Signs of spinal dysraphism, kyphoscoliosis
- Unusual body odor: Inborn error of metabolism
- Abdomen: Hepatosplenomegaly, palpable bladder
- Cardiovascular and respiratory system examination: Murmurs, features of bronchiectasis in ataxia telangiectasia.

Motor System Examination

Around the age of 4-6 years, most children with normal intelligence will take part in motor system examination as done for an older child and adult. However, many obstacles may arise while evaluating the motor system in infants and toddlers and it can be a challenging task. Here again, observation plays a pivotal role while doing the motor evaluation. One should inspect for any asymmetry in the movements of arms and legs and differences in muscle bulk or limb length discrepancies. Early hand preference (before the age of 2 years) may indicate that the child has hemiparesis. One must also make a note of any involuntary movements noticed at this stage of examination of the child as they may point towards extrapyramidal disease.

A. Examination of tone
B. Examination of power
C. Examination of reflexes
   - Developmental reflexes
   - Deep tendon reflexes
   - Superficial reflexes
   - Allied reflexes
D. Examination of gait

Examination of Tone

Test	Method	Inference
Inspection	Posture and attitude "Pithed frog" attitude in the supine position (position of limpness) Lower limbs are abducted and externally rotated at hips such that the lateral aspect of the thigh touches the surface on which the child is placed.	Indicates hypotonia
	Decorticate/decerebrate posturing	Hypertonia
	One arm is flexed at elbow and adducted, persistent fisting, thumb adducted against palm. One lower limb on the same side is adducted	Hemiparesis

Contd...

Contd...

Test	Method	Inference
	Dislocation of the hip and multiple joint contractures present at birth	Hypotonia of intrauterine onset
	Pectus excavatum	Long standing weakness of chest wall muscles
	Occipital Plagiocephaly (Flattening of occiput) and hair loss on the posterior portion of the scalp	Hypotonic weak infants who are in constant contact with the surface
Step 2: Palpation of the muscle	The muscle appears flabby in a hypotonic child. Hypertonic muscle appears rigid. Caution: One must not mistake subcutaneous fat for muscle mass and the muscle beneath the fat must be carefully palpated.	
Step 3: Passive movements to assess tone	Gently shake the arms and legs about the various joints: 1. Pronation and supination 2. Tucking of thumbs under the fingers resulting in fisting 3. Difficulty in separating the hips when changing the diaper indicates spasticity 4. When the child is held in vertical suspension, scissoring or crossing of the lower limbs and standing on toes when feet touch the surface indicates spasticity.	Indicates hypertonia

Contd...

Contd...

Test	Method	Inference
	5. In horizontal suspension, there is a backward curve of the extended head, neck and back.	
Traction test	When pulled to sit, significant head lag and rounded back indicates hypotonia.	Normally (infants more than 33 weeks), the infant pulls back against the traction and there is flexion at the elbows, knees and ankles. Head lag should be minimal. More than minimal head lag and failure to counter traction by flexion of extremities indicates hypotonia
Vertical suspension	Place both hands in the axillae and without holding the chest, lift the infant straight up	Normally, the shoulders press down on the examiners hands, the head is erect in the midline and there is flexion of hips, knees and ankles. Hypotonia: Head falls forward, legs hang loosely and the child appears to slip through the examiners fingers
Horizontal suspension	Place the infant on the palm and hold In this position	Normal: infant lifts head up intermittently, back is straight and there is flexion of elbows, hips, knees and ankles. A hypotonic child will hang limply like a "rag doll" over the examiners hands.
	180° flip test is useful for assessing tone	

Examination of Power Estimation

It is not practical testing individual groups of muscles to assess power in infants and young children unlike in older children and adults. Spontaneous movements against gravity provide ample information regarding muscle power. The examiner must make use of every opportunity available to test the muscle strength using different maneuvers. Only with repeated examination will one gain adequate experience to distinguish the usual level of resistance offered by a child to overcome a movement.

Assessing power of the lower extremities

- A young uncooperative child can be placed on the floor. Eventually, he will make a attempt to get up and as he arises, one can assess the proximal muscle strength in the legs. Simultaneously one can observe for Gower's sign (use of the arms to help the child climb up the legs)
- A 3-year-old should be able to stand on one leg for a brief period of time
- Try to entice kids with interesting toys and make them reach for it to assess whether they can stand on their toes
- Observation of the child's gait may provide information regarding the presence or absence of proximal muscle weakness: Trendelenburg sign indicates weakness of the hip abductors. Children with myopathies have a waddling gait
- By asking the child to stoop down to pick up an object, one can assess any weakness of the leg muscles if present
- Different groups of muscles can be tested by asking the child to hop, " duck walk" and walk on toes and heels
- A more formal testing of muscle power as done in an adult is recommended for a school aged child.

Assessing power in the upper extremities

- Proximal muscle power can be assessed by lifting the infant or toddler with the hands placed below the axilla without grasping the thorax. A child with normal power will be able to push down on the examiners hands with his shoulders and prevent himself from slipping through
- Tempting a child with a toy and asking him to pull it with his hands is a useful measure to assess distal muscle strength
- "Wheelbarrow race": The child is placed on the floor and the examiner grasps the feet such that the child assumes a wheelbarrow position. This will help in gauging the strength of the shoulder girdle and the arms
- Another method to assess arm and shoulder girdle strength is by making the child lean against the wall with his feet a few inches away from the wall edge and arms outstretched and palms pushing against the wall. By this maneuver, one can also observe for scapula winging if present
- More formal testing of individual muscle groups to assess power is recommended in an older child.

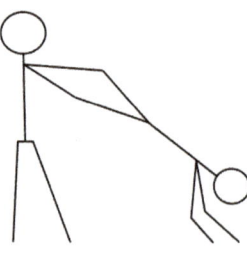

'Wheelbarrow position'

Muscle power is graded as follows:

Grade 5	Normal power
Grade 4	Inability to maintain position against moderate resistance
Grade 3	Inability to maintain position against gravity
Grade 2	Active movement with gravity eliminated
Grade 1	Trace of contraction
Grade 0	No contraction

Pearls

1. Asking the child to outstretch his hands as if to catch raindrops and observing for drifting or pronation is a good indicator of mild muscle weakness.
2. One should test muscles which are more likely to be affected earlier and are more sensitive indicators of weakness. These include deltoids ("holding out your arms as if flying"), wrist extensors (Holding out your hands as if to stop the traffic like a policeman") hamstrings ("pulling your foot back towards the buttock") and ankle dorsiflexors (flexing the feet as though pointing to the head").
3. Biceps, quadriceps, handgrip and gastrocnemius are stronger muscles which are affected in the later stage of the disease.
4. Asking the child to walk or run is useful to assess ataxia or asymmetry of posture, arm swing or foot orientation.

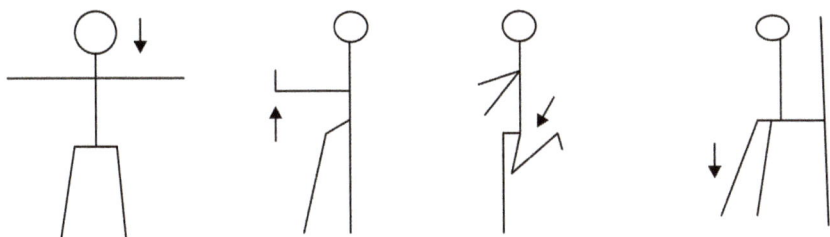

Examination of Reflexes

Developmental/Primitive reflexes

These reflexes are useful in assessing the general neurological development of a child but have minimal localizing value. They form an important aspect of neurological examination in all children below the age of one year. One should carefully examine the child for the abnormal persistence of a reflex that is expected to disappear at a particular age, asymmetric response or absent response. Table 18.1 outlines the method of eliciting each reflex and the time when it is expected to appear and disappear.

Table 18.1: Methods of eliciting various reflexes and the time when they are expected to appear and disappear.

Reflex and method	Normal response	Appearance age	Disappearance age	Inference
Moro's reflex: Place the child supine on the surface. The head is lifted at 30° angle with respect to the horizontal plane and allowed to drop on the examiners hand	Extension and abduction of the arms with extension of fingers followed by flexion and adduction accompanied by the child emitting a cry	Birth (after 34 weeks gestation)	3–4 months (the adduction phase is greatly attenuated by 2 months of age)	Abnormal Moro's indicates CNS depression. Severe spasticity can also cause limitation of Moro's reflex. Asymmetric Moro's may be due to Erb's or Klumpke's palsy or fracture of the ipsilateral clavicle or humerus
Grasp reflex: Keeping the head in the midline, introduce an object or your finger into the palm of the baby's hand from the ulnar aspect. A similar response can be elicited in the foot by stroking the sole behind the toes	Fingers flex and grip the object (Caution: Do not touch the dorsum of the hand otherwise the opposite reflex is stimulated and the hand will open)	At birth	6 months: Palmar grasp 9–10 months: Plantar grasp	Excessively strong grasp reflex is seen in spastic cerebral palsy and kernicterus. Asymmetric grasp is seen in hemiplegia
Crossed extension reflex: One leg is held firmly with the knee extended and firm pressure is applied on the sole	The free leg flexes, adducts and then extends as if pushing away the stimulus	Birth	1 month	
Placing reflex: The anterior aspect of the ulna or tibia is made to touch against the table edge.	Lifting of the leg to step on the table or lifting the arm to place the hand on the table	Birth in term babies weighing > 1,800 g		

Contd...

Contd...

Reflex and method	Normal response	Appearance age	Disappearance age	Inference
Walking reflex: the baby is held upright on the table such that the sole presses on the table	Alternate flexion and extension of the legs simulating walking	Birth	5–6 weeks. This reflex can also be seen in preterm babies who walk on their toes. It can be elicited in older babies after 6 weeks by extending their head	
Galant's reflex: By holding the child in ventral suspension, stimulate the back lateral to the spine	The trunk flexes towards the side the stimulus is applied			
Perez reflex: Keeping the child prone or in ventral suspension, apply firm pressure upwards from the sacrum along the spine towards the head	Flexion of the arms and legs, extension of the neck followed by a cry			
Asymmetrical tonic neck reflex: With the child lying supine, his head is turned to one side	Extension of ipsilateral arm and leg and flexion of the contralateral knee. ("Fencing Position")	Birth	2–3 months but can be positive up to 6 months of age	In cerebral palsy, there is persistence of the reflex and it may be exaggerated. This reflex disappears when the child starts to roll over
Symmetric tonic neck reflex: Place the child in the prone or kneeling position and raise the head	Extension of the arms and flexion of the legs. On flexing the neck, the opposite response is seen with flexion of the arms and extension of the legs	Birth	Disappears when the child learns to crawl	Exaggerated in cerebral palsy

Contd...

Contd...

Reflex and method	Normal response	Appearance age	Disappearance age	Inference
Neck righting reflex: Turn the head to one side	Turning of the head is followed by movement of the body as a whole	Birth	6 months	
Body righting reflex: With the patient supine, head in the midline and arms and legs extended, turn the head to one side	Body rotates as a whole	6 months	18 months	
The Landau reflex	When the child is in ventral suspension, the neck, spine and legs extend. When the head is flexed, the hip, knees and elbows flex	10 months	2 years	Absent Landau reflex is seen in motor weakness and cerebral palsy
The parachute reflex: Hold the child in ventral suspension and suddenly lower him towards the couch	The arms flex as if to protect himself from falling	6–9 months	Persists throughout life	Absent in cerebral palsy and asymmetric in hemiplegia
Sucking and swallowing reflexes		Full-term babies at birth		
Rooting reflex: Lightly touch the corner of the baby's mouth	Eversion of the lower lip and tongue moves towards the side of stimulation			

Deep tendon reflexes

The easiest reflexes to elicit in infants are the biceps jerk, knee jerk and supinator jerks. These reflexes are exaggerated in pyramidal tract disease. By flexing and abducting the hip, flexing the knee and rapidly but gently dorsiflexing the ankle, one can elicit the ankle clonus. The presence of an ankle clonus does not necessarily imply any disease and only means there is increase in the muscle tone and the child may be re-examined in a month or two. One cannot diagnose cerebral palsy on an isolated finding of a brisk knee jerk or the presence of an ankle clonus. A combination of clinical signs are needed to make an accurate diagnosis.

Knee reflex (L3, L4): It is best tested by sitting opposite the child and placing the child's feet on the examiner's knees. The angle at the knees should be approximately 120°. One should tap just below the patella to elicit the reflex. It is preferable to use knee hammers with a wheel at the top while eliciting deep tendon reflexes.

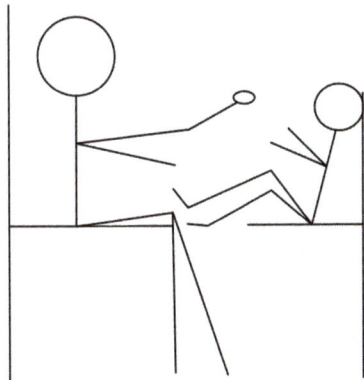

Ankle reflex (S1, S2): The foot is held at an angle of 90° with the thumb on the plantar surface and the other fingers supporting the dorsum of the foot. The child can be made to kneel on the chair with the heels over the edge. The Achilles tendon is tapped to elicit the reflex.

Supinator reflex (C5, C6): With the arm flexed on the abdomen, a finger is placed on the radial tuberosity and the finger is struck with the knee hammer. Watch for contraction of the brachioradialis muscle.

Triceps reflex (C7): With the arm drawn across the chest and elbow flexed at 90°, the triceps tendon is struck with the knee hammer. The triceps contracts and there is extension response at the elbow.

Allied reflexes

Hoffmann reflex: The terminal phalanx of the child's middle finger is flicked downward between the examiner's finger and thumb. The tips of other fingers flex and there is flexion and adduction of the thumb. If unilateral, it may indicate early pyramidal tract involvement.

Wartenburg's sign: The child's hand is supinated and fingers are slightly flexed and with the examiner's hand pronated, he forms a link between his flexed fingers and the patient's. Both the patient and the examiner then flex their fingers further against one another's resistance.

Normal response: Extension of the thumb although there may be a slight flexion of the terminal phalanx. In corticospinal tract lesions, the thumb adducts and flexes against the resistance offered.

Rossolimo's reflex: This is elicited in the lower limb and is considered equivalent to the Hoffmann's reflex discussed earlier. The patient lies supine with the knee extended and foot slightly dorsiflexed and the ball of the big toe is struck with the knee hammer or the toe is flicked upwards. Flexion response of other toes may indicate pyramidal tract lesion.

Superficial reflexes

A. *Plantar reflex*: It is tested in an infant using the finger which should be applied to the distal half of the outer side of the foot. The prerequisites before testing for this reflex are:
   1. Child should be supine
   2. Head should be in the midline to abolish asymmetric tonic neck reflex (ATNR)
   3. Knee is extended
   4. Foot is at right angles to the plane of the body.

   Response: The plantar response in early infants is extensor and not flexor. Normally, there is flexion of all toes. In pyramidal tract lesions, there is extension of the big toe and fanning of the other toes (positive Babinski's response). In older infants up to 2 years of age, the response can be extensor.

   Caution: The finger should not be taken across the sole of the foot, otherwise the grasp reflex will be stimulated. Never use a key to test plantar response in infants.

   Inference: Extensor response in older children indicates pyramidal tract disease.

   False extensor response is elicited by flexing the hips. False flexor response by extending the stimulus across the sole.

   Other methods: Stroking the tibia (Oppenheim's sign), squeezing the gastrocnemius (Gordon's sign), flexing hip against resistance, stroking abdomen, neck or thorax.

B. *Abdominal reflex (T8 – T12):* With the child lying supine, stroke from the lateral aspects of the abdominal quadrants towards the umbilicus, as if to draw a pinwheel.

   Normal response: Umbilicus moves towards the side stimulated. It is absent in pyramidal tract disease.

C. *Cremasteric reflex (L1, L2)*: The inner aspect of the thigh is stroked from below upwards.

Response: Retraction of testes on the same side. Absent in corticospinal tract lesions.
D. *Anal reflex (S3, S4, S5)*: The skin around the anus is scratched
Response: Contraction of the anal ring. Absent in pyramidal tract lesions and conus lesions.

Examination of Gait

Observing the gait of the child forms a very important part of neurological examination. One should make the child walk back and forth in a corridor preferably and up and down the stairs. One should also be aware of the normal gait in children as it changes as the child grows older. One must look for symmetric reciprocal movements of the arms and legs and presence of wide based gait or toe walking. It is always advisable to make the child run as any neurological impairment is exaggerated when the child is made to run. When testing for gait, the lower limbs should always be exposed and the child should be made to walk barefoot on a flat surface. The examiner should also make the child walk on his heels (dorsiflexors), on his toes (plantar flexors) and to stand on one leg (gluteus medius).

The normal gait of a child varies according to the age of the child. A complete walk cycle consists of a *stance* phase (foot on the ground propelling the body forward) and a *swing* phase (foot off the ground) with simultaneous swinging of the arms.

It may be useful to examine the child's shoes as excessive wearing of one sole or part of a sole can indicate an abnormal gait.

Gait at various stages of development
1. 11-13 months: The child "cruises" or walks with support and gait abnormalities can be detected at this stage. Usually, he walks with wide based, short irregular steps and flexed elbows. There is no reciprocal arm movement. Foot and heel are placed simultaneously on the ground. Child may often fall when he starts walking after a few steps. There is hesitancy and unsteadiness when he walks.
2. 15 months: Starts walking independently with frequent falls. Crawls upstairs
3. 18 months- Walks better. Runs stiffly. Walks upstairs holding one hand.
4. 2 years: Walks with greater speed and step length. Runs well. Walks up and downstairs, one step at a time.
5. 30 months: Jumps
6. 36 months: After three years the gait pattern of a child approaches that of an adult. Goes upstairs with alternating feet. Can stand on one leg for a brief period of time.
7. 48 months: Hops on one foot, climbs well
8. 60 months: Skips
9. 7 years: Adult pattern of walking

Types of gait
- Toe walking: This can be normal in a toddler or can be seen in children with spastic diplegia
- Spastic paraplegic gait: Bilateral shuffling gait with the tendency for the child to pull his legs together as in adduction (scissoring).
- Waddling gait: Seen in muscular dystrophies, developmental dysplasia of the hip (bilateral), slipped capital femoral epiphysis (bilateral), proximal muscle weakness
- Foot drop: Peripheral neuropathy
- Staggering gait/ataxic gait: Cerebellar lesions
- Circumduction gait: Spastic hemiplegia
- Commando crawl: Dragging of lower limbs and pulling the body forward with the help of upper limbs: Spastic diplegia.

Cortical Functions

General Remarks

1. Frontal lobes: Motor aphasia is seen in children greater than 6–7 years of age if Broca's area in the dominant hemisphere is damaged. An irritative lesion in the frontal lobe (e.g. Seizure) causes the eyes to deviate away from the side of the lesion. On the other hand, a destructive lesion causes the eyes to deviate towards the side of the lesion. If the anterior aspect of the frontal lobe is involved, it would cause irritability, behavior abnormalities or lethargy. Spincter incontinence may develop and there may be re- appearance of primitive reflexes like sucking, rooting and grasp reflex.
2. Temporal lobe: Lesions in this lobe also affect the personality. Wernickes aphasia results from damage to the superior and middle gyri. Involvement of the nondominant lobe causes distorted perception of spatial relationships and a change in musical appreciation. Temporal lobe dysfunction can cause memory impairment, homonymous superior quadrantinopia and aggressive behavior. Learning difficulties can arise from bilateral hippocampal involvement.
3. Parietal lobes: Dysfunction of parietal lobes results in abnormalities in sensory perception (two point discrimination, graphesthesia, appreciation of size, shape and texture). Lesion in parietal lobe results in impairment of awareness on the opposite side. Parietal lobe lesions also result in apraxia or the inability to perform a series of tasks although every individual component can be completed by the individual. In small children, parietal lobe damage affects growth of the affected side, e.g. smaller hand in a child with hemiparesis indicates damage to the parietal lobe.
4. Occipital lobe: Bilateral damage results in cortical blindness. If unilateral, it causes homonymous visual field defects.

To assess spatial perception, one can ask the child to copy few geometric figures.

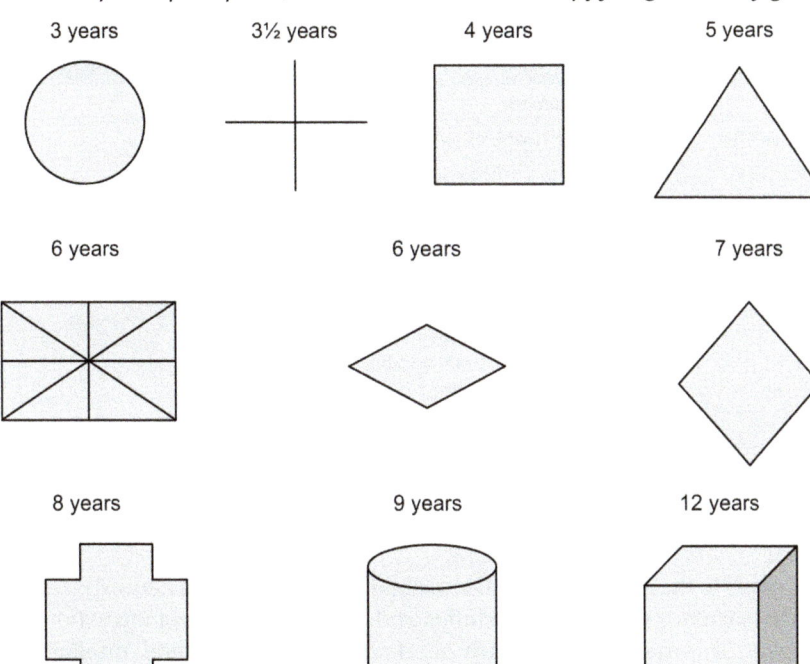

Higher Mental Functions Examination

The approach to mental status evaluation should be adjusted to the age of the baby. Up to approximately age six months, mental status is assessed through (a) review of the history and, (b) observation of the early developmental milestones.

1. Attention: The baby's attentiveness and awareness of the environment as well as his or her responsiveness to social stimulation (e.g. response to rattle, sound or light) is noted. Response of a child to a rattle at different age is shown in Table 18.2.

Table 18.2: Response of a child to a rattle at different ages.

Age	Response
4 months	Tries to reach the object but overshoots it
5 months	Reaches out for objects and plays
6–7 months	Transfers objects in one hand to the other

2. Language: After six months mental status is evaluated by determining the level of development of language and adaptive behavior. These are determined by review of the developmental history provided by the parents and by observation of the baby in spontaneous activity and in response to the parents or examiner.

Table 18.3 gives briefly about the age at which language development occurs.

Table 18.3: Age at which language development occurs.

Age	Development
3–4 months	Cooing–vowel like sounds
7 months	Babbling–1 syllable sounds
10 months	Responds to name
11–12 months	Speaks at least one word responds to simple commands such as "no"
18 months	Speaks more than three words knows two or three body parts
2 years	• Has two to three word sentence • Follows two or three word commands • Points to pictures as requested
3 years	• Speaks three or four word sentences • Uses pronouns and plurals • Knows age, sex and full name • Asks questions

Adaptive Behavior

This refers to the faculties that reflect a child's ability to initiate new experiences and to learn from them. This includes understanding, concept formation and imagery. This measure has a fairly good correlation with overall intelligence. This ability is also estimated by review of the history provided by the parent and by the observation of spontaneous or elicited behaviors and functions at the time of examination.

There are several accessories that will be useful for the examination. This includes several one inch building blocks of different colors, toys of interest to a child including ones with which he or she can interact (e.g. doll, truck), a book with pictures and simple text and a container into which the child can put a pellet or other object. Table 18.4 gives the adaptive behavior development at different age.

Table 18.4: Adaptive behavior development at different ages.

Age	Behavior
6 weeks	Smiles responsively
12 weeks	Follows visually 180°
4 months	Reach for object
7–8 months	Holds one block/toy in each hand
9 months	Has stranger awareness/anxiety
12 months	Waves bye-bye, plays peek a boo, finds object hidden in presence
15 months	Places one block on top of another, throws items
1.5 years	Mimics examiner, finger feeds self, helps undress self
2 years	Copies vertical line, builds tower of 6–7 blocks, turns single book pages
2.5 years	Copies horizontal line, imitates train with chimney using blocks
3 years	Mostly dresses self, copies circle, builds tower with nine blocks, imitates building of bridge

Cranial Nerve Examination

- Olfactory nerve examination can be done in older children.
- Optic nerve:
  - Materials required: Red ring, thread/string to dangle the ring, Torch
  - Visual acuity:
    - Testing of visual acuity in children depends on the age and cooperation of the child. Immaturity and inability to vocalize prevents the usage of regular Snellen chart in children. Monocular testing cannot be done up to 42 months
    - In younger children visual acuity is assessed by analyzing the ability of the baby to fixate and follow a light or interesting object such as dangling red ring.
    - A dangling red ring held 8-10 inches from the baby can be used. The distance, the baby follows the moving object depends on the age of the baby which is given in the following table:

Age	Inference
1 month	Follows the red ring in a range of 90°
3 months	Follows the red ring in a range of 180°
6 months	Adjusts his position to see objects (bending back or crouching)

    - Poor or absent fixation to the test indicates macular dysfunction or severe visual impairment. Decreased vision results in photophobia, nystagmus and roving eye movements. Severe visual impairment results in hyperkinetic and rhythmic eye movements along with grimacing and other facial contortions.
    - Infants aged 1 year and above are tested by offering small interesting objects.
    - 2-3 years: Miniature toys are used. The child has one set and the examiner has an identical set. Examiner hold up a toy standing 10 feet away from the child. Child has to match the examiners toy with his own set.
    - Snellen's E chart can be used from 3 years of age
    - Peripheral vision: This can be tested from 1 year onwards . Child is distracted with a toy in front, while bringing a red toy from behind the infants peripheral field of vision. A child with normal vision should respond as soon as the toy reaches a perpendicular to the outer canthus of the eye.
    - Color vision is tested from three years onwards using modified Ishihara tests suitable for children.
    - Accommodation: Not developed well until 2 months. Dangling red ring can be used to check accommodation from 3 months

- Pupillary response: To open eyes in very young babies circumoral region is stimulated. Torch is used to stimulate the pupillary response
- Fundoscopy: The parent holds the baby so that the baby is looking over one of the parents shoulder. The examiner gently holds the baby's head, and views the fundus.

3. III, IV and VI cranial nerves:
   - Dolls eye reflex is used in age 3 months. In dolls eye reflex, movement of head to one direction results in movement of the eyeballs to opposite direction.
   - The eye lags behind head movement in babies lesser than 3 months.
   - 5 months—rattle can be used to check the movements of the eyes.

4. V cranial nerve:
   - Masseter muscle is felt when the baby is breastfeeding. A sterilized tongue depressor is kept between the gum of the infant. When infant tries to bite the depressor the masseter muscle can be palpated.
   - Jaw reflex: To elicit the reflex tap the chin of the baby with the index finger when the mouth is slightly open. The reflex results in jaw closure. This maneuver can be used in babies up to 4–5 months.
   - Corneal reflex: Cornea is touched with a wisp of cotton, which is brought to the eye from the side, outside the field of vision resulting in blinking of the eye.

5. VII cranial nerve:
   - Facial nerve innervates the muscles of the face. Observation of the face allows good assessment of this nerve. Assessment is best done when baby cries or smiles. Look for any asymmetry in wrinkles over the forehead and the angle of the mouth.
   - Corneal reflex tested also assesses 7th nerve as it is the efferent nerve for the reflex. Taste sensation cannot be assessed in children.

6. VIII cranial nerve:
   - Risk factors for development of hearing defect are as follows: Preterm babies, cerebral palsy, kernicterus, rubella or CMV infections during Pregnancy, syndromes (Treachers Collin, Klippel-Feil, Pendred, Kallman) congenital deafness in the family
   - In newborn period baby responds to sound by startle response, blinking, and crying
   - Baby quietens when crying to sound
   - Distraction test: Baby sits on mothers lap facing forward. Mother distracts the baby with a toy (no noisy toy). The examiner then makes soft noise standing behind the mother and the baby and outside the baby's field of vision. Bell, or a noise making rattle can be used. The response to the sound at different age groups are given in Table 18.5:

Table 18.5: Response to sound at different age groups.

Age	Response to sound
3 months	Turns head to the side of the sound
3–4 months	Turns head and eyes towards the side of the sound
5–6 months	Turns the head to the side and then downwards if the sound is made below the level of the ear
6 months and above	Turns the head to the side and then upwards if the sound is made above the level of the ear
6–8 months	Turns the head in a curving arc towards the sound source
8–10 months	Turns the head diagonally and directly towards the sound

- If the baby fails to respond to the sound on 2 separate occasions 1 month apart then the baby should be subjected to audiological testing (BERA or OAE)
- Rinne and Webers tuning fork test can be used in children above 6 years.

7. IX and X cranial nerve:
   - Testing of these cranial nerve are limited only to questionnaire and observation
   - Ask for regurgitation of milk through the nose
   - When baby cries during the course of examination observe the palatal movements and note any nasal twang to the voice
   - Gag reflex is examined in the same steps as in older children.
8. XI cranial nerve: Baby is placed in supine position. The shoulders are supported but not the head, the head is pushed laterally. The child will resist the movement, and the examiner can palpate the sternomastoid muscle.
9. XII cranial nerve: Examination of this nerve is limited to observation of the tongue when the mouth is open.

Examination of the Coordination

- The principle function of the cerebellum is coordination of the voluntary movements. The ability to experience cerebellar dysfunction depends upon the maturity of the motor system supported by the cerebellum. This implies that cerebellar examination can be done as the motor (gross and fine) functions mature.
- Stability of the trunk and coordination while walking is predominantly the function of the midline of the cerebellum. While testing of the fine motor coordination of the extremities is the function of the cerebellar hemispheres.
- Truncal stability and coordination while walking is assessed by the following:
    - Observing the child get in and out of sitting position
    - Noting stability in sitting and standing position

- Watching child walk (Examination of gait is discussed elsewhere in the chapter)
    - Perform age appropriate skills like hopping, tandem walking, standing on one leg
- Expected age dependent capabilities are as follows:
    - Child pulls to sit from supine position: 10 months
    - At around 1 year of age child walks with wide based gait
    - Stands on one foot: 3 years
    - Tandem walking: 3-4 years
    - Skips on one foot: 4 years
    - Skips on both foot: 5 years
- Standard test to assess the appendicular (extremities) coordination are repetitive finger and foot tapping, front to back hand tapping, finger nose test, heel to shin test.
- These tests should be modified to perform in babies: The child is asked to press the penlight bulb with the index finger or great toe. This test can be performed in children 18 months and above.

Sensation

- A tracing wheel with blunt edges can be used
- Child is distracted with a toy the examiner then runs the tracing wheels on the legs or the arms
- A child with normal sensation will immediately look at the site of simulation
- This test can be used from 9 months onwards.

BIBLIOGRAPHY

1. Bale JF Jr, Bonkowsky JL, Filloux FM, Hedlund GL, Nielsen DM, Larsen PD. Pediatric neurology: a color handbook. 201 Manson Publishing.
2. Goldbloom RB. Pediatric clinical skills. Elsevier publications, 4th edition; 2010.
3. Illingworth RS. The normal child, 10th edition; Elsevier publications; 1997.
4. Kulakarni ML. Clinical methods in paediatrics. Jaypee publications; 2005.
5. Nair MKC, Russel P, (Eds). Illingworth's The development of the infant and young child normal and abnormal, 10th edition. Elsevier publications; 2012.
6. Swaiman KF, Ashwal S, Ferriero DM, Schor NF. Swaiman's pediatric neurology- principles and practice, 5th edition. Elsevier publications; 2012.

Index

Page numbers followed by *b* refer to box, *f* refer to figure, *fc* refer to flowchart, and *t* refer to table.

A

Abdomen 478
Abdominal reflex 300*f*, 488
Abducens nerve 105
Abduction force 447
Abductor pollicis brevis 261, 262
   anatomy of 261*f*
   testing of 262*f*
Abductor pollicis longus 261, 262
   anatomy of 261*f*
   testing of 262*f*
Aberrant reinnervation 135
Abetalipoproteinemia 362
Acalculia
   primary 29
   secondary 29
Acanthocytosis 361, 373
Accommodation 493
Acetylcholine 61
Acid maltase deficiency, adult onset 204
Acoustic aura 382
Acquired immunodeficiency syndrome 70
Acquired metabolic causes of chorea 362*b*
Acromioclavicular joint 295, 437
   disorder 439*f*
Acromion 437
Adduction force 447
Adductor 306
   longus, brevis 268
   magnus 268
   reflex 302, 304
Adductor pollicis
   anatomy of 263*f*
   testing of 263*f*
Adenoma sebaceum 478
Adie's pupil 123
Adipose tissue 420
Adrenergic innervation, tests of 411
Adson's test 423
Agnosia 31, 32, 32*f*, 34
   apperceptive 31, 33, 33*f*, 34*f*
   color 35
   landmark 36
   tactile 33
   verbal auditory 36
Agraphia 16, 17
Akathisia 374
Akinesia, unilateral 382
Akinetic mutism 73
Alcohol 362, 409
Alexander's law 389, 390, 395
Alexia 16, 17
Alpha-gamma coactivation 214
Alzheimer's disease 79, 368, 369
American Autonomic Society 412
American College of Rheumatology 451
Aminoacidopathy 362
Aminoacidurias 357
Amnesia
   anterograde 43
   retrograde 43
Amphetamine 362
Amusia 32, 36
   apperceptive 36
Amygdala 40, 77, 381
Amyotrophy 360
Anal reflex 489
   superficial 307, 308
Anemia 356
Angiomas 478
Anhydrosis 409
Anisocoria 125*fc*
   pathological 124
Ankle 218, 306
   clonus 337
   jerk 302, 305
   plantar flexion 275
      against gravity, testing of 275*f*
      plantar flexors, anatomy of 275*f*
   reflex 304, 487
Anomia 9
Anomic aphasia 16, 17
Anosmia 77-79
   bilateral 79
Antecubital fossa 295
Anterolateral system 293
Anteromedial thalamus 40
Anthropometry 478
Anticholinergics 362
Anti-epileptic drugs 362
Antipsychotics 372
Aphasia 9, 382, 383
   conduction 15, 17
   global 14, 17, 19*f*

thalamic 16
transcortical
   mixed 15, 17
   motor 15, 17
   sensory 15, 17
Apley's scratch test 438, 438f
Apneusis 66f
Apraxia 9, 19
   buccofacial 21
   causes of 25b
   constructional 21, 23, 24, 25
   dressing 21, 23, 25
   evaluation of 22t
   ideational 21, 22, 23, 26
   ideomotor 21, 22, 23
   localization 25
   network, simplified 21f
   orofacial 22, 24, 25
   speech 17
   types of 22
Archimedes spiral drawing 351
Argyll Robertson pupil 128
Arm 217
   abduction test 422
   drift 286
   dropping test 217
   pain, examination of 417, 418
   recoil 464
   swing, exaggerated 337
   traction 466
Arnold-Chiari malformation 159b, 398
Arterioles 420
Arthritis 361
Arytenoid muscle 195
Ashleaf macules 478
Ashworth scale 218
Asymmetric binocular nystagmus, causes of 159b
Ataxia 342
   spinocerebellar 361
   telangiectasia 361, 362
Ataxic breathing 66f
Ataxic gait 490
Athetoid 461
Athetosis 357
Atlantoaxial subluxation 343
Atonic seizure 381
Atrophy 436
Attention deficit disorder 373
Auditory agnosia 31
   general 31, 36
Auditory aura 379
Auditory comprehension 12
Auditory orientation 462
Auditory pathway 181f
Autistic spectrum disorders 372
Autoimmune encephalopathies 369

Automotor seizure 381, 386
Autonomic aura 379, 382
Autonomic dysfunction 409
Autonomic function tests, specific bedside 411
Autonomic nervous system 407
Autonomic neuropathy 131
Autonomic signs 424
Autonomic system 379
Axial myoclonus 367
Axial trunk muscle extensor action 215
Axillary freckling 478
Axillary line, contralateral 466

B

Babinski's buck reflex hammer 300f
Babinski's hammer 300f
Babinski's reflex 310f
Babinski's response 488
Babinski's sign 305, 309, 310f, 311-313
Babinski's tonus test 217
Basal forebrain 61
Basal ganglia 21, 142, 142f
   circuits 340f
   lesions 17
   stroke 447
Bat wing appearance 356
Batten's disease 102
Bedside orthostatic test 412
Beighton score 411
Bell's phenomenon 69, 178, 179
Biceps brachii 236, 244, 245f
   anatomy of 244f
Biceps femoris 272
Biceps reflex 302, 303
Biceps tendon 437
Binswanger's disease 336
Bitemporal hemianopia 81
Blepharospasm 354
Blind spot, enlarged 90
Blink reflex 172
Blood
   pressure, diastolic 412
   vessels, abnormalities of 100
Body righting reflex 486
Bouncing gait 337
Brachialis 244
Brachioradialis 244
   reflex 303
Bradykinesia 348
Brain
   injury, hypoxic 460
   iron accumulation 361
   levels of 66f
Brainstem 62, 164f, 182f, 366t
   axial myoclonus, causes of 369
   centers 143
   cross-section of lower 194f

functions 63
lesions 128, 198, 369
levels of 67f
myoclonus 364, 367
nuclei 155f
reticular formation, neurons of 61f
saccadic centers 139f
Break test 225
Breathing 65
  deep 411
Broca's aphasia 13-15, 17
Broca's area 17
Bucket test 390, 391, 392f
Bulbocavernosus reflex 307, 308
Burst neurons 140

C

Cafe au lait spots 460, 478
Cajal, interstitial nucleus of 139, 140, 145, 394
Calcium channel blockers 362
Calibrated finger rub auditory screening test 183
Callosal lesion 27
Caloric tests 187
Caloric vestibulo-ocular reflex 72
Camel gait 337
Carbamazepine 372
Carbon monoxide 372
Cardiovagal innervation, tests of 411
Carditis 361
Carotid sinus 197
Carotid thrombosis 136f
Cataract 478
Catatonia 73, 343
Celiac disease 342, 369
Cerebellar ataxia 287, 361b
Cerebellar disease 322
  bilateral 325
  unilateral 326
Cerebellar dysfunction, mild 330
Cerebellar eye movement abnormalities 152t
Cerebellar influence 143f
Cerebellar lesion 403, 490
  contralateral 151
Cerebellar signs 348, 360, 368
Cerebellar truncal tremor 337
Cerebellopontine-angle tumors 396
Cerebellum 143, 321
  nuclei of 320f
  physiological systems of 320f
Cerebral
  injury, parasagittal 473
  ptosis 135
  spasticity 219
Cerebrocerebellum 321
Ceroid lipofuscinosis 362
Cervical
  dystonia 343b

  retrocollis 357
  spine 418f, 437
  torticollis 357
Cherry red spot 369, 478
Cheyne-Stokes respiration 65, 66f
Chiasmal body 81
Chiasmal lesions 127
Chorea 337, 342, 359, 361b, 362b, 373, 374
  etiology of 359fc
  examination of 359
  rheumatic 372
Choreoacanthocytosis 361
Chorioretinitis 478
Chromosomal disorders 372, 373
Ciliary ganglion 120
Ciliospinal reflex 69
Cingulate 77
  gyrus 4
Claudication
  distance 434
  neurogenic 434, 434t
  vasogenic 434, 434t
Clonic seizure 380
Clonic tics 371
Clostridium tetani 220
Cluster breathing 66f
Coat hanger 421
  distribution pain 409
Cocaine 372
Cockayne syndrome 102
Collateral ligament
  lateral 443, 447
  medial 443, 447
Colliculus, inferior 182
Collier's sign 128
Coma 73t
  examination of 60
  metabolic 68
    causes of 74t
  structural causes of 74t
Compression test 441, 442f
Connect standard electrocardiography 412
Consciousness
  impaired 373
  level of 64
  loss of 409
  state of 74
  system, components of 61f
Contrast sensitivity charts 84
Convergence insufficiency 153
Convergence spasm 153
Coprolalia 373
Copropraxia 373
Coracoacromial arch 439f
Corneal reflex 69, 172, 179, 494
Coronary artery bypass graft 19

Corpus callosum 21
Cortex, dorsolateral
    frontal 8
    prefrontal 4, 5, 141
Cortical amnestic syndrome 43
Cortical control 141
Cortical functions 490
Cortical interactions 142
Cortical lesions 198
Cortical myoclonus 364
    causes of 369
Corticobasal degeneration 342
Corticobasal ganglionic degeneration 368, 369
Corticospinal tracts 215
    anterior 215
    lateral 215
Cover-uncover test 113
Cramping pain 434
Cranial nerve 67, 76, 104, 105, 200f, 201, 208f, 473, 474, 477, 494, 495
    accessory 200
    course of 208f
    examination 64, 66, 473, 493
    nucleus of 139, 164f, 194f
    spinal branches of 201f
Cranium, auscultation of 478
Cremasteric reflex 307, 309, 488
Creutzfeldt-Jakob disease 368, 369
Cribriform plate 77
Cricoarytenoids, lateral 195
Cross-arm test 438
Cruciate ligament
    anterior 443, 447
    posterior 443, 447
Cry, nature of 462

D

Deafness, congenital 494
Dementia 57, 362b, 368
Demyelinating optic neuropathy 90
Dentatorubral-pallidoluysian atrophy 361, 362
Dentatorubrothalamic pathway 349
Depression 343
    generalized 91f
Dermatomes 429, 430f
Desmin myopathy 204
Dialeptic seizure 380
Diencephalic dysfunction, bilateral 68
Diffuse forebrain damage 66f
Diplopia 106, 108
    chart 113, 114
Disc disease 419f
Distal interphalangeal flexion, testing of 254
Distraction test 441, 441f, 494
Dix-Hallpike maneuver 398f, 399, 401
Dizziness, bedside evaluation of 402
Dopamine 61

agonists 362
receptor blockers 372
Dopa-responsive dystonia 338
Dorsal midbrain syndrome, part of 153
Down's syndrome 372
Drawer test
    anterior 447, 448f
    posterior 448f
Dressing 47
Drop test 442, 443f
Dubowitz scheme 459
Duchenne muscular dystrophy 372, 373
Dynamic sensitivity 402
Dysarthria 9
Dysdiadochokinesis 322, 329
Dysequilibrium 322
Dyskinesia 317
    paroxysmal kinesigenic 354
Dysmetric saccades 145
Dysphasia 9
Dysplastic ears, abnormal 478
Dyssynergia 322, 327
Dystonia 341, 342, 353, 356, 357, 360, 361b, 373, 374
    classification 354
    diurnal variation of 357
    fixed 355
    fluctuating 357
    oromandibular 360
    paradoxical 355
    paroxysmal exercise-induced 354
    plus 354
    primary 342, 356, 372
    secondary 356
    truncal 337
Dystonic attacks 357
Dystonic hand posturing 382
Dystonic tics 355, 357, 371
Dystonic tremor 349

E

Ears 478
    abnormal placement of 478
Echolalia 373
Echopraxia 373
Edema 101, 409
Edinger-Westphal nucleus 104, 120
Ehlers-Danlos syndrome 415
Elbow
    extension 246
    flexion 244, 245f
Electrocardiography 417
Elliptical pendular nystagmus 161
Empty can test 440
Encephalitis 372
Encephalopathy
    metabolic 369

neonatal 458
paraneoplastic 369
Enophthalmos 133
Entorhinal cortex 77
Epidural fibrofatty tissue 420
Epigastric aura 379, 382, 386
Epilepsy 378
    childhood absence 384
    clinical evaluation of 376
    focal 382*t*
    maternal 459
    myoclonic 368
    paracentral 385
    parieto-occipital lobe 385
    progressive myoclonic 369
    specific report 383
Epileptic seizures 377, 385t
Episodic memory 41
Equines gait 337
Esotropia 108
Ewald's first law 389
Ewald's second law 389, 395
Ewald's third law 389
Exercise 355, 409
Exotropia 108
Expanded Medical Research Council Scale for manual muscle testing 227
Extensor carpi radialis longus 251
    and brevis, anatomy of 251*f*
Extensor carpi ulnaris 251
    anatomy of 251*f*
Extensor digiti minimi 255
Extensor digitorum 255
    brevis 281
    longus 281
Extensor hallucis longus 281
Extensor indicis 255
Extensor muscles 215
Extensor pollicis brevis 260
    anatomy of 260*f*
    testing of 260*f*
Extensor pollicis longus 260, 261
    anatomy of 260*f*
Extrafusal fibers 214
Extraocular muscles 107*f*
    actions of 106*t*
Extrapyramidal disease 330
Extrapyramidal signs 424
Extrapyramidal system 216
Eye 478
    closure 69
        effect of 287
    field
        frontal 141
        supplementary 141
    movement
        conjugate 150
        downward 149*f*
        examination of 390, 393
        generation 155*f*
        spontaneous 69, 74
        tests of 110
        upward 149*f*
    parasympathetic innervation of 121*f*
    position, spontaneous 60*f*
    resting position of 69
    torsion of 391
Eyelid 67, 133
    examination 133
    opening, apraxia of 22, 24, 343

F

Face
    and jaw 346
    sensory innervation of 168*f*
Facet joint 423, 426, 427*f*
Facial colliculus 177
Facial dystonia 343
Facial nerve 176, 177, 494
Facial nuclei, anatomy of 176*f*
Facial palsy 179
Fasciculus, superior longitudinal 21
Fastigial nucleus and vermis 141
Fatiguing 342
Feet dystonia 337
Ferritin associated basal ganglia disease 362
Fever 409
Fibromyalgia 451, 456*f*
Figure of 4 sign 382
Fine distal movements 21
Finger
    abduction 256, 257
    abductors
        anatomy of 256*f*, 257*f*
        testing of 257*f*, 258*f*
    flexion 306
        reflex 302, 303
    flexors, long 258
    identification 30, 58
    metacarpophalangeal extension 255
    nose test, variations of 327
Finger-to-finger test 327
Finger-to-nose test 327, 347
Flexor carpi radialis 249
    anatomy of 249*f*
Flexor carpi ulnaris 249
    anatomy of 249*f*
Flexor digitorum
    brevis 280
    longus 280
    profundus 253, 253*f*
        testing of 254*f*
    superficialis 253, 254
        anatomy of 253*f*
        testing of 254*f*

Flexor halluces
  brevis 279
  longus 280
Flexor pollicis brevis 259
  anatomy of 259f
  testing of 259f
Flexor pollicis longus 259, 259f, 260
  testing of 259f
Floppy infant syndrome 458
Flunarizine 362
Fluoxetine 362
Focal epilepsy, benign 384
Focal myoclonus 367
Focal seizures 343
Foot
  angle 333
  dorsiflexion 276
    testing of 276f
  dorsiflexors, anatomy of 276f
  drop 490
    differential diagnosis of 434t
  eversion 278
    testing of 278f
  evertors, anatomy of 278f
  inversion 277
  invertors
    anatomy of 277f
    testing of 277f
Forearm pronation 248
  anatomy of 248f
Forearm supination 247
  anatomy of 247f
Forearm and hand, examination of 244
Forehead wrinkling 133
Formainal compression test 422
Fragile X syndrome 372
Frenzel's glasses 393, 395-398
Friedreich's ataxia 361
Froment's maneuver 217
Froment's sign 348
Frontalis overaction 133
Fukuda test 390
Fundoscopy 494
Funduscopic examination 74
Funiculus, dorsolateral 284, 285

G

Gabaergic Purkinje neurons 155
Gaenslen's test 440, 441f
Gait 332, 489
  apraxia of 23, 26
  assessment 332
  cerebellar 336
  circumduction 490
  cock 337
  cycle 332, 333f
    typical 333f
  disorder 337
    psychogenic 338
  dromedary 337
  duck 337
  examination of 332, 489
  flail 337
  high stepping 337
  military 337
  spastic 336
    ataxic 337
    paraplegic 490
  staggering 490
  stamping 337
  types of 490
  waddling 337, 490
Galant's reflex 485
Gamma aminobutyric acid 61
Gangliosidosis 362
Gasserian ganglion 166
Gastrocnemius 275
Gaucher's disease 369
Gaze disorders, examination of 138
Gaze palsy, horizontal 396
Gaze paretic nystagmus 155
Gaze-evoked nystagmus 394
Gelastic seizure 382
Genetic diseases 100
Genetic syndromes 459
Geniculate body, medial 183
Geniculate nucleus, lateral 121
Genioglossus pushes 211
Gerstmann syndrome, part of 30
Gerstmann-Sträussler-Scheinker syndrome 151
Gestes antagonistes 353
Gestural comprehension 21
Gestural production 21
Glabellar reflex 172
Glasgow coma score 64, 65t
Glenohumeral joint 437
Globe, rotational axis of 107f
Glossopharyngeal nerve 191
  anatomy of 192f
  nuclei of 191f
Gluteus maximus 267
Gluteus medius and minimus 269, 271
Gnosis 31
Grand mal epilepsy 384
Grasp reflex 315, 484
Great toe
  ball of 310f
  dorsiflexion of 310f
Gunn phenomenon 135
Gustatory aura 379, 382
Gustatory sweating 409

H

Hair
  cells 182, 183
  light colored 478
  loss of 409
  tuft of 460
Hallpike maneuver 190
Hamstring reflex 302
  lateral 304
  medial 304
Harlequin syndrome 129
Hashimoto's encephalopathy 369
Hawkins test 438, 439f
Head 346, 478
  and eye version 382
  dropping test 217
  heave test 390, 393, 404
  impulse test 402, 402f
  injury 372
  lag 468, 468f
  position 355
  rotation, direction of 403
  shaking nystagmus 396
  syndrome
    causes of dropped 204
    dropped 343
  thrust 133, 187
    test 187
  tilt 110
Headedness, light 409
Head-shaking nystagmus 395
Hearing
  evaluation of 478
  loss
    conductive 185
    sensorineural 185
Heart disease
  rheumatic 373
  valvular 373
Heart rate 412
  response to breathing 411
Heel-knee-toe test 328
Heel-to-ear maneuver 467
Hemangiomas 460, 478
Hemidystonia 354
Hemiplegia
  left 314
  spastic 490
Hemorrhage 62
  disc 101
  subhyaloid 74
Hennebert's sign 398
Hepatic disease 356
Hereditary chorea, benign 362
Hereditary sensory 131
Hering's law 108f, 113
Heschl's gyrus 10

Heterochromia iridis 124, 130
Heterophoria 108
Heterotropia 108
Hip
  abduction 269
    anatomy of 269f
    testing of 269f
  adduction 268
  adductors
    anatomy of 268f
    testing of 268f
  extension 267
    testing of 267f
  extensors, anatomy of 267
  external rotation 270
    anatomy of 270f
    testing of 270f
  flexion 266
  flexors
    anatomy of 266f
    testing of 266f
  internal rotation 271, 271f
    testing of 271f
Hirschberg test 112
Histamine 61
Hoffa's fat tissue 444
Hoffmann reflex 487
Hormone 362
  melanin concentrating 61
Horner's pharmacology 129f, 130t
Horner's syndrome 123, 124, 129, 131, 134, 135
  localization of 130f
  painful 135
Hot environment 409
Hot water bath 409
Human immunodeficiency virus 362
Human musculoskeletal system 223f
Humphrey's visual field
  analyzer 87
  test 88f
Huntington's disease 342, 361, 362, 372, 373
Hutchinson's pupil 69
Hydrocephalus 337
Hyperekplexia 369
Hyperglycemia 362
Hyperhydrosis 409
Hyperkinetic disorders 342
Hyperkinetic motor disorders, types of 374t
Hyperkinetic movement disorders 342fc
Hypermetria 327
Hyperopia 126
Hyperosmia 77
Hyper-reflexia 305
Hyperthermia 409
Hypertonia 218
Hypertropia 108
Hyperventilation 396, 409

Hypoglossal nerve palsy, right 211
Hypoglycemia 362
Hypokinetic disorders 342
Hypometria, unilateral 327
Hypomotor 380
Hypoparathyroidism 204
Hyporeflexia 305, 348
Hyposmia 77
Hypothalamic-midbrain damage 65
Hypothalamus 382
    lateral 61
Hypothermia 409
Hypothyroidism 204, 343
Hypotonia 218, 322, 360
    central 473
    distribution of 473
    neuromuscular 473
Hypotropia 108
Hysterical ptosis 135

I

Ictal
    eye blinking 382
    nystagmus 382
    speech 382
    spitting 382
    testing 383
    vomiting 382
Iliacus 266
Iliopsoas muscle 454*f*
Iliopsoas trigger points 454*f*
Impaired pursuit defect, bilateral 151
Infarct 62
Inflammatory demyelinating polyneuropathy, chronic 204
Inflammatory myopathies 204
Infraspinatus 242
Insula 77
Insular region 382
Interossei, dorsal 256
Interphalangeal joints 280*f*
Interphalanges flexion, distal 280
Intervertebral foramen 426
Intracranial bruits 478
Intrafusal fibers 214
Intransitive gestures 23
Involuntary movements 459, 460
Ipsilateral axillary line 466
Ipsilateral dorsolateral tract 293
Ipsilateral nipple line 466
Ipsilateral tilt 337
Iris ischemia 126
Ischemic optic neuropathy, anterior 101
Ishihara color
    charts 86*f*
    test 85
Ishihara test 85
Isometric muscle testing 444

J

Jargon speech 10
Jaw jerk 172, 302, 306, 424
Jaw weakness, bilateral 173
Jerky movements 342
Joint
    contractures 460
    hyperextensibility 411
    position sensation 287
    sacroiliac 440
Jugular foramen 198
Juvenile Huntington's disease 369
Juvenile myoclonic epilepsy 369, 384, 386

K

Kayser-Fleischer ring 356, 373
Kearns-Sayre syndrome 102
Keiser-Fleischer ring 348
Ketogenic diet 362
Kinesthesia 284
Kinetic tremor 345, 347
Klinefelter syndrome 372
Knee 218, 306
    endorotation of 445*f*, 446*f*
    exorotation of 445*f*, 446*f*
    extension 273
        anatomy of 273*f*
        testing of 274*f*
    flexion 272
        against gravity, testing of 272*f*
    flexors
        anatomy of 272*f*
        reciprocal inhibition of 301*f*
    jerk 302
    joint 443
    reflex 304, 305, 487
Kollner's rule 85
Krabbe's disease 369
Kyphoscoliosis, sign of 478
Kyphosis 431

L

Lambert-Eaton myasthenic syndrome 204
Lamotrigine 362, 372
Landau reflex 486
Language 9, 57, 491
    assessment 9
        interpretation of 14
    dependent functions 50
    development occurs 492*t*
    disorders 9
    network, dual stream model of 10*f*
Laryngeal nerve
    recurrent 195, 198
    superior 195, 198
Larynx 197
Laterodorsal tegmental nucleus 61

Latissimus dorsi 237
   anatomy of 237f
   isolation of 238
   testing of 238f, 239f
Leaky neural integrator 156f
Leber's hereditary 100
Leg
   action myoclonus of 337
   length, measure 431
   movements, causes of involuntary 337
   recoil 467, 467f
   rolling 218
   traction 467
   tremor 349
Lennox-Gastaut syndrome 384
Lesch-Nyhan syndrome 362, 372
Lesion
   central 403
   left frontal 27
   peripheral 403
Leukomalacia, periventricular 473
Levator dehiscence disinsertion 134
Levodopa 362, 372
Lexical semantics 9
Lhermitte's test 423
Lid
   examination of 117
   retraction 135
Ligaments 420, 427
Light near dissociation 123, 126, 128, 128t
Lights and glare, interior 85
Limb
   ataxia 287
   coordination 390
   dystonia 343
   flexors 214
   kinetic apraxia 21, 23, 24, 25
   position sense 284
   tone of 459
Lippman's test 440
Lissauer tract 293
Lithium 362
Little finger opposition 265
Liver disease signs 360
Lobe
   epilepsy, frontal 384
   frontal 490
Locked-in syndrome 73
Locomotor center 332
Locus coeruleus 61
Longitudinal fasciculus, medial 121, 139, 145, 155, 182, 391
Lordosis, loss of 431
Low back pain, examination of 426
Lower limb
   muscles, power of 266
   placing reflex 470
   tremor 348

Lower motor nerve 179
   facial palsy 179
Lower pontine tegmental
   damage 65
   lesion 66f
Lower trapezius fibers 233
   muscle 202f
Lumbar spine 428f
Lumbar vertebrae 426
Lumbosacral segments 285
Lumbricals 252
   against gravity, testing of 253f
Luria alternating sequence test 6
Luria test 8

M

Macrosaccadic oscillations 146
Macrosquare wave jerks 146
Macular disease 85
Malformations, congenital 460
Mandibular nerve 170f
Manganese toxicity 337
Mastication, muscles of 165f
Maternal neuromuscular illnesses 459
Maxillary nerve 169, 170f
McGill reflex 300f
McLeod's syndrome 361, 362
Medial prefrontal circuit, syndrome of 4
Medulla, dorsomedial part of 66f
Medullary dysfunction 65
Meissner's corpuscles 291
Memory 38, 58
   classification of 39fc
   long-term 40, 42
   nonverbal 42
   types of 39f
   verbal 41
   working 41
Ménière's disease 189, 397
Ménière's syndrome 190
Meniscus
   lateral 447
   medial 447
Mental functions
   assessment of higher 1
   examination, higher 491
   higher 477
Mental status
   examination 1
   function 3f
Merkel discs 291
Mesial temporal sclerosis 386f
Metacarpophalangeal extension 252
   testing of 253f
Metacarpophalangeal joints 255f
Metatarsophalangeal joints 279f
Methylphenidate 362, 372

Michael's glasses 393, 395-398
Midbrain lesion 135
Midclavicular line 295, 296
Mimic shoulder abduction 240
Mini-cog test 42
Mini-mental status examination 2, 51
Mitochondrial disease 342, 361, 362, 368, 369
Mobile dystonia 355
Mollaretz's triangle 365*f*
Mono-ocular diplopia 115*fc*
   interpretation of 115
Montreal cognitive assessment 2
Moro reflex 470, 472, 484
Morpheme 9
Motor
   activity 379
   area, supplementary 382
   function 177
      examination, interpretation of 173
   neuron disease 204
   nucleus 166
      dorsal 194
   seizure 380
      complex 381
      simple 380
   skill, complex 332
   system 64, 212, 477
      examination 479
   tics 371
Movement assessment, range of 438
Movement disorder 339, 340, 340*f,* 342*t,* 343*b,* 357, 362*b*
   broad classification of 342*b*
   combinations of 342
   examination of 339
Mucocutaneous junction 297
Mueller's muscle 136
Multiple system atrophy 342, 369
Murmurs 478
Muscle 231, 232
   antigravity 473
   belly 451
   contralateral 219
   diseases 135
   intrinsic and extrinsic 209
   paravertebral 420
   power
      assessment of 223
      testing, rules of 224
   spasm 431
   spindles 214
   strength
      assessment 177
      grading of 226
   testing 223
      specific rules of 225
   tone 74, 212*f,* 214

weakness 226
   functional assessment of 227
   proximal 373
   yoked pairs of 106*t,* 107*f*
Myasthenia 135, 459
   gravis 204
Myoclonus 342, 357, 364, 364*fc,* 365, 368, 373, 374
   diagnosis of 369
   dystonia 354, 369
   horizontal 70
   post anoxic 369
   symptomatic palatal 368
   vertical 70
Myopathies, congenital 473
Myopia 126
Myotomes 428, 429*t*
   of lower limbs, complex 429*f*
Myotonia 221, 343
   dystrophica 459
Myotonic disorders 221
Myotonic dystrophy 204

N

Nasal reflex 197
Natural light, mild 85
Nausea 409
Neck 217
   and back, midline of 478
   extensor myopathy, isolated 204
   level, lower 198
   pain
      examination of 417
      non-radiating 421
   righting reflex 486
Neer's test 438, 439*f*
Neocerebellum 321, 324*f,* 325
Nerve
   hypoglossal 206
   musculocutaneous 303
   palsy 123
   peripheral 473
   roots 420, 427
   supply 229, 231, 234
Nervous systems, sympathetic 408*f*
Nervus intermedius 177
Neural integrator 154, 155
Neuroacanthocytosis 361, 362, 372
Neurodegenerative disease 372
Neurogenic hyperventilation, central 66*f*
Neuroleptics 362
Neuromyotonia 343
Neuronal ceroid lipofuscinoses 368, 369
Neurons
   excitatory burst 140
   second order 182, 183

Neuropathy
  peripheral 360, 361b, 490
  peroneal 434
Neuroretinitis 100
Neurosyphilis 372
Neurovascular examination 444, 447
Nevus flammeus 460
Niemann-Pick disease 362
Nocturia 409
Nodules, myofascial 431
Non-jerky movements 342
Non-Wilsonian hepatolenticular degeneration 362
Nose-to-finger test 327
Nucleus
  central 104
  prepositus hypoglossi 145
  solitarius 194
  superior vestibular 156, 182
Nystagmus 154, 188, 287, 326, 390
  beating 396
  brun's 162, 395
  causes of
  bilateral symmetric 159b
    gaze-evoked 161b
    mono-ocular 159b
    periodic alternating 160b
    vertical 161b
  central 189, 189t, 402t
    positional 399
  clinical classification of 158fc
  congenital 155
  convergence 160
  divergence 160
  downbeat 156, 161
  horizontal jerk 162
  hyperventilation-induced 396
  infantile 161
  jerky convergence-retraction 160
  pendular 155, 161
    convergence 160
  periodic alternating 155, 157, 161, 395
  peripheral 189, 189t
  positional 398
  recovery 396
  spontaneous 188
  symmetric gaze paretic 161
  types of 154, 157f
  upbeat 156, 161
  Valsalva-induced 397, 398
  vibration-induced 397

O

Oblique muscles 107f
Obturator nerve 304
Ocular
  bobbing, reverse 70

  counter rolling reflex 156
  dipping, reverse 70
  flutter 146
  misalignment 390, 391
  motility 74
  motor
    nerves 104
    palsy 109, 109f
      interpretation of 115
    system, physiologic basis of 106
    tilt reaction 390, 390f, 391
Oculomotor nerve 104
  compression 69
Oculomotor nucleus complex 104
Olfactory aura 379, 382
Olfactory cortex 77
Olfactory nerve 76, 76f
  examination 493
Olfactory nucleus, anterior 77
Olfactory tubercle 77
Ophthalmic nerve 169f
Ophthalmoscope 96f, 459
Oppenheim's sign 488
Opponens digiti minimi, testing of 265f
Opponens pollicis
  anatomy of 264f
  testing of 264f
Opsoclonus 146, 369
  causes of 146b
  myoclonus syndrome 369
Optic
  aphasia 31, 35
  atrophy 369
  chiasm 81
  disc 91
    examination 94
  nerve 80, 93f, 493
    disease 85
    lesion 128
    neuritis 84, 100
    neuropathy 102
  tract
    lesions 127
    nucleus of 156
Optociliary shunts 101
Oral contraceptive pills 362
Oral reflexes, primitive 317
Orbicularis oculi reflex 178, 179
Orbicularis oris reflex 178
Orbitofrontal circuit, syndrome of 5
Orthostatic tremor 337
Oscillator, central 344, 349
Oscillopsia 161
Oval pupil 124
Pain
  and temperature 292
    pathways 292

assessment 293
distribution 417f
location of 434
maneuvers aggravating 434
musculoskeletal 421t
myofascial 451, 452
pattern of 454f

P

Painful arc sign 440
Palatal myoclonus 365f, 368, 369
Palatal reflex 193, 197
Palate 197
Paleocerebellum 321
Palilalia 373
Palipraxia 373
Palmar erythema 478
Palmar grasp 470
    reflex 471, 471f
Palmar interossei 257
Palmomental reflex 318, 424
Palpable myofascial trigger points 454f
Palpate peripheral pulses 431
Palsy, sympathetic 135
Pancoast syndrome 129
Panencephalitis, subacute sclerosing 368
Papilledema 74, 90, 101, 101t, 478
    stages of 99
Parachute reflex 486
Paralysis
    convergence 153
    divergence 153, 154
Paramedian pontine reticular formation 140
Paramyotonia 221
Paraneoplastic state 132
Paraphasia 9, 13
Parapontine reticular formation 139, 145
Parasympathetic nervous systems 408f
Parasympathetic palsy, postganglionic 132t
Paratonia 219
Paresthesia, unilateral 382
Parietal copy test 286
Parietal cortex, posterior 141
Parietal lobule, inferior 28f
Parkinson's disease 79, 335, 341, 351
Parosmia 77
Paroxetine 362
Paroxysmal positional vertigo
    benign 398f
    lateral canal benign 405b
Pars interna 359
Patellar
    instability 449
    reflex generation 301f
    stability 447
    subluxation test 449

Patellofemoral
    compression test 449, 449f
    grinding test 449
Pectoral nerves
    lateral 302
    medial 302
Pectoralis 306
    major 241
        anatomy of 241f
        clavicular head, testing of 241f
    reflex 302
Pediatric neurological examination 477
Pedunculopontine 332
Pelizaeus-Merzbacher disease 161
Pellagra 369
Pelli-Robson charts 84, 84f
Pemoline 372
Pendular jerks 155, 360
Perez reflex 485
Peri-ictal urinary urge 382
Periosteum 420
Peripheral vision 493
Perirolandic region 382
Peroneus longus 278
Pharyngeal reflex 193, 197
Pharynx 197
Phenobarbitone 372
Phenylketonuria 478
Phenytoin 362, 372
Phonagnosia 32, 36
Phonic tics 371
Piano playing movements 286
Ping-pong gaze 70
Piriform cortex 77
Plantar reflex 309, 488
    normal 310
    physiological basis of 310f
Platysma activation 177
Pontine
    lateral 69
    tegmental lesions 69
Pontocerebellum 325
Pontomesencephalic junction 332
Popliteal angle 466, 466f
Popliteal fossa 297
Port-wine stain 460
Postganglionic fibers 120
Postictal nose-rubbing 382
Postictal paresis 382
Postural equilibrium, control of 323
Postural tremor 345, 349
Posture 460
Pout reflex 317, 424
Power estimation, examination of 481
Praxis 57
Prefrontal cortex 3f, 4, 43
Prepositus hypoglossi 140

Pressure hydrocephalus, normal 336
Prion diseases 361
Pronator quadratus 248
Pronator teres 248
Proptosis 110
Prosopagnosia 31, 35
Pseudoathetosis 286, 287, 343
Pseudo-Babinski sign 312
Pseudopapilledema 98, 101, 101t
Pseudoptosis 134
Psoas major 266
Psychic aura 379
Pterygoids 166f
Ptosis 110, 343
   mimicking 134
   myasthenic 134
   nonfatigable 134
Pupil 110, 119
   autonomic innervations of 119f
   examination 67, 117
   reactivity 74
   size 74
      measurement of 122f
   sympathetic innervation of 119f
Pupillary abnormalities 68f, 126f
Pupillary reaction, normal 68
Pupillodilator muscle 120
Pupillo-visual dissociation 127
Purkinje cell 325, 397
Pursuit system 148
Pyramidal disease 326, 330

Q

Q angle 449
Quadratus lumborum muscle 455f

R

Rabot test 449
Radial nerve 303
Radiating neck pain 421
Rebound test 330
Recent language network model 10
Rectus femoris 273
Rectus muscles 107f
Reflex 177, 299, 306, 344, 348, 459, 460, 470, 477
   developmental 479, 483
   examination of 172, 479, 483
   eye movements 71, 74
   frontal release 178
   hammer 459
   oculocephalic 71, 187
   overflow 305
   pathologic 314
   primitive 314, 315, 483
   spread 305
   superficial 307, 479, 488
      abdominal 307
   types of 471
Refractive errors 478
Refsum's disease 102
Reliability index 88
Relief sign 422
Remote memory 40
Renal failure 362
   signs 361
Rent test 437
Respiratory rate, increased 74
Reticular activating system, ascending 2, 62
Reticular formation, lesion of 66f
Reticular myoclonus 368, 368t
Retina 80, 95
   abnormalities of 100
Retinal angiomas 478
Retinal exudates 101
Retinitis pigmentosa 369
Retinopathy, pigmentary 102
Retrieval system 43
Retrochiasmal pathways 81
Retrogeniculate lesions 127
Retropharyngeal abscess 343
Rhomboid
   major 234
   minor 234
   muscles
      anatomy of 234f
      testing of 234f
Rinne test 184
Romberg's sign 324
Romberg's test 186, 286, 287, 390
Rooting reflex 317, 486
Rossolimo's reflex 488
Rostral interstitial nucleus 139, 140, 145, 155
Rotator cuff
   muscles of 437f
   tendonitis 439f
Roving eye movements 70

S

Saccades 139
   abnormalities of 145t
   hypermetric 141
   mechanics of 140f
Saccadic control, general organization of 139f
Sacral dimples 460
Sacroiliac tenderness 431
Sandifer syndrome 343
Sarcoid lesion 136f
Sarcoidosis 100
Scalene trigger points 454f
Scalp tenderness 424
Scapula 437
   elevators of 231f
   range of movement of 229f

Scapular
    adduction 232-234
    depression 233
    elevation 231
    motions 228*f*
    movements 228
    nerve, dorsal 234
    position, symmetry of 229*f*
    winging 202
Scarf sign 465, 465*f*
Schirmer's test 410
Schizophrenia 372
Schwabach's test 184
Sciatic nerve
    palsy 434
    tibial component of 304
Sclerosis, tuberous 372, 373
Scoliosis 431
Scotoma
    central 89
    junctional 81, 81*f*, 91
Seated straight leg raise 433
See-saw nystagmus 156, 156*f*, 162
Seizure 360, 381
    absence 380
    clinical evaluation of 376
    myoclonic 381
    neonatal 458
    non-epileptic 377, 385*t*
    semiology 378, 386
Semantic memory 40
Semicircular canal
    anatomy 389*f*
    function, tests of 390
    horizontal 388*f*, 395
    physiology 389*f*
    posterior 398, 398*f*
Semiology 386
Semitendinosus 272
Senile gait 338
Sensation 496
    tactile 291
Sensory
    ataxia 287, 337
    dysfunction, interpretation of 172
    examination 424
    function 177, 178, 197
        examination of 172
    level 424
    loss, segmental localization of 294
    portion 167
    system 478
        examination of 283
    tricks 353, 355
Sentence repetition 12
Serratus anterior 229*f*
    power of 230*f*
Shagreen patches 478

Shopping cart sign 434
Shoulder 217
    abduction 239
        against gravity, testing of 240*f*
    abductors, anatomy of 239*f*
    adduction 241
    extension 237
    external rotation 242, 242*f*
    flexion 235
        testing of 235*f*
    flexors, anatomy of 235*f*
    internal rotation 243
        testing of 243*f*
    joint 436
        pain 436
    shaking test 217
Sialidosis 368
Side-lying test 399
Simultanagnosia 31
    dorsal 35
Single word comprehension defect 17
Sinuvertebral nerves 421
Sjögren's syndrome 132
Skew deviation comitance 391
Skin 420
    and hair 478
    lesions 373
Skull 295
    shape of 478
Small cell lung cancer 361
Smell perception tests 77
Smell recognition tests 77
Smooth pursuit circuit 148*f*, 150
Snellen's chart 83, 84*f*, 493
Snout reflex 317, 424
Somatic
    afferent, general 194
    efferent, general 194
Somatosensory aura 379
    unilateral 382
Spastic disorders 216*b*
Spasticity, pathogenesis of 213*f*
Special somatic afferent 194
Special visceral
    afferent 194
    efferent 194
Speech 287
    apraxia of 22, 26
    areas, isolation of 15
    initiation defects, isolated 17
    morphology 9
    slurred 409
    spontaneous 11, 13, 14
Spinal canal
    central 426
    stenosis 434*t*
        chronic degenerative 432*f*

Spinal cord 427
   injury 473
      classification of 294
Spinal deformities 337, 460
Spinal dysraphism, sign of 478
Spinal extension 432*f*
Spinal flexion 432*f*
   withdrawal response 310
Spinal myoclonus 365, 366*t*
Spinal nerve 429*f*
   roots 418*f*
Spinal segmental control 212*f*, 214
Spinal spasticity 219
Spinal tract, nucleus of 194
Spinocerebellum 322*f*, 323
   integrity of 326
Spirography 351
Spoken speech processing 10
Spurling's sign 433
Spurling's test 422, 423, 424*f*
Square wave jerks 145
Square window, angle of 465*f*
Squint 478
Standardized mini-mental state examination 51
Startle myoclonus 368
Static encephalopathies 372
Static perimetry 87
Stenosis, lateral recess 434*t*
Sternoclavicular joints 437
Stiff person syndrome 220
Stimuli 64
Strabismus
   comitant 108
   noncomitant 108
Straight leg
   raise, reverse 433
   raising test 431, 432
Stride length 333, 334
Stroke 372
   thalamic 337
Strychnine 221*f*
Subnucleus, lateral 104
Subscapularis, anatomy of 243*f*
Sucking reflex 317, 470, 471, 486
Sudomotor tests 411
Superficial flexion reflex, normal 310
Superior colliculus 141, 142
Superselective serotonin reuptake inhibitors 362
Supinator reflex 302, 303, 487
Supranuclear gaze palsy, vertical 369
Supranuclear palsy, progressive 369
Swelling 437
Swollen disc 98
   bilateral 101
   unilateral 100, 101*t*

Sydenham's chorea 361
Symmetric spontaneous jerk nystagmus, bilateral 160*b*
Syntax 9
Syringobulbia 159
Syringomyelia 204

T

Tachycerebrale 478
Tactile sensation, ascending pathways of 290
Taut band 451
Taut piriformis muscle 451
Taut scalene muscles 451
Taylor hammer 300*f*
Tegmental lesion, dorsolateral 66*f*
Telangiectasia 478
Temporal artery tenderness 424
Temporal lobe 382, 490
   dominant 382
   epilepsy 384
Temporomandibular joint tenderness 424
Temporo-occipital junction 382
Tendon reflexes 287, 306*t*
   deep 299, 305, 424, 470, 472, 473, 479, 487
Tensor fascia latae 271
Teres major 237
Teres minor 242
Tetanus 220
   toxin, action of 221*f*
Thigh thrust test 442*f*
Thoracic nerve, long 229
Thoracic vertebrae 426
Thumb
   abduction 261
   adduction 263
   extension 260
   flexion 259
   motions of 258*f*
   movements 258
   opposition 264
   rule of 97, 226
Thyroarytenoids 195
Thyroid ophthalmopathy 136
Thyrotoxicosis 362
   sign of 348
Tibial nerve 304
Tibialis
   anterior 276
   posterior 277
Tics 342, 357, 371, 372
   classification of 371
   complex 371, 372
   disorder 372
   etiology of 372
   simple 371
Tiger-eye appearance 356
Tissue, subcutaneous 420

Toe
    dorsiflexion 281
        testing of 281f
    dorsiflexor, anatomy of 281f
    fanning of 310f
    flexors
        anatomy of 279f, 280f
        testing of 280f
    metatarsophalangeal flexion 279
    plantar 280
    walking 490
Tomahawk hammer 300f
Tone 460, 464
    examination of 479
Tonic neck reflex
    asymmetric 464, 470, 472, 472f, 485, 488
    symmetric 485
Tonic posturing, bilateral 382
Tonic pupil 128
Tonic seizure 380
Tonic spasms 343
Tonic tics 371
Tonic-clonic seizure 380, 386
    asymmetric termination of 382
    generalized 382, 386
Topographagnosia 31
Topography 345, 355, 359, 366
Torch 459
Torticollis, congenital 343
Tourette's syndrome 372, 373f
Toxins 372
Tract, lateral vestibulospinal 215
Traction test 423
Trail making test 6, 8
Transient tic disorder 372
Trapezius 231, 232, 306
    against gravity, power of 231f
    lower fibers of 233, 233f
    middle fibers of 232f
    reflex 302
Trauma, acute 451
Tremor 342, 344, 357
    action 345
    classification of 344fc
    plus dystonia 340
    rating scale, essential 345
Triceps reflex 302, 303, 487
Tricyclic antidepressants 362
Trigeminal nerve 76, 163, 167, 194, 302
    examination of 171
Trigger points 423, 456
    complex 452f
    examination of 451
Trigger zones 431
Trismus 343
Trochlear nerve palsy 105, 391
Troemner hammer 300f

Trunk, tone of 459
Tullio's phenomenon 190
Tumarkin otolithic catastrophe 190
Tuning fork tests 185t

U

Unterberger-Fukuda stepping test 187
Unverricht-Lundborg disease 342
Upper limb 346, 470
Upper motor nerve 179
    facial palsy 179
Upper neck level 198
Upper temporal field loss 91f
Upper trapezius muscle fibers 202f
Utricular function, tests of 390
Uvula 197
Uvulonodular lesions 160b

V

Vagal nerve lesions 198
Vagus nerve 194
    branches of 196f
Valgus stress test 448f
Valsalva maneuver 397, 411, 414, 423
Valsalva test 423
Varus stress 447
Vasculitis 362, 478
Vasomotor instability, sign of 478
Veins 420
Ventral tegmental tract 156
Vergence system 152
Versive seizure 381
Vertebrae 426
Vertical nystagmus, mechanism of 157f
Vertigo
    central 189
        and peripheral 189t
    examination of 388
    peripheral 189
Vestibular disease 326
Vestibular lesion 188, 337, 403
Vestibular nerve 185
Vestibular nucleus
    inferior 182
    lateral 182
    medial 145, 182
Vestibular system examination 388
Vestibulocerebellum 321f
    integrity of 326
Vestibulocochlear nerve 181
Vestibulo-ocular reflexes 152, 154, 187, 390, 402
Vestibulo-ocular tests 390
Vestibulospinal reflexes 185
Vestibulospinal tests 390
Vestibulospinal tract 215
    medial 215

Vibration 287
Visceral
　afferent, general 194
　efferent, general 194
Vision
　central 82
　color 85, 101, 493
Vistech chart 84
Visual acuity 85, 110, 478, 493
　test
　　dynamic 404
　　steps of 83
Visual agnosia 31, 35
　mild degrees of 34*f*
　testing 33
Visual aura 379
　complex 382
　simple 382
Visual blurring 409
Visual cancellation 404
Visual field 87
　assessment 86
　defect 92*f*, 101
　map 88, 89*f*
　testing, methods of 87
　types of 89
Visual fixation 154
Visual impairment 51
Visual orientation 462
Visual pathway 80*f*
　lesions 126
Vital signs 478
Vocal tics 360
Voice 197, 346
Voluntary automatic dissociation 23
Voluntary saccades circuit 148*f*

Voluntary suppression 355
Vomiting 197

W

Walking 390
　ability 334
　backwards 355
　on heels 431
　reflex 485
Wartenberg's pendulum test 218
Wartenburg's sign 488
Weakness
　etiology of 473
　neonatal 458
　neuromuscular 343
　peroneal 337
Weber's test 184, 185
Wernicke's aphasia 13-17
Wernicke's area 10, 17
Wernicke's encephalopathy 153
West syndrome 384
Whipple's disease 161
Willebrand's knee 81
Wilson's disease 342, 360-362, 372, 373
Wing beating tremor 347*f*
Wrist extension 251
　examination of 252*f*
Wrist flexion 249
　against gravity 250*f*
Writer's cramp 353, 354
Writing tremor, primary 349

X

Xiphisternum 296, 466

Y

Yergason's test 440

EU GSPR Authorised Reprsentative
Logos Europe, 9 rue Nicolas Poussin
1700, La Rochelle, France
Phone: +33 (0) 6 67 93 73 78
E-mail: contact@logoseurope.eu

www.ingramcontent.com/pod-product-compliance
Ingram Content Group UK Ltd.
Pitfield, Milton Keynes, MK11 3LW, UK
UKHW050427150426
5217IPUK00019B/1277